BEYOND THE
HIPAA PRIVACY RULE

Enhancing Privacy, Improving Health Through Research

Sharyl J. Nass, Laura A. Levit, and Lawrence O. Gostin, *Editors*

Committee on Health Research and the Privacy of Health Information:
The HIPAA Privacy Rule

Board on Health Sciences Policy

Board on Health Care Services

INSTITUTE OF MEDICINE
OF THE NATIONAL ACADEMIES

THE NATIONAL ACADEMIES PRESS
Washington, D.C.
www.nap.edu

THE NATIONAL ACADEMIES PRESS   500 Fifth Street, N.W.   Washington, DC 20001

NOTICE: The project that is the subject of this report was approved by the Governing Board of the National Research Council, whose members are drawn from the councils of the National Academy of Sciences, the National Academy of Engineering, and the Institute of Medicine. The members of the committee responsible for the report were chosen for their special competences and with regard for appropriate balance.

The project is sponsored by the National Institutes of Health and the National Cancer Institute, the Robert Wood Johnson Foundation, American Cancer Society, American Heart Association/American Stroke Association, American Society for Clinical Oncology, Burroughs Wellcome Fund, and C-Change. Any opinions, findings, conclusions, or recommendations expressed in this publication are those of the author(s) and do not necessarily reflect the views of the organizations or agencies that provided support for the project.

Library of Congress Cataloging-in-Publication Data

Beyond the HIPAA privacy rule : enhancing privacy, improving health through research / Committee on Health Research and the Privacy of Health Information, the HIPAA Privacy Rule ; Sharyl J. Nass, Laura A. Levit, and Lawrence O. Gostin, editors.
   p. ; cm.
Includes bibliographical references and index.
ISBN 978-0-309-12499-7 (pbk.)
   1. United States. Health Insurance Portability and Accountability Act of 1996. 2. Medical records—Access control—United States 3. Health—Research—United States 4. Privacy, Right of—United States. I. Nass, Sharyl J. II. Levit, Laura A. III. Gostin, Lawrence O. (Lawrence Ogalthorpe) IV. Institute of Medicine (U.S.). Committee on Health Research and the Privacy of Health Information, the HIPAA Privacy Rule.
   [DNLM: 1. United States. Health Insurance Portability and Accountability Act of 1996. 2. Medical Records--legislation & jurisprudence—United States—Guideline. 3. Privacy—legislation & jurisprudence--United States--Guideline. 4. Confidentiality—legislation & jurisprudence--United States--Guideline. 5. Research—methods—United States—Guideline. WX 173 B573 2009]
   R864.B49 2009
   651.5'04261—dc22
                              2009003375

Additional copies of this report are available from the National Academies Press, 500 Fifth Street, N.W., Lockbox 285, Washington, DC 20055; (800) 624-6242 or (202) 334-3313 (in the Washington metropolitan area); Internet, http://www.nap.edu.

For more information about the Institute of Medicine, visit the IOM home page at: **www.iom.edu.**

Suggested citation: IOM (Institute of Medicine). 2009. *Beyond the HIPAA Privacy Rule: Enhancing Privacy, Improving Health Through Research.* Washington, DC: The National Academies Press.

*"Knowing is not enough; we must apply.
Willing is not enough; we must do."*
—Goethe

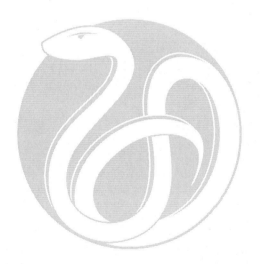

INSTITUTE OF MEDICINE
OF THE NATIONAL ACADEMIES

Advising the Nation. Improving Health.

THE NATIONAL ACADEMIES
Advisers to the Nation on Science, Engineering, and Medicine

The **National Academy of Sciences** is a private, nonprofit, self-perpetuating society of distinguished scholars engaged in scientific and engineering research, dedicated to the furtherance of science and technology and to their use for the general welfare. Upon the authority of the charter granted to it by the Congress in 1863, the Academy has a mandate that requires it to advise the federal government on scientific and technical matters. Dr. Ralph J. Cicerone is president of the National Academy of Sciences.

The **National Academy of Engineering** was established in 1964, under the charter of the National Academy of Sciences, as a parallel organization of outstanding engineers. It is autonomous in its administration and in the selection of its members, sharing with the National Academy of Sciences the responsibility for advising the federal government. The National Academy of Engineering also sponsors engineering programs aimed at meeting national needs, encourages education and research, and recognizes the superior achievements of engineers. Dr. Charles M. Vest is president of the National Academy of Engineering.

The **Institute of Medicine** was established in 1970 by the National Academy of Sciences to secure the services of eminent members of appropriate professions in the examination of policy matters pertaining to the health of the public. The Institute acts under the responsibility given to the National Academy of Sciences by its congressional charter to be an adviser to the federal government and, upon its own initiative, to identify issues of medical care, research, and education. Dr. Harvey V. Fineberg is president of the Institute of Medicine.

The **National Research Council** was organized by the National Academy of Sciences in 1916 to associate the broad community of science and technology with the Academy's purposes of furthering knowledge and advising the federal government. Functioning in accordance with general policies determined by the Academy, the Council has become the principal operating agency of both the National Academy of Sciences and the National Academy of Engineering in providing services to the government, the public, and the scientific and engineering communities. The Council is administered jointly by both Academies and the Institute of Medicine. Dr. Ralph J. Cicerone and Dr. Charles M. Vest are chair and vice chair, respectively, of the National Research Council.

www.national-academies.org

JOY PRITTS, Health Policy Institute, Georgetown University, Washington, DC
ED WAGNER, Director of the W.A. MacColl Institute for Healthcare Innovation, Center for Health Studies, Group Health Cooperative of Puget Sound, Seattle, WA
ALAN WESTIN, Privacy Consulting Group, Teaneck, NJ

Study Staff

SHARYL NASS, Study Director and Senior Program Officer
LAURA LEVIT, Associate Program Officer (Christine Mirzayan Science and Technology Policy Graduate Fellow, December 2006 to March 2007)
CATHERINE REYES, Christine Mirzayan Science and Technology Policy Graduate Fellow (September 2006 to November 2006)
MARY ANN PRYOR, Senior Program Assistant (until August 2007)
MICHAEL PARK, Senior Program Assistant (from September 2007)
ROGER HERDMAN, Director, Board on Health Care Services
ANDREW POPE, Director, Board on Health Sciences Policy
JULIE WILTSHIRE, Financial Associate (until July 2007)
PATRICK BURKE, Financial Associate (from July 2007)

Reviewers

This report has been reviewed in draft form by individuals chosen for their diverse perspectives and technical expertise, in accordance with procedures approved by the National Research Council's Report Review Committee. The purpose of this independent review is to provide candid and critical comments that will assist the institution in making its published report as sound as possible and to ensure that the report meets institutional standards for objectivity, evidence, and responsiveness to the study charge. The review comments and draft manuscript remain confidential to protect the integrity of the deliberative process. We wish to thank the following individuals for their review of this report:

CLARA D. BLOOMFIELD, Distinguished University Professor, The Ohio State University Comprehensive Cancer Center and James Cancer Hospital and Solove Research Institute, Columbus
ALEXANDER M. CAPRON, Professor of Law and Medicine, Gould School of Law, University of Southern California, Los Angeles
ANN CAVOUKIAN, Information and Privacy Commissioner of Ontario, Office of the Information and Privacy Commissioner, Canada
DEBORAH COLLYAR, President, PAIR: Patient Advocates in Research, Danville, CA
EDWARD GOLDMAN, Associate Vice President and Deputy General Counsel, University of Michigan Health System, Ann Arbor

EMMETT B. KEELER, Senior Mathematician, Pardee RAND Graduate School, University of California–Los Angeles School of Public Health, Los Angeles

BETSY KOHLER, Executive Director, North American Association of Central Cancer Registries, Springfield, IL

MELISSA L. MARKEY, Associate, Hall, Render, Killian, Heath & Lyman, P.L.L.C., Troy, MI

DEVON McGRAW, Director, Health Privacy Project, Center for Democracy & Technology, Washington, DC

LYNNE WARNER STEVENSON, Director, Cardiomyopathy and Heart Failure Program, Brigham and Women's Hospital, Cardiovascular Division, Boston, MA

MARCY WILDER, Partner, Hogan & Hartson, L.L.P., Washington, DC

Although the reviewers listed above have provided many constructive comments and suggestions, they were not asked to endorse the conclusions or recommendations nor did they see the final draft of the report before its release. The review of this report was overseen by **Neal A. Vanselow, M.D.,** Chancellor Emeritus and Professor Emeritus of Medicine at the Tulane University Medical Center, and **Bradford H. Gray, Ph.D.,** Editor, *The Milbank Quarterly*, and Principle Research Associate, The Urban Institute. Appointed by the National Research Council and the Institute of Medicine, they were responsible for making certain that an independent examination of this report was carried out in accordance with institutional procedures and that all review comments were carefully considered. Responsibility for the final content of this report rests entirely with the authoring committee and the institution.

Acknowledgments

The Committee is grateful to many individuals who provided valuable input and information for the study, either through formal presentations or through informal communications with study staff and Committee members. Contributors to the study include: Joan E. Bailey-Wilson (National Institutes of Health), Marianna Bledsoe (National Institutes of Health, Office of Science Policy), Stefan Brands (Credentica), Suanna Bruinooge (American Society of Clinical Oncology), Robert Califf (Duke Translational Medicine Institute), Fred H. Cate (Indiana University School of Law), Janlori Goldman (Columbia University, Mailman School of Public Health), Elizabeth Goss (American Society of Clinical Oncology), Sarah Greene (HMO Research Network), Christina Heide (Department of Health and Human Services, Office for Civil Rights), David Helms (Academy-Health), James Hodge (Johns Hopkins Bloomberg School of Public Health), Judd Hollander (Society for Academic Emergency Medicine), Holly Howe (North American Association of Central Cancer Registries), International Pharmaceutical Privacy Consortium, Katherine Kahn (University of California, Los Angeles), Murat Kantarcioglu (University of Texas at Dallas), Anthony Knettel (Association of Academic Health Centers), Elizabeth Mayer-Davis (University of South Carolina), Roberta Ness (University of Pittsburgh), Rachel Nosowsky (Miller, Canfield, Paddock and Stone, PLC), Ann O'Mara (National Cancer Institute, Community Clinical Oncology Program), John Pandiani (The Bristol Observatory), Wendy Patterson (National Cancer Institute), Deborah Peel (Patient Privacy Rights), Joy Pritts (Georgetown Health Policy Institute), John Ring (American Heart Association), Kristin Rosati (Coppersmith Gordon Schermer & Brokelman,

PLC), Mark Rothstein (University of Louisville), Elaine Rubin (Association of Academic Health Centers), Richard Schilsky (University of Chicago), Frank L. Silver (Registry of the Canadian Stroke Network), Lana Skirboll (National Institutes of Health, Office of Science Policy), Penelope Solis (American Heart Association), Ed Wagner (HMO Research Network), Alan Westin (Privacy Consulting Group), Marcy Wilder (Hogan & Hartson, L.L.P.), and Marsha Young (Booz Allen Hamilton).

Contents

Summary

BEYOND THE HIPAA PRIVACY RULE:
ENHANCING PRIVACY, IMPROVING
HEALTH THROUGH RESEARCH

Ethical health research and privacy protections both provide valuable benefits to society. Health research is vital to improving human health and health care—and protecting individuals involved in research from harm and preserving their rights is essential to the conduct of ethical research. The primary justification for protecting personal privacy is to protect the interests of individuals. In contrast, the primary justification for collecting personally identifiable health information for health research is to benefit society. But it is important to stress that privacy also has value at the societal level because it permits complex activities, including research and public health activities, to be carried out in ways that protect individuals' dignity. It is also important to note that health research can benefit individuals, for example, when it facilitates access to new vaccines, therapies, improved diagnostics, and more effective ways to prevent illness and deliver care.

The U.S. Department of Health and Human Services (HHS) developed a set of federal standards for protecting the privacy of personal health information under the Health Insurance Portability and Accountability Act of 1996 (HIPAA).[1] The HIPAA Privacy Rule set forth detailed regulations

---

[1] The HIPAA Privacy Rule ("Standards for Privacy of Individually Identifiable Health Information: Final Rule") can be found at 45 Code of Federal Regulations (C.F.R.) parts 160 and 164. http://www.hhs.gov/ocr/AdminSimpRegText.pdf (accessed August 2, 2008). A summary of the HIPAA Privacy Rule, prepared by the HHS Office for Civil Rights, is available at http://www.hhs.gov/ocr/privacysummary.pdf (accessed August 2, 2008).

regarding the types of uses and disclosures of individuals' personally identifiable health information—called "protected health information"—permitted by "covered entities" (health plans, health care clearinghouses, and health care providers who transmit information in electronic form in connection with transactions for which HHS has adopted standards under HIPAA).[2] A major goal of the HIPAA Privacy Rule is to ensure that individuals' health information is properly protected while allowing the flow of information needed to promote high-quality health care. The HIPAA Privacy Rule also set out requirements for the conduct of health research.

The Institute of Medicine Committee on Health Research and the Privacy of Health Information (the committee) was charged with two principal tasks[3]: (1) to assess whether the HIPAA Privacy Rule is having an impact on the conduct of health research, defined broadly as "a systematic investigation, including research development, testing and evaluation, designed to develop or contribute to generalizable knowledge"[4]; and (2) to propose recommendations to facilitate the efficient and effective conduct of important health research while maintaining or strengthening the privacy protections of personally identifiable health information.

The committee's conclusion is that the HIPAA Privacy Rule does not protect privacy as well as it should, and that, as currently implemented, the HIPAA Privacy Rule impedes important health research. The committee found that the Privacy Rule (1) is not uniformly applicable to all health research, (2) overstates the ability of informed consent to protect privacy rather than incorporating comprehensive privacy protections, (3) conflicts with other federal regulations governing health research, (4) is interpreted differently across institutions, and (5) creates barriers to research and leads to biased research samples, which generate invalid conclusions. In addition, security breaches are a growing problem for health care databases. In developing its recommendations to improve this situation, the committee was guided by three overarching goals: (1) improve the privacy and data security of health information; (2) improve the effectiveness of health research; and (3) improve the application of privacy protections for health research. A summary of the committee's recommendations is presented in Box S-1.

---

[2] 45 C.F.R. § 160.103 (2006).

[3] The study was funded by the National Institutes of Health, the National Cancer Institute, the Robert Wood Johnson Foundation, the American Cancer Society, the American Heart Association/American Stroke Association, the American Society for Clinical Oncology, the Burroughs Welcome Fund, and C-Change.

[4] 45 C.F.R. § 164.510 (2006).

RECOMMENDATION I. DEVELOP A NEW APPROACH TO PROTECTING PRIVACY IN ALL HEALTH RESEARCH

The committee's first and foremost recommendation (Recommendation I) is that Congress should authorize HHS and other relevant federal agencies to develop a new approach to protecting privacy in health research that would apply uniformly to all health research. When this new approach is implemented, HHS should exempt health research from the HIPAA Privacy Rule. The new approach should enhance privacy protections through improved data security, increased transparency of activities and policies, and greater accountability, while also allowing important health research to be undertaken with appropriate oversight. The new approach should do all of the following:

- Apply to any person, institution, or organization conducting health research in the United States, regardless of the source of data or funding.
- Entail clear, goal-oriented, rather than prescriptive, regulations.
- Require researchers, institutions, and organizations that store health data to establish strong data security safeguards.
- Make a clear distinction between the privacy considerations that apply to interventional research and research that is exclusively information based.
- Facilitate greater use of data with direct identifiers removed in health research, and implement legal sanctions to prohibit unauthorized reidentification of information that has had direct identifiers removed.
- Require ethical oversight of research when personally identifiable health information is used without informed consent. HHS should develop best practices for oversight that should consider:
  o Measures taken to protect the privacy, security, and confidentiality of the data;
  o Potential harms that could result from disclosure of the data; and
  o Potential public benefits of the research.
- Certify institutions that have policies and practices in place to protect data privacy and security in order to facilitate important large-scale information-based research for clearly defined and approved purposes, without individual consent.
- Include federal oversight and enforcement to ensure regulatory compliance.

BOX S-1
Summary of the Committee's Recommendations

The committee's foremost recommendation is the following:

I. Congress should authorize HHS and other relevant federal agencies to develop a new approach to protecting privacy that would apply uniformly to all health research. When this new approach is implemented, HHS should exempt health research from the HIPAA Privacy Rule.
→ Apply privacy, security, transparency, and accountability obligations to all health records used in research.

If national policy makers choose to continue to rely on the HIPAA Privacy Rule rather than adopt a new federal approach (Recommendation I), the committee recommends the following:

II. HHS should revise the HIPAA Privacy Rule and associated guidance.

A. HHS should reduce variability in interpretations of the HIPAA Privacy Rule in health research by covered entities, Institutional Review Boards (IRBs) and Privacy Boards through revised and expanded guidance and harmonization.

1. HHS should develop a dynamic, ongoing process to increase empirical knowledge about current "best practices" for privacy protection in responsible research using protected health information (PHI), and promote the use of those best practices.
2. HHS should encourage greater use of partially deidentified data called "limited datasets" and develop clear guidance on how to set up and comply with the associated data use agreements more efficiently and effectively, in order to enhance privacy in research by expanding use and usability of data with direct identifiers removed.
3. HHS should clarify the distinctions between "research" and "practice" to ensure appropriate IRB and Privacy Board oversight of PHI disclosures for these activities.
4. HHS guidance documents should simplify the HIPAA Privacy Rule's provisions regarding the use of PHI in activities preparatory to research and harmonize those provisions with the Common Rule, in order to facilitate appropriate IRB and Privacy Board oversight of identification and recruitment of potential research participants.

B. HHS should develop guidance materials to facilitate more effective use of existing data and materials for health research and public health purposes.

1. HHS should develop guidance that clearly states that individuals can authorize use of PHI stored in databases or associated with biospecimen banks for specified future research under the HIPAA Privacy Rule with IRB/Privacy

Board oversight, as is allowed under the Common Rule, in order to facilitate use of repositories for health research.
2. HHS should develop clear guidance for use of a single form that permits individuals to authorize use and disclosure of health information in a clinical trial and to authorize the storage of their biospecimens collected in conjunction with the clinical trial, in order to simplify authorization for interrelated research activities.
3. HHS should clarify the circumstances under which DNA samples or sequences are considered PHI, in order to facilitate appropriate use of DNA in health research.
4. HHS should develop a mechanism for linking data from multiple sources so that more useful datasets can be made available for research in a manner that protects privacy, confidentiality, and security.

C. HHS should revise provisions of the HIPAA Privacy Rule that entail heavy burdens for covered entities and impede research without providing substantive improvements in patient privacy.

1. HHS should reform the requirements for the accounting of disclosures of PHI for research.
2. HHS should simplify the criteria that IRBs and Privacy Boards use in making determinations for when they can waive the requirements to obtain authorization from each patient whose PHI will be used for a research study, in order to facilitate appropriate authorization requirements for responsible research.

Regardless of whether Recommendation I or II is implemented, the following recommendations, which are independent of the Privacy Rule, should be adopted:

III. Implement changes necessary for both policy options above (Recommendations I and II).

A. All institutions (both covered entities and non-covered entities) in the health research community should take strong measures to safeguard the security of health data.
→ HHS should also support the development and use of new security technologies and self-evaluation standards.

B. HHS—or, as necessary, Congress—should provide reasonable protection against civil suits for members of Institutional Review Boards and Privacy Boards who serve in good faith to encourage service on IRBs and Privacy Boards.
→ But no protection for willful or wanton misconduct.

C. HHS and researchers should take steps to provide the public with more information about health research by:

1. Disseminating research results to study participants and the public.
2. Educating the public about how research is done and what value it provides.

Informative examples for such an approach include Ontario's Personal Health Information Protection Act (PHIPA)[5] and a similar model recently proposed in the United Kingdom.[6] Ontario's PHIPA shares a number of similarities with the HIPAA Privacy Rule. In general, both rules require the holder of personally identifiable health data to get informed consent (referred to as authorization in the Privacy Rule) before using those data for a purpose other than providing services directly related to the health care of the patient. If a researcher wishes to use personally identifiable health data without getting informed consent, both rules require the researcher to obtain a waiver of informed consent approved by an independent ethics board before the study begins.

However, the HIPAA Privacy Rule and PHIPA do have some key differences. One major difference is that unlike the HIPAA Privacy Rule, which applies privacy obligations unevenly across the health care sector, PHIPA applies to health information custodians (HICs; e.g., providers, hospitals, and pharmacies) that collect, use, and disclose personally identifiable health information, as well as to non-HICs that receive personally identifiable health information from a HIC. Thus, the privacy protections follow the data.

Another important difference is that PHIPA permits HICs to disclose personally identifiable health information without consent to "prescribed persons or entities" that have in place privacy practices, policies, and procedures approved by Ontario's Information and Privacy Commissioner. The prescribed persons or entities may then disclose information to researchers either in deidentified form, or in identifiable form with approval of a Research Ethics Board (Canadian equivalent of an Institutional Review Board [IRB] or Privacy Board). Consistent with the principle of transparency, a prescribed entity must also make public a description of its functions and a summary of its practices, policies, and procedures. A similar approach was recommended in a report commissioned by the United Kingdom's Prime Minister on secondary uses of personal information. This report suggested the creation of "safe harbors," which have three defining characteristics: (1) they provide a secure environment for processing personally identifiable health data, (2) they are restricted to "approved researchers" who meet relevant criteria, and (3) they implement penalties and allow for criminal sanctions against researchers who abuse their access to personally identifiable data. The committee believes that such an approach, combined with strong security measures, offers adequate privacy protections for personally

---

[5] Personal Health Information Protection Act, Statutes of Ontario 2004, Ch. 3, Schedule A; Ontario Regulation 329/04.

[6] In a report commissioned by the United Kingdom's Prime Minister on secondary uses of personal information.

identifiable health information in information-based health research, while greatly expanding research opportunities.

The committee's new framework entails a two-part practical approach to protecting health information privacy because there are fundamental differences between information-based research (e.g., using medical records or stored biological samples) and direct, interventional human subjects research. Applying the same human subjects protections in these two different scenarios is neither appropriate nor justifiable. Promoting individual autonomy is essential when a person's health care or participation in clinical research is considered. The purpose of informed consent in this type of research is mainly to protect research participants from physical harm by providing a description of the potential risks and benefits of the study. In contrast, in information-based research that relies solely on medical records and stored biospecimens, the research participant faces no risk of direct physical harm. In this context, informed consent (authorization) is intended to ensure that individuals are able to exercise control over their personal information that is held by third parties, and to give individuals the right to determine whether their personal information can be used in a particular research project (or a series of such projects, if consent for future research is permitted). Because of these fundamental differences between information-based research and direct, interventional human subjects research, the committee makes a clear distinction between the privacy considerations that apply to interventional research and research that is exclusively information based.

First, the committee recommends that all interventional research, regardless of funding source and support, should be required to comply with the Common Rule,[7] and all researchers who gain access to personally identifiable health information as part of the interventional research should be required to protect that information with strong security measures. Research participants should be allowed to provide consent for future research uses of data and biological materials collected as part of the interventional study as long as an IRB reviews and approves the future uses, ensuring that the new study is not incompatible with the original consent.

Second, the committee recommends that HHS and other relevant federal agencies develop a new approach to uniform, goal-oriented oversight of information-based research, with a focus on best practices in privacy, security, and transparency as in PHIPA and the proposed United Kingdom model. This new approach should include a mechanism by which some programs or institutions could be certified by HHS or another accrediting body, similar to a prescribed entity as in PHIPA or a safe harbor as in

---

[7]The "Common Rule" is the term used by 18 federal agencies who have adopted the same regulations governing the protection of human subjects of research.

the United Kingdom model. Such entities could then collect and analyze personally identifiable health information for clearly defined and approved purposes, without individual consent. Because of the administrative requirements in becoming certified, this option is most appropriate for disease registries and other very large scale research databases. Certified entities could also aggregate personally identifiable data from multiple sources, and then provide data to researchers with direct identifiers removed, under strict security requirements. This would facilitate greater use of data with direct identifiers removed in research because the aggregated datasets would be more complete and thus would lead to more accurate conclusions. To further protect privacy, unauthorized reidentification of information that has had direct identifiers removed should be prohibited by law, and violators should face legal sanctions.

In cases where researchers cannot use data with direct identifiers removed, and personally identifiable health information is needed for research, approval and oversight by an ethics oversight board should be required, partially analogous to what is now done under the HIPAA Privacy Rule and PHIPA. This board could perhaps entail a new body specifically formulated to review medical records research, rather than relying on traditional IRBs that were created to review interventional research. If researchers seek a waiver of patient consent, an ethics oversight board should consider the measures the researchers propose to take to protect the privacy and confidentiality of the data, the potential harms that could result from disclosure of the data, and the potential public benefits of the proposed research study. In order to facilitate consistent application of this option, HHS will need to develop clear guidance and best practices on how to assess the potential harm, the proposed measures to protect privacy and confidentiality, and the potential public benefits of a research study, as has been done under PHIPA.

Although expectations regarding privacy vary among different demographic groups, public opinion polls suggest that a significant portion of the American public would like to control all access to their medical records for research via an individual consent mechanism. However, obligations to implement comprehensive privacy protections—such as security, transparency, and accountability—are independent of patient consent. Moreover, the committee concluded, based on considerable testimony and other evidence, that a universal requirement for informed consent can lead to invalid results because of significant differences between patients who do or do not grant consent, and missed opportunities to advance medical science because it can be prohibitively costly and difficult to obtain consent for studies that require analysis of very large datasets. As a result, the committee's new framework includes two alternatives to consent that can be used in certain circumstances (e.g., disclosure to a certified entity and waiver of informed consent by an ethics review board), which are intended to facilitate research that is socially beneficial and to protect privacy through increased security, transparency, and accountability.

If society seeks to derive the benefits of medical research in the form of improved health and health care, information should be shared to achieve that greater good, and governing regulations should support the use of such information, with appropriate oversight. In the committee's proposed new framework, the greater emphasis on ensuring the security protections of personally identifiable health information (as in the committee's Recommendation III.A), facilitating research using data with direct identifiers removed, and ensuring the scientific merits of any proposed research in the new framework should help to foster its acceptability. Nonetheless, effective communication with the public about how health research is done and the value it provides (the committee's Recommendation III.C) will be important to address concerns and gain acceptance.

RECOMMENDATION II. REVISE THE PRIVACY RULE AND ASSOCIATED GUIDANCE

If this comprehensive new approach is not implemented (or, for the interim while the new framework is being developed), the committee proposes as an alternative that HHS revise the current HIPAA Privacy Rule and the associated guidance. These revisions would address some of the problems uncovered during the course of this study.

Recommendation II.A. The committee recommends that HHS develop guidance materials to reduce variability among IRBs and Privacy Boards in their interpretation of the HIPAA Privacy Rule as applied to research. One of the weaknesses in the current privacy protection system is that there is extreme variability in the regulatory interpretations and approval decisions among IRBs and Privacy Boards. Regulatory language often is not easily understandable and is subject to wide interpretation. Thus local IRBs and Privacy Boards interpret state and federal regulations independently, resulting in a great deal of variation in how the regulations are implemented. To address this problem, the committee developed four specific recommendations.

First, HHS should develop a dynamic, ongoing process to increase empirical knowledge about current "best practices" for privacy protection in responsible research using protected health information (PHI), and promote use of those best practices. To accomplish this, HHS should regularly convene consensus development conferences in collaboration with health research stakeholders to collect and evaluate current practices in privacy protection.

Second, HHS should encourage greater use of partially deidentified data called "limited datasets" and develop clear guidance on how to set up and comply with the associated data use agreements (DUAs) more efficiently and effectively. Currently, there is pervasive confusion regarding the conditions of DUAs and how recipients may meet those conditions. As a result, in some health care settings, the burden of establishing a DUA prevents research from going forward. At the other extreme, some covered entities sign DUAs as a matter of course, providing little meaningful privacy protection to the patient.

Third, HHS should clarify the somewhat artificial distinction it has made between "research" and "practice" to ensure appropriate IRB and Privacy Board oversight of PHI disclosures for these closely related activities. This will require HHS to consult with relevant stakeholders to develop standard criteria for IRBs and Privacy Boards to use when making distinctions between health research and related endeavors, such as public health practice and quality improvement practices. These criteria should be evaluated regularly by HHS to ensure that the criteria are helpful and producing the desired outcomes.

Fourth, HHS should simplify the guidance regarding the use of PHI in activities preparatory to research and harmonize these provisions with the Common Rule. The committee recommends that all researchers (including those internal to a covered entity) be required to obtain IRB approval (as required under the Common Rule) prior to contacting potential research participants. When making a decision about whether to approve research projects, the IRB should review and consider the investigator's plans for contacting patients, and ensure that the information will be used only for research projects approved by the IRB and will not be disclosed elsewhere.

Recommendation II.B. The committee recommends that HHS develop guidance materials to facilitate more effective use of existing data and materials for health research and public health purposes. Many institutions create and maintain databases with patient health information or repositories with biological materials collected from patients. These databases and biospecimen banks are used for many types of health research, including studies to understand diseases or to compare patient outcomes following different treatments. Current interpretations of provisions of the HIPAA Privacy Rule sometimes make it difficult to effectively use these valuable resources for health research. The committee developed four specific recommendations to facilitate important health research by maximizing the usefulness of patient data associated with biospecimen banks and in research databases, thereby allowing novel hypotheses to be tested with existing data and materials as knowledge and technology improve. The recommendations would align interpretation of the HIPAA Privacy Rule with the Common Rule on several points, simplify or clarify the relevant processes in research, and develop new tools for data aggregation.

First, the committee recommends that HHS develop guidance which clearly states that individuals can authorize use of PHI stored in databases or associated with biospecimen banks for specified future research under the HIPAA Privacy Rule with IRB oversight, as is allowed under the Common Rule. Future uses should be described in sufficient detail to allow individuals to give informed consent, and researchers should be required to have IRBs determine that the new research is not incompatible with the initial consent. Second, the committee recommends that HHS develop clear guidance for use of a single form that permits individuals to authorize use and disclosure of health information in a clinical trial and to authorize the storage of their biospecimens collected in conjunction with the clinical trial. This will simplify the authorization process for interrelated research activities by integrating all relevant information into one simple document.

Third, the committee recommends that HHS clarify the circumstances under which DNA samples or sequences are considered PHI. Genetic information does not itself identify an individual in the absence of other identifying information. However, in some circumstances, a person's genetic code could be construed as a unique identifier in that it could be used to match a sequence in another biospecimen bank or databank that does include identifiers. The committee advocates a focus on strong security measures and the adoption of strict prohibitions and legal sanctions against the unauthorized reidentification of individuals from DNA sequences, by anyone.

Fourth, HHS should develop a mechanism for linking data from multiple sources so that more useful datasets can be made available for research in a manner that protects privacy, confidentiality, and security. One way this could be accomplished, for example, might be through data warehouses that are certified for the purpose of linking data from different sources. The organizations responsible for such linking would be required to use strong security measures and would maintain the details about how the linkage was done, should another research team need to recreate the linked dataset.

Recommendation II.C. The committee recommends that HHS revise provisions of the HIPAA Privacy Rule that currently hinder research but do not provide substantive privacy protections. First, HHS should reform the requirements for the accounting of disclosures (AOD) of PHI made for research and public health purposes. Until technology advances make automatic AOD tracking feasible, affordable, and widely available, the HIPAA Privacy Rule should permit covered entities to inform patients in advance that PHI might be used for health research with IRB/Privacy Board oversight or for public health purposes. As an alternative to AOD, to ensure transparency, institutions should maintain a list, accessible to the public, of all studies approved by an IRB/Privacy Board.

In addition, HHS should simplify the criteria that IRBs and Privacy Boards use in determining whether to waive the requirement that researchers obtain authorization from each patient whose PHI will be used in a research study. If HHS decides to retain the current waiver criteria, HHS should provide clear and reasonable definitions to the vague terms used in the waiver criteria (i.e., what constitutes "minimal risk" to the privacy of individuals and what constitutes "impracticable"), as well as providing specific case examples. This would be especially helpful for multi-institutional studies, which fall under the jurisdiction of multiple IRBs or Privacy Boards.

RECOMMENDATION III. IMPLEMENT CHANGES NECESSARY FOR BOTH POLICY OPTIONS ABOVE (RECOMMENDATIONS I AND II)

The committee's last set of recommendations do not directly relate to the HIPAA Privacy Rule, but should be adopted in order to achieve the committee's overarching goals under both policy options described above (the new framework or revisions to the HIPAA Privacy Rule and associated guidance).

Recommendation III.A. The committee recommends that all health research institutions improve the security of personally identifiable health information. For example, institutions could: appoint a security officer responsible for assessing data protection needs and implementing solutions and staff training; make greater use of encryption and other techniques for data security; include data security experts on IRBs; implement a breach notification requirement, so that patients may take steps to protect their identity in the event of a breach; and implement layers of security protection to eliminate single points of vulnerability to security breaches. In addition, the federal government should support (1) the development and use of genuine privacy-enhancing techniques that minimize or eliminate the collection of personally identifiable data, and (2) standardized self-evaluations and security audits and certification programs to help institutions achieve the goal of safeguarding the security of personal health data.

Recommendation III.B. The committee also recommends that HHS—or, as necessary, Congress—provide reasonable protection against civil suits brought pursuant to state or federal laws for members of IRBs and Privacy Boards for decisions made within the scope of their responsibilities under the HIPAA Privacy Rule and the Common Rule. The limitation on liability should not include protection for willful and wanton misconduct in reviewing the research, but should instead be reserved for good-faith decisions, backed by minutes or other evidence. Effective oversight of health research depends on the recruitment of qualified and knowledgeable volunteers to serve on IRBs and Privacy Boards. But the increasing workload and complexity of IRB and Privacy Board service have made it difficult to recruit and retain knowledgeable IRB members and to ensure time for the ethical reflection necessary to make appropriate decisions about human research projects. Moreover, because of the growth over the past decade of lawsuits naming individual IRB members as defendants, fear of penalties and civil suits can be a significant deterrent in recruiting qualified volunteers to serve on IRBs and Privacy Boards.

Recommendation III.C. Finally, the committee recommends that HHS and researchers take steps to provide the public with more information about health research. Surveys indicate that the vast majority of Americans believe health research is important, and they are interested in the findings of research studies. Yet patients often lack information about how health research is conducted and are rarely informed about research results that may have a direct impact on their health. The committee recommends that researchers inform interested research participants (who granted authorization for a particular study) with a simplified summary of the results at the conclusion of a research study. HHS should also encourage researchers to register their trials and other studies in public databases, particularly when the research is being conducted under a waiver of authorization. In addition, HHS and the health research community should work to educate the public about how research is done, and what value it provides. These recommendations could be accomplished without any changes to HIPAA or the Privacy Rule by making them a condition of funding for research grants from HHS and other research sponsors, and by providing additional funds to cover the cost.

Overview of Conclusions
and Recommendations

Ethical health research and privacy protections both provide valuable benefits to society. Health research is vital to improving human health and health care—and protecting individuals involved in research from harm and preserving their rights is essential to the conduct of ethical research. The primary justification for protecting personal privacy is to protect the interests of individuals. In contrast, the primary justification for collecting personally identifiable health information for health research is to benefit society. But it is important to stress that privacy also has value at the societal level because it permits complex activities, including research and public health activities, to be carried out in ways that protect individuals' dignity. It is also important to note that health research can benefit individuals, for example, when it facilitates access to new therapies, improved diagnostics, and more effective ways to prevent illness and deliver care.

The U.S. Department of Health and Human Services (HHS) developed a set of federal standards for protecting the privacy of personal health information under the Health Insurance Portability and Accountability Act of 1996 (HIPAA).[1] The HIPAA Privacy Rule set forth detailed regulations regarding the types of uses and disclosures of individuals' personally identifiable health information—called "protected health information"—permitted by "covered entities" (health plans, health care clearing houses, and health care providers who transmit information in electronic form in connection with transactions for which HHS has adopted standards under

---

[1] The HIPAA Privacy Rule can be found at 45 Code of Federal Regulations (C.F.R.) parts 160 and 164 (2006).

HIPAA).[2] A major goal of the Privacy Rule is to ensure that individuals' health information is properly protected while allowing the flow of information needed to promote high-quality health care. The Privacy Rule also set out requirements for the conduct of health research.

The Institute of Medicine (IOM) Committee on Health Research and the Privacy of Health Information (the committee) was charged with two principal tasks[3]: (1) to assess whether the HIPAA Privacy Rule is having an impact on the conduct of health research, defined broadly to include biomedical research, epidemiological studies, and health services research, as well as studies of behavioral, social, and economic factors that affect health; and (2) to propose recommendations to enable the efficient and effective conduct of important health research while maintaining or strengthening the privacy protections of personally identifiable health information (Box O-1).

The committee's conclusion is that the HIPAA Privacy Rule does not protect privacy as well as it should, and that, as currently implemented, the Privacy Rule impedes important health research. The committee found that the Privacy Rule (1) is not uniformly applicable to all health research, (2) overstates the ability of informed consent to protect privacy rather than incorporating comprehensive privacy protections, (3) conflicts with other federal regulations governing health research, (4) is interpreted differently across institutions, and (5) creates barriers to research and leads to biased research samples, which generate invalid conclusions. In addition, security breaches are a growing problem for health care databases. In this report, the committee presents its analysis and findings, along with several recommendations for accomplishing the dual goals of protecting health privacy while facilitating responsible and beneficial research.

DEFINITIONS

Definition of Privacy and Why Privacy Is Important

The term "privacy" is used frequently, yet there is no universally accepted definition of the term, and there is considerable confusion about the meaning, value, and scope of the concept. The focus of the HIPAA Privacy Rule and the IOM committee's report are on the privacy of personal health information. In this context, privacy pertains to the collection, storage, and use of personal information and addresses the question of who

---

[2] 45 C.F.R. § 160.103 (2006).

[3] The study was funded by the National Institutes of Health, the National Cancer Institute, the Robert Wood Johnson Foundation, the American Cancer Society, the American Heart Association/American Stroke Association, the American Society for Clinical Oncology, the Burroughs Wellcome Fund, and C-Change.

BOX O-1
Committee Statement of Task

An Institute of Medicine committee will investigate the effects on health research of the Privacy Rule regulations implementing the Health Insurance Portability and Accountability Act of 1996 (HIPAA) section on Administrative Simplification and prepare a report. In conducting the study, the committee will:

1. Consider the range of study types, such as clinical trials, epidemiologic designs, research using tissue repositories and databases, public health research, and health services research, to the extent that available data and evidence allow;
2. Consider research carried out by the full range of sponsors: government, public and private academic, and for-profit sectors, including the pharmaceutical, biotechnology, and medical device industries;
3. Review provisions of the Privacy Rule relevant to health research, including those dealing with authorizations and accounting of disclosures of personal health information, deidentification of data, reviews preparatory to research, and others, and on reviewing them, may identify provisions that merit priority attention and analysis;
4. Consider issues of interpretation and implementation of the Privacy Rule, as well as of harmonization with overlapping provisions of the Common Rule and Food and Drug Administration regulations, which have existed much longer;
5. Examine the potential impact of the Rule on public health research, on the recruitment of research subjects for studies, on carrying out research internationally, and on research using data and biomaterials in databases and tissue repositories; and
6. Consider the needs for privacy of identifiable personal health information and the value of such privacy to patients and the public.

As data and evidence allow, the needs and benefits of patient privacy will be balanced against the needs, risks, and benefits of identifiable health information for various kinds of health research. The committee will formulate recommendations for alterations or retention of the status quo accordingly.

---

has access to personal information and under what conditions. Issues of privacy include whether specific types of data about an individual can be collected at all, as well as the justifications, if any, under which data collected for one purpose can be used for another purpose. Another important issue in privacy analysis is whether an individual has authorized particular uses of his or her personal information.

Although privacy is often used interchangeably with the terms "confidentiality" and "security," they have distinct meanings. Confidentiality, though closely related to privacy, refers to the obligations of those who receive information in the context of an intimate relationship to respect the privacy interests of those to whom the data relate and to safeguard that information. Confidentiality addresses the issue of whether to keep information exchanged in that relationship from being disclosed to third parties. Thus, for example, confidentiality requires physicians not to disclose information shared with them by a patient in the course of a physician–patient relationship. Unauthorized or inadvertent disclosures of data gained as part of an intimate relationship are considered breaches of confidentiality.

Security, as defined by Turn and Ware in 1976, is "the procedural and technical measures required to (a) prevent unauthorized access, modification, use, and dissemination of data stored or processed in a computer system, (b) prevent any deliberate denial of service, and (c) to protect the system in its entirety from physical harm."[4] Currently existing, commonly deployed security measures help keep health records safe from unauthorized use, although no security measure can prevent an invasion of privacy by individuals who have authority to access a health record.

American society places a high value on a private sphere protected from intrusion, and the bioethics principle of nonmaleficence[5] requires safeguarding personal privacy. Breaches of an individual's privacy and confidentiality may affect a person's dignity and cause irreparable harm. When personally identifiable health information[6] is disclosed to an employer, insurer, or family member, for example, the disclosure can result in stigma, embarrassment, and discrimination. Safeguarding privacy and confidentiality are also important for both individuals and society. Individuals are less likely to participate in health research or other socially and individually beneficial activities, including candid and complete disclosures of sensitive information to their physicians, if they do not believe their privacy is being protected. However, it should also be noted that perceptions of privacy vary among individuals and groups. Information that is considered intensely private by one person may not be by others. The concept of privacy is also context specific, and acquires a different meaning depending on the stated reasons for the information being gathered, the intentions of the parties involved, as well as the politics, convention, and cultural expectations.

The bioethics principle of respect for persons places importance on individual autonomy or self-determination, which allows individuals to make decisions for themselves about matters that are important to their own wellbeing. U.S. society also places a high value on individual autonomy, and one

---

[4]Turn, R., and W. H. Ware. 1976. Privacy and security issues in information systems. *The RAND Paper Series*. Santa Monica, CA: The RAND Corporation.

[5]The ethical principle of doing no harm, based on the Hippocratic maxim, primum non nocere, first do no harm.

[6]This term may encompass a broad range of information, including personal and family health history, physician notes and orders, test results, medication and immunization records, and documentation of surgeries or hospitalizations.

way to respect individuals is to ensure that they can make the choice about when, and whether, personal information (particularly sensitive information) can be shared with others.

Many statutory and regulatory protections of privacy have attempted to incorporate these values and concerns through emphasis on the principles of fair information practices,[7] which have been adopted in various forms at the international, federal, and state levels. The principles of fair information practices address issues such as data quality, limitations on collection and use, specification of purpose, security safeguards, openness of practices and policies, individual participation, and accountability. They reflect a broad consensus about the need for standards to protect individual privacy and to facilitate information flows in an increasingly technology-dependent, global society.

Definition of Health Research and Why Health Research Is Important

Under both the HIPAA Privacy Rule and a federal regulation known as the Common Rule,[8] "research" is defined as "a systematic investigation, including research development, testing and evaluation, designed to develop or contribute to generalizable knowledge." This is a broad definition that may include biomedical research, epidemiological studies,[9] and health services research,[10] as well as studies of behavioral, social, and economic factors that affect health.

Perhaps the most familiar form of health research is the clinical trial in which patients volunteer to participate in studies to test the efficacy of new medical interventions. Today, though, an increasingly large portion of health research is information based. More and more research entails the analysis of data and biological samples that were initially collected for one purpose and are now being used for another purpose such as research.[11]

---

[7] The concept of fair information practices originated with the 1973 report of the Secretary's Advisory Committee on Automated Personal Data Systems, reporting to the Secretary of the U.S. Department of Health, Education, and Welfare, titled *Records, Computers and the Rights of Citizens*, http://epic.org/privacy/hew1973report/ (accessed August 3, 2008).

[8] The Common Rule is a federal policy for the protection of human subjects adopted by 18 federal agencies and offices. 45 C.F.R. part 46, http://www.hhs.gov/ohrp/policy/common.html (accessed August 3, 2008).

[9] Epidemiology is the study of the occurrence, distribution, and control of diseases in populations.

[10] Health services research has been defined as a multidisciplinary field of inquiry, both basic and applied, that examines the use, costs, quality, accessibility, delivery, organization, financing, and outcomes of health care services to increase knowledge and understanding of the structure, processes, and effects of health services for individuals and populations.

[11] The National Committee on Vital and Health Statistics has noted that the term "secondary uses" of health data is ill defined and therefore urged abandoning it in favor of precise description of each use. Consequently, the IOM committee has chosen to minimize use of the term in this report.

In the fields of epidemiology, health services research, and public health research, the use of existing data to conduct research is common. Existing data are analyzed to identify patterns of occurrences, determinants, and the natural history of disease; to evaluate health care interventions and services; to perform drug safety surveillance; and to perform some genetic and social studies.

A prime example of the benefits of research using existing biological samples and patients' records is the development of Herceptin® (trastuzumab), a revolutionary new treatment for some kinds of breast cancer. In addition, many findings from research using patients' medical records have changed the practice of medicine. Examples of how health research based on data from medical records has informed and influenced national and other policy decisions abound. Just to cite a few: Research based on data from medical records underlies the estimate that tens of thousands of Americans die each year from medical errors in the hospital and has provided valuable information for reducing these medical errors by implementing health information technology, such as e-prescribing. Medical records research has documented that disparities and lack of access to care in inner cities and rural areas results in poorer health outcomes, and has demonstrated that specific preventive services (e.g., mammography) substantially reduce mortality and morbidity at reasonable costs. Furthermore, such research has established a causal link between the nursing shortage and patient health outcomes by documenting that patients in hospitals with fewer registered nurses are hospitalized longer and are more likely to suffer complications, such as urinary tract infections and upper gastrointestinal bleeding. As the use of electronic medical records increases, the pace of medical records research is accelerating, and the opportunities to use these records to generate new knowledge about what works in health care are expanding.

The varying methods of health research provide complementary insights. Although clinical trials can provide important information about the efficacy and adverse effects of medical interventions by controlling the variables that could impact the results of the study, feedback from real-world clinical experience is also crucial for comparing and improving the use of drugs, vaccines, medical devices, and diagnostics. The Food and Drug Administration's (FDA's) approval of a drug for a particular indication, for example, is based on a series of controlled clinical trials, often with a few hundred to a few thousand patients. After a drug has received the FDA's approval for marketing, however, it may be used by millions of people in many different contexts. Thus tracking clinical experience with the drug is important for identifying relatively rare adverse effects and for determining the effectiveness in different populations or circumstances.

Like privacy, all of these health-related activities provide high value to society. Collectively, these activities can provide important information about disease trends and risk factors, outcomes of treatment or public health interventions, functional abilities, patterns of care, and health care costs and utilization. They have led to significant discoveries, the development of new therapies, and a remarkable improvement in health care and public health.[12] Thus, they provide a sense of hope for people with chronic, life-threatening, or fatal conditions. If the health research enterprise is impeded, or if it is less robust, important societal interests are adversely affected.

THE HIPAA PRIVACY RULE

The U.S. Congress passed HIPAA in 1996 with the primary goals of making health care delivery more efficient and increasing the number of Americans with health insurance coverage.

The HIPAA Privacy Rule was developed by HHS under HIPAA's administrative simplification provisions, which mandated the creation of privacy standards for "protected health information" (PHI) in the absence of federal legislation. A major goal of the HIPAA Privacy Rule is to ensure that individuals' health information is properly protected while allowing the flow of information needed to promote high-quality health care. Recognizing that patients' health records also play an important role in health research, Congress wanted to ensure that the implementation of HIPAA would not impede health researchers' continued access to data from health records. Responding to this objective, HHS attempted to create a system that mandates privacy protection for individually identifiable health information while allowing important uses of the information in health care and research.

The HIPAA Privacy Rule sets forth detailed regulations regarding the types of uses and disclosures of "protected health information," defined as "individually identifiable health information" that is held or transmitted by a "covered entity." Covered entities are health plans, health care clearinghouses, and health care providers who transmit information in electronic form in connection with a transaction for which HHS has developed a standard under HIPAA.[13] A covered entity may not use or disclose PHI except either (1) as the Privacy Rule permits, or (2) as the individual who is the subject of the information (or the individual's personal representative) authorizes in writing. The Privacy Rule applies not only to health information exchanged or stored electronically, but also to PHI held by a

---

[12] See Standards for Privacy of Individually Identifiable Health Information: Proposed Rule, 64 Fed. Reg. 59918, 59967 (1999) for a discussion on the benefits of health records research.

[13] 45 C.F.R. § 160.103 (2006).

covered entity in any form or media, including electronic, paper, and oral communications.[14]

Although the HIPAA Privacy Rule applies to information uses and transactions necessary for the provision of health care, it is also applicable to a great deal of information used in health research. As already explained, the data in individuals' medical records may be important or essential to some types of health research. When obtaining PHI from a covered entity to use in their research, health researchers are required to follow the provisions of the HIPAA Privacy Rule. The Privacy Rule permits a covered entity to use and disclose PHI for research purposes without an individual's authorization if the covered entity obtains either (1) documentation that an alteration or waiver of the individual's authorization for the use or disclosure of the information has been approved by an IRB or Privacy Board, or (2) specified representations from the researchers that the PHI is being used or disclosed solely for purposes preparatory to research, or for research using only the PHI of decedents. A covered entity may also use or disclose PHI without an individual's authorization if the PHI is contained as part of a "limited dataset" from which specified direct identifiers have been removed, and the researcher enters into a data use agreement with the covered entity.

THE COMMITTEE'S CHARGE AND THE
OVERARCHING GOALS OF THE RECOMMENDATIONS

The sponsors of this study asked the IOM to assess whether the HIPAA Privacy Rule implemented by HHS is impacting the conduct of health research, and requested that the IOM committee propose recommendations to facilitate the efficient and effective conduct of important health research while maintaining or strengthening the privacy protections of personally identifiable health information. To undertake this task, the IOM appointed a 15-member committee (Committee on Health Research and the Privacy of Health Information) with a broad range of expertise and experience covering various fields of health research; privacy of health information; health law, regulation, and ethics; human research protections; health center administration; use and protection of electronic health information; and patient advocacy.

As the study progressed and committee members began thinking about potential recommendations, they identified three general methods for improving the current system for safeguarding health information privacy:

---

[14]Under the HIPAA Privacy Rule protected health information excludes education records covered by the Family Educational Rights and Privacy Act, as amended, 20 U.S.C. 1232(g), records described at 20 U.S.C. 1232(g)(a)(4)(B)(iv), and employment records held by a covered entity in its role as employer.

(1) the provision of guidance from HHS and its Office for Civil Rights to Institutional Review Boards (IRBs), Privacy Boards, institutions, and other participants and stakeholders, which is the easiest way to achieve changes; (2) regulatory changes to the HIPAA Privacy Rule provisions, which can be done via HHS, but is more difficult than providing new guidance; and (3) statutory changes in HIPAA or other legislation at the federal or state level, which is the most difficult to accomplish, but may be necessary. The committee members decided to be as modest as possible in proposing recommendations to facilitate the efficient and effective conduct of important health research while maintaining or strengthening the privacy protections of personally identifiable health information, with the goal of making it easier to effect change if policy makers agree with the proposals.

Ultimately, committee members agreed to make two sets of recommendations. First, the committee proposes a bold, innovative, and more uniform approach to the dual challenge of protecting privacy while supporting beneficial and responsible research.[15] Although a totally new approach may be harder to implement in the short term than more incremental changes, it might help to stimulate fresh ideas about the best ways to protect privacy and improve health research as the nation seeks the best way to support these two interconnected values over the next several years. Second, in the event that policy makers decide that HIPAA was—and continues to be—the most useful model for how to safeguard privacy in health research, the committee proposes a series of detailed proposals to improve the HIPAA Privacy Rule and associated guidance.

There is no question that the goals of safeguarding privacy and enhancing health research are sometimes in tension. Stringent measures to safeguard privacy can make it harder to conduct high-quality research, and research itself can pose a threat to privacy. Yet the committee believes that there is a synergy between the two, that promoting both is desirable, and that it is possible to strengthen certain privacy protections while still facilitating important health research.

For that reason, the committee's intent in developing its recommendations was to advance both privacy and health research interests to the extent possible. The committee understands that the lines are not neat, the questions are complex, and the challenges are formidable. Nevertheless, our recommendations are aimed at strengthening health research regulations and practices that effectively safeguard personally identifiable health information, while changing provisions of the HIPAA Privacy Rule or its interpretations that the committee found to be mostly formalistic or

---

[15] Responsible health research is methodologically sound, is scientifically valid, protects the rights and interests of study subjects, and addresses a question or problem relevant to improving human health.

ineffective. They also aim to facilitate data collection and use for beneficial and high-quality health research, with appropriate oversight, to advance knowledge about human health.

To facilitate beneficial health research while still ensuring adequate protection of patient privacy, the committee grounded its recommendations in three fundamental goals: (1) improve the privacy and data security of health information; (2) improve the effectiveness of health research; and (3) improve the application of privacy protections for health research (Box O-2). These three basic goals are discussed further below.

BOX O-2
Three Goals Underlying the Committee's Recommendations

1. Improve the privacy and data security of health information.
2. Improve the effectiveness of health research.
3. Improve the application of privacy protections for health research.

Improve the Privacy and Data Security of Health Information

In the context of health research, the privacy goal is the commitment to handle personal information of patients and research participants in accordance with meaningful privacy protections. These protections should include strong security measures, disclosure of the purposes for which personally identifiable health information is used (transparency), and legally enforceable obligations to ensure information is secure and used appropriately (accountability). This commitment extends to everyone who collects, uses, or has access to personal information of patients and research participants.

Practices of security, transparency, and accountability take on extraordinary importance in the health research setting. Researchers and other data users should disclose clearly how and why personal information is being collected, used, and secured, and should be subject to legally enforceable obligations to ensure that personal information is used appropriately and securely. In this manner, privacy protection will help to ensure research participant and public trust and confidence in medical research.

Improve the Effectiveness of Health Research

Research discoveries are central to achieving the goal of extending the quality of healthy lives. Research into causes of disease, methods for prevention, techniques for diagnosis, and new approaches to treatment has increased life expectancy, reduced infant mortality, limited the toll of infectious diseases, and improved outcomes for patients with heart disease, cancer, diabetes, and other diseases. Patient-oriented clinical research that tests new ideas makes medical and public health progress possible.

Today the rate of discovery is accelerating, and science is at the precipice of a remarkable period of investigative promise made possible by new knowledge about the genetic underpinnings of disease. Genomic research is opening new possibilities for preventing illness and for developing safer, more effective medical care that may eventually be tailored for specific individuals. Further advances in relating genetic information to predispositions to disease and responses to treatments will require use of large amounts of existing health-related information and stored biological specimens. The increasing use of electronic medical records will further facilitate the generation of new knowledge through research and accelerate the pace of discovery. These efforts will require broad participation of patients in research and broad data sharing to ensure that the results are valid and applicable to different segments of the population. Collaborative partnerships among communities of patients, their physicians, and teams of researchers to gain new scientific knowledge will bring tangible benefits for people in this country and around the world.

Improve the Application of Privacy Protections for Health Research

The HIPAA Privacy Rule was written to provide consistent standards in the United States for the use and disclosure of PHI by covered entities, including the use and disclosure of such information for research purposes. In its current state, however, the HIPAA Privacy Rule is difficult to reconcile with other federal regulations, including HHS regulations for the protection of human subjects (the Common Rule), FDA regulations pertaining to human subjects protections,[16] and other applicable federal or state laws.

For example, inconsistencies in federal regulations governing the deidentification of personal health information, obtaining individual consent for future research, and the recruitment of research volunteers make it challenging for health researchers to undertake important research activities while seeking to comply with all these regulations. In addition, there is substantial variation in the way in which institutions interpret and apply the Privacy Rule. For example, the way in which IRBs and Privacy Boards interpret the provisions when making decisions about authorization requirements varies across institutions, and often is quite conservative. Especially for multisite research and studies that are reviewed by both IRBs

---

[16]21 C.F.R. parts 50 and 56 (1988).

and Privacy Boards, the inconsistent interpretation and application of the HIPAA Privacy Rule's provisions pertaining to research can create barriers to research and even lead to the discontinuation of ongoing research studies, which squanders the contributions of research participants. Adding yet another layer of complexity and variability for health researchers is a lack of clarity in the way the HIPAA Privacy Rule applies to various types of health research or closely related health care practices. Moreover, there are significant gaps in who and what is covered by current federal research regulations. Whether a research activity is subject to the provisions of the Privacy Rule or the Common Rule depends on a number of factors, including the source of funding, the source of the data, and whether the researcher meets the definition of a covered entity.

The situation in the United States is in stark contrast to the situation in most other countries, where uniform regulations apply to all research conducted in the country. The committee believes a new direction is needed, with a more uniform approach to patient protections, including privacy, in health research. Improved clarity, harmonization, and uniform application of regulations governing health research are needed to align the interests and understandings of the research community, the custodians of PHI, and other stakeholders such as patients, so that implementation of the privacy protections in health research can be achieved with acceptability to all.

THE COMMITTEE'S RECOMMENDATIONS

The IOM Committee on Health Research and the Privacy of Health Information developed several recommendations with the intent of strengthening the privacy protections of personally identifiable health information and facilitating the efficient and effective conduct of beneficial health research. A summary of the committee's recommendations is presented in Box O-3.

The committee's first and foremost recommendation (Recommendation I) is that Congress should authorize HHS and other relevant federal agencies to develop a new approach to ensuring privacy that would apply uniformly to all health research in the United States. When this new approach is implemented, HHS should exempt health research from the HIPAA Privacy Rule. This new approach, separate from the HIPAA Privacy Rule, should ensure privacy in health research by emphasizing security, accountability, and transparency while also allowing important health research to be undertaken with appropriate oversight. If national policy makers decide that the HIPAA Privacy Rule has been, and continues to be, a useful model for safeguarding privacy in health research, the committee also proposes as an alternative that HHS revise the current HIPAA Privacy Rule and the associated guidance. These revisions, which could also be implemented in the interim while a new, comprehensive approach is being developed, would address many of the problems uncovered during the course of this study. HHS should develop guidance materials to reduce variability among IRBs and Privacy Boards in their interpretation of the HIPAA Privacy Rule as applied to research (Recommendation II.A); develop guidance materials to facilitate more effective use of existing data and materials for health research and public health purposes (Recommendation II.B); and revise some provisions of the HIPAA Privacy Rule that currently hinder research but that do not provide meaningful privacy protections (Recommendation II.C). The committee's last set of recommendations, though not directly related to the HIPAA Privacy Rule, should be adopted in order to achieve the committee's overarching goals. The committee recommends that all health research institutions improve the security of personally identifiable health information (Recommendation III.A), that HHS—or, as necessary, Congress—provide reasonable protection to IRB and Privacy Board members for good faith decisions to encourage service on IRBs (III.B), and that HHS and researchers take steps to disseminate health research results more broadly, and to inform the public about the nature of health research and its value to individuals and society as a whole (Recommendation III.C). Adopting this set of recommendations will be important regardless of whether Option I or II is implemented.

In the remaining pages of this overview, the abbreviated recommendations of the IOM committee, shown in Box O-3, are presented in fuller detail.

I. Develop a New Approach to Protecting Privacy in All Health Research

Background

The primary justification for including research provisions in the HIPAA Privacy Rule was to remedy perceived shortcomings of federal privacy protections in health research under the Common Rule, but the HIPAA Privacy Rule has numerous limitations of its own. In proposing the Privacy Rule, HHS acknowledged that, ideally, it would have preferred to regulate health researchers directly by extending the protections of the Common Rule to research that is not federally supported and by imposing additional criteria for the waiver of patient authorization for the use of personally identifiable health information in research.[17] But HHS recognized that it did not have the authority to do this. For that reason, HHS attempted to protect the health information released to researchers indirectly (but within the scope

---

[17]U.S. Secretary of Health and Human Services, *Recommendations on the Confidentiality of Individually-Identifiable Health Information to the Committees on Labor and Human Resources* (1997), and Standards for Privacy of Individually Identifiable Health Information: Proposed Rule, 64 Fed. Reg. 59918, 59968 (1999).

BOX O-3
Summary of the Committee's Recommendations

The committee's foremost recommendation is the following:

I. Congress should authorize HHS and other relevant federal agencies to develop a new approach to protecting privacy that would apply uniformly to all health research. When this new approach is implemented, HHS should exempt health research from the HIPAA Privacy Rule.
→ Apply privacy, security, transparency, and accountability obligations to all health records used in research.

If national policy makers choose to continue to rely on the HIPAA Privacy Rule rather than adopt a new federal approach (Recommendation I), the committee recommends the following:

II. HHS should revise the HIPAA Privacy Rule and associated guidance.

A. HHS should reduce variability in interpretations of the HIPAA Privacy Rule in health research by covered entities, IRBs, and Privacy Boards through revised and expanded guidance and harmonization.

1. HHS should develop a dynamic, ongoing process to increase empirical knowledge about current "best practices" for privacy protection in responsible research using protected health information (PHI), and promote the use of those best practices.
2. HHS should encourage greater use of partially deidentified data called "limited datasets" and develop clear guidance on how to set up and comply with the associated data use agreements more efficiently and effectively, in order to enhance privacy in research by expanding use and usability of data with direct identifiers removed.
3. HHS should clarify the distinctions between "research" and "practice" to ensure appropriate IRB and Privacy Board oversight of PHI disclosures for these activities.
4. HHS guidance documents should simplify the HIPAA Privacy Rule's provisions regarding the use of PHI in activities preparatory to research and harmonize those provisions with the Common Rule, in order to facilitate appropriate IRB and Privacy Board oversight of identification and recruitment of potential research participants.

B. HHS should develop guidance materials to facilitate more effective use of existing data and materials for health research and public health purposes.

1. HHS should develop guidance that clearly states that individuals can authorize use of PHI stored in databases or associated with biospecimen banks for specified future research under the HIPAA Privacy Rule with IRB/Privacy

Board oversight, as is allowed under the Common Rule, in order to facilitate use of repositories for health research.

2. HHS should develop clear guidance for use of a single form that permits individuals to authorize use and disclosure of health information in a clinical trial and to authorize the storage of their biospecimens collected in conjunction with the clinical trial, in order to simplify authorization for interrelated research activities.

3. HHS should clarify the circumstances under which DNA samples or sequences are considered PHI, in order to facilitate appropriate use of DNA in health research.

4. HHS should develop a mechanism for linking data from multiple sources so that more useful datasets can be made available for research in a manner that protects privacy, confidentiality, and security.

C. HHS should revise provisions of the HIPAA Privacy Rule that entail heavy burdens for covered entities and impede research without providing substantive improvements in patient privacy.

1. HHS should reform the requirements for the accounting of disclosures of PHI for research.

2. HHS should simplify the criteria that IRBs and Privacy Boards use in making determinations for when they can waive the requirements to obtain authorization from each patient whose PHI will be used for a research study, in order to facilitate appropriate authorization requirements for responsible research.

Regardless of whether Recommendation I or II is implemented, the following recommendations, which are independent of the Privacy Rule, should be adopted:

III. Implement changes necessary for both policy options above (Recommendations I and II).

A. All institutions (both covered entities and non-covered entities) in the health research community should take strong measures to safeguard the security of health data.

→ HHS should also support the development and use of new security technologies and self-evaluation standards.

B. To encourage service on Institutional Review Boards, HHS—or, as necessary, Congress—should provide reasonable protection against civil suits for members of Institutional Review Boards and Privacy Boards who serve in good faith.

→ But no protection for willful or wanton misconduct.

C. HHS and researchers should take steps to provide the public with more information about health research by:

1. Disseminating research results to study participants and the public.

2. Educating the public about how research is done and what value it provides.

of its limited authority) by imposing restrictions on information disclosures by covered entities. The National Committee on Vital and Health Statistics (NCVHS) and others have noted the limitations of the HIPAA Privacy Rule and have called for stronger protections of health privacy—notably, by expanding the purview of the Privacy Rule beyond the current covered entities.

The IOM committee believes an even bolder change is needed. The number of studies using medical records to address important questions about health and disease is likely to increase with the growing availability of electronic records. As the volume and importance of digital personal health data increase exponentially, the public can be expected to heighten demands for a legal framework that provides meaningful safeguards to protect personally identifiable health information in the health research setting. Thus, the IOM committee recommends developing a new framework to both protect individuals' privacy and facilitate responsible and beneficial health research.

> **Recommendation I: Congress should authorize HHS and other relevant federal agencies to develop a new approach to protecting privacy in health research that would apply uniformly to all health research. When this new approach is implemented, HHS should exempt health research from the HIPAA Privacy Rule. The new approach should enhance privacy protections through improved data security, increased transparency of activities and policies, and greater accountability while also allowing important health research to be undertaken with appropriate oversight. The new approach should do all of the following:**
>
> - **Apply to any person, institution, or organization conducting health research in the United States, regardless of the source of data or funding.**
> - **Entail clear, goal-oriented, rather than prescriptive, regulations.**
> - **Require researchers, institutions, and organizations that store health data to establish strong data security safeguards.**
> - **Make a clear distinction between the privacy considerations that apply to interventional research and research that is exclusively information based.**
> - **Facilitate greater use of data with direct identifiers removed in health research, and implement legal sanctions to prohibit unauthorized reidentification of information that has had direct identifiers removed.**
> - **Require ethical oversight of research when personally identifiable health information is used without informed consent. HHS should develop best practices for oversight that should consider:**

- o Measures taken to protect the privacy, security, and confidentiality of the data;
- o Potential harms that could result from disclosure of the data; and
- o Potential public benefits of the research.
- Certify institutions that have policies and practices in place to protect data privacy and security in order to facilitate important large-scale information-based research for clearly defined and approved purposes, without individual consent.
- Include federal oversight and enforcement to ensure regulatory compliance.

Rationale

The committee concluded that the HIPAA Privacy Rule impedes important health research and does not protect privacy as well as it should. Rather than offering an effective and comprehensive approach to solving the real problems of protecting privacy while ensuring the vitality of the national research agenda, the Privacy Rule often focuses on formalistic issues. A new approach to protecting the privacy of personally identifiable information used in health research should both provide strong and effective protection for often-sensitive personally identifiable health information and facilitate scientific discovery and medical innovation necessary to save lives and enhance the quality of the public's health. It should do so in a way that does not burden individuals with a flurry of health privacy notices and consent forms, or burden our health care system with a new level of bureaucracy and expense.

A new framework developed by HHS and other relevant agencies that emphasizes privacy, security, accountability, and transparency and is applicable to all health research in the United States would eliminate confusion, reduce variability, facilitate responsible research, and enhance trust in the research enterprise. Clear and simple regulations that are less subject to varying interpretation by ethical oversight boards, as well as federal oversight and enforcement of regulatory compliance, will be important to consistently and efficiently ensure privacy and instill trust while enabling important research.

The committee favors an approach in which both ethical health research and privacy protections are supported. Informative examples for such an approach include Ontario's Personal Health Information Protection Act (PHIPA)[18] and a similar model recently proposed in the United

---

[18]Personal Health Information Protection Act, Statutes of Ontario 2004, Ch. 3, Schedule A; Ontario Regulation 329/04.

Kingdom.[19] Ontario's PHIPA shares a number of similarities with the HIPAA Privacy Rule. In general, both rules require the holder of personally identifiable health data to obtain informed consent (referred to as authorization in the Privacy Rule) before using those data for a purpose other than providing services directly related to the health care of the patient. If a researcher wishes to use personally identifiable health data without obtaining informed consent, both rules require the researcher to obtain a waiver of informed consent approved by an independent ethics board before the study begins.

However, the HIPAA Privacy Rule and PHIPA do have some key differences. One major difference is that unlike the HIPAA Privacy Rule, which applies privacy obligations unevenly across the health care sector, PHIPA applies to health information custodians (HICs; e.g., providers, hospitals, and pharmacies) that collect, use, and disclose personally identifiable health information, as well as to non-HICs that receive personally identifiable health information from a HIC. Thus, the privacy protections follow the data.

Another important difference is that PHIPA permits HICs to disclose personally identifiable health information without consent to "prescribed persons or entities," who must have in place practices, policies, and procedures approved by Ontario's Information and Privacy Commissioner to protect the privacy and confidentiality of personally identifiable health information it receives and maintains. The prescribed persons or entities may then disclose information to researchers either in deidentified form, or in identifiable form with approval of a Research Ethics Board (Canadian equivalent of an IRB or Privacy Board). Consistent with the principle of transparency, a prescribed entity must also make public a description of its functions and a summary of its practices, policies, and procedures. A similar approach to prescribed entities was recommended in a report commissioned by the United Kingdom's Prime Minister on secondary uses of personal information. This report suggested the creation of "safe harbors," which have three defining characteristics: (1) they provide a secure environment for processing personally identifiable health data, (2) they are restricted to "approved researchers" who meet relevant criteria, and (3) they implement penalties and allow for criminal sanctions against researchers who abuse their access to personally identifiable data. The committee believes that such an approach, combined with strong security measures, offers adequate privacy protections for personally identifiable health information in information-based health research, while greatly expanding research opportunities.

---

[19] In a report commissioned by the United Kingdom's Prime Minister on secondary uses of personal information.

Health research increasingly relies on the review of information about patients' actual experiences with treatments to determine the risks and benefits of drugs and other therapies, in addition to traditional interventional and comparative clinical trials with patients. Regulations under a new approach to ensuring privacy in health should acknowledge the fact that research based exclusively on information (e.g., using medical records or stored biological samples) is not the same as direct, interventional human subjects research. For that reason, applying the same human subjects protections in these two different scenarios is neither appropriate nor justifiable. Promoting individual autonomy is essential when a person's health care or participation in clinical research is considered. The purpose of informed consent in this type of research is mainly to protect research participants from physical harm by providing a description of the potential risks and benefits of the study. In contrast, in information-based research that relies solely on medical records and stored biospecimens, the research participant faces no risk of direct physical harm. In this context, informed consent (authorization) is intended to ensure that individuals are able to exercise control over their personal information that is held by third parties, and to give individuals the right to determine whether their personal information can be used in a particular research project (or a series of such projects, if consent for future research is permitted).

Because of these fundamental differences between information-based research and direct, interventional human subjects research, the committee suggests a two-part practical approach to protecting health information privacy. First, all interventional research, regardless of funding source and support, should be required to comply with the Common Rule and all researchers who gain access to personally identifiable health information as part of the interventional research should be required to protect that information with strong security measures. Research participants should be allowed to provide consent for future research uses of data and biological materials collected as part of the interventional study as long as an IRB reviews and approves the future uses, ensuring that the new study is not incompatible with the original consent.

Second, a new approach to uniform, goal-oriented oversight of information-based research should be developed by HHS and other relevant federal agencies, with a focus on best practices in privacy, security, and transparency as in PHIPA and the proposed United Kingdom model. This new approach should include a mechanism by which some programs or institutions could be certified by HHS or another accrediting body, similar to a prescribed entity as in PHIPA or a safe harbor as in the United Kingdom model. Such entities could then collect and analyze personally identifiable health information for clearly defined and approved purposes, without individual consent. Because of the administrative requirements in becoming certified, this option is most appropriate for disease registries and other very large scale research databases. Certified entities could also aggregate personally identifiable data from multiple sources, and then provide data to researchers with direct identifiers removed, under strict security requirements. This would facilitate greater use of data with direct identifiers removed in research because the aggregated datasets would be more complete and thus would lead to more accurate conclusions. To further protect privacy, unauthorized reidentification of information that has had direct identifiers removed should be prohibited by law, and violators should face legal sanctions.

In cases where researchers cannot use data with direct identifiers removed, and personally identifiable health information is needed for research, approval and oversight by an ethics oversight board should be required, partially analogous to what is now done under the HIPAA Privacy Rule and PHIPA. This oversight board could perhaps entail a new body specifically formulated to review medical records research, rather than relying on traditional IRBs that were created to review interventional research. If researchers seek a waiver of patient consent, an ethics oversight board should consider the measures to be taken to protect the privacy and confidentiality of the data, the potential harms that could result from disclosure of the data, and the potential public benefits of the proposed research study. In order to facilitate consistent application of this option, HHS will need to develop clear guidance and best practices on how to assess the potential harm, the proposed measures to protect privacy and confidentiality, and the potential public benefits of a research study, as has been done under PHIPA.

There is a great deal of variability in whether and how IRBs and other ethical oversight boards consider the public benefit and scientific merit of research proposals. But the first rule of ethical research is that the research must have scientific value—meaning that it addresses an important question of human health and is designed and conducted using methodology that is appropriate and rigorous. The scientific merit of research varies by project, just as the potential risk to privacy of research varies across different protocols. The committee believes that when making decisions about whether a research protocol that entails the disclosure of personally identifiable information should go forward, ethical oversight boards should take all of these factors—potential risks/harms to research participants' privacy as well as scientific merit and potential public benefit of the research proposal—into consideration.

A previous IOM committee on Assessing the System for Protecting Human Research Subjects recommended that "human research participant protection programs" use distinct mechanisms for initial reviews of scientific merit and that these reviews should precede and inform the comprehensive ethical review of research studies. Ethical oversight board members themselves may not have the expertise to assess the merit of diverse research studies, but they should have access to evaluations by scientific review committees or funder peer review panels, which would help them assess the anticipated benefits of a proposed research project.

Although expectations regarding privacy vary among different demographic groups, public opinion polls suggest that a significant portion of the American public would like to control all access to their medical records for research via an individual consent mechanism. However, obligations to implement comprehensive privacy protections—such as security, transparency, and accountability—are independent of patient consent. Moreover, the committee concluded, based on considerable testimony and other evidence, that a universal requirement for informed consent can lead to invalid results because of significant differences between patients who do or do not grant consent, and to missed opportunities to advance medical science because it can be prohibitively costly and difficult to obtain consent for studies that require analysis of very large datasets. As a result, the committee's new framework includes two alternatives to consent that can be used in certain circumstances (e.g., disclosure to a certified entity and waiver of informed consent by an ethics review board), which are intended to facilitate research that is socially beneficial and to protect privacy through increased security, transparency, and accountability.

If society seeks to derive the benefits of medical research in the form of improved health and health care, information should be shared to achieve that greater good, and governing regulations should support the use of such information, with appropriate oversight. In the committee's proposed new framework, the greater emphasis on ensuring the security protections of personally identifiable health information, facilitating research using data with direct identifiers removed, and ensuring the scientific merits of any proposed research in the new framework should help to foster its acceptability. Nonetheless, effective communication with the public about how health research is done and the value it provides (the committee's Recommendation III.C below) will be important to address concerns and gain acceptance.

The committee's proposal for a new approach to ensuring privacy in health research that is uniformly applicable to all health research in the United States is especially timely because Congress has shown considerable interest in producing new legislation to facilitate the implementation of a nationwide health information technology system. Such a system has been hailed as a means of addressing rising health care costs and improving the quality and efficiency of health care, but privacy concerns are emerging as a primary obstacle to the implementation of such a nationwide system. Some legislative proposals would follow the HIPAA model of privacy protections, while others would require different or additional approaches to ensure the privacy of electronic health records. A nationwide health information technology system has the potential to accelerate health research by making large amounts of health data available to study and thus could lead to major advances in medicine. Nevertheless, caution is warranted in developing new regulations because the adoption of new, restrictive regulations might actually impede health research, to the great detriment of patients and society.

If Recommendation I is not implemented and the nation continues to rely on the HIPAA Privacy Rule for protecting privacy in health research, the committee proposes an alternative set of recommendations (Recommendations II.A–C) that could address some of the problems uncovered during the course of this study, by improving the HIPAA Privacy Rule and associated guidance.

II. Revise the Privacy Rule and Associated Guidance

Recommendation II.A: HHS should reduce variability in interpretations of the HIPAA Privacy Rule in health research by covered entities, IRBs, and Privacy Boards through revised and expanded guidance and harmonization.

Background

One of the weaknesses in the current privacy protection system is that there is extreme variability in the regulatory interpretations and approval decisions among IRBs and Privacy Boards. Regulatory language often is not easily understandable and is subject to wide interpretation. Thus local IRBs and Privacy Boards interpret state and federal regulations independently, resulting in a great deal of variation in how the regulations are implemented. For example, projects that are similar in design and intent may be granted a waiver of individual authorization by some IRBs and Privacy Boards, but not others, on the basis of differing interpretations of the Privacy Rule's waiver criteria. In addition, some IRBs and Privacy Boards may conflate the Common Rule and Privacy Rule, or apply the research provisions of the Privacy Rule to activities for which they are not applicable, such as public health practice or the operation of cancer registries.

Furthermore, in the case of the HIPAA Privacy Rule, covered entities that disclose PHI are regulated, not the health researchers who receive the information. As a result, covered entities, as well as IRBs and Privacy Boards, may be reluctant to permit disclosures of PHI that would allow health research to go forward, even in situations where it is ethically and legally justified. Lacking sufficient guidance from HHS, IRBs and Privacy Boards sometimes interpret the HIPAA Privacy Rule too conservatively out of concern that a particular health research activity might result in institutional noncompliance with the Privacy Rule.

HHS intended to allow IRBs and Privacy Boards to have some local control in implementing and interpreting the HIPAA Privacy Rule as it applies to the use and disclosure of PHI for research. The committee's recommendations below are intended not to reduce the decision-making powers and flexibility of local IRBs and Privacy Boards, but rather to make it easier for IRBs and Privacy Boards to review research proposals fairly and quickly. Additional guidance and clarification from HHS on the specific points listed below, along with specific case examples to help delineate what is or is not permissible under the Privacy Rule, would make it easier for IRBs and Privacy Boards to make the appropriate review decisions.

> **Recommendation II.A.1: HHS should develop a dynamic, ongoing process to increase empirical knowledge about current "best practices" for privacy protection in responsible research using PHI, and promote use of those best practices.**

- **HHS should regularly convene consensus development conferences in collaboration with health research stakeholders to collect and evaluate current practices in privacy protection in order to identify and disseminate best practices.**
- **Stakeholders can then enable and encourage researchers to use these best practices in designing and conducting research involving the use of PHI.**

Rationale

There are many diverse approaches to health research. The broad array of methods and data sources for such research presents a challenge to IRBs and Privacy Boards that must determine how various state and federal regulations apply to each research protocol. Uncertainty about how the various regulations apply to a given protocol can lead to overly conservative decisions by these boards, making it more difficult for some important health research to go forward. For example, some covered entities misinterpret the Privacy Rule by requiring researchers to obtain authorization from next of kin in order to access the PHI of decedents, which is not required under the provisions. Such factors contribute to the tremendous variability in the decisions made by IRBs and Privacy Boards.

Current guidance from HHS addresses only what is permissible under the HIPAA Privacy Rule; the guidance does not identify best practices. A dynamic, ongoing process for the identification and dissemination of best practices in privacy protection for various types of health research by HHS would facilitate reviews by IRBs and Privacy Boards and lead to more consistent and appropriate decisions. HHS guidance materials with best practices and models or templates for things such as the patient authorization form, waiver of authorization form, data use agreements, and business associate agreements would make it easier for investigators to appropriately design research projects and put institutions at ease about decisions their IRBs and Privacy Boards make with regard to privacy concerns. Such guidance materials should be written as clearly and simply as possible, using an inclusive, dynamic, and transparent development process, and should override all prior guidance documents.

The committee believes that a proactive role by HHS in disseminating guidance changes to IRBs and Privacy Boards is essential. This endeavor could perhaps be accomplished as an activity of the National Institutes of Health Roadmap for Medical Research under the direction of the HHS Office for Civil Rights. An informative precedent for the dissemination efforts might be the Health Resources and Services Administration's development of the *National Practitioner Data Bank (NPDB) Guidebook*,[20] an activity established through Title IV of the Healthcare Quality Improvement Act of 1986. The *NPDB Guidebook*, which is frequently updated, provides many case examples of what should be done in various situations.

Stakeholders—including researchers; research institutions, IRBs, and Privacy Boards; sponsors of research; public health practitioners and agencies; patient and consumer organizations; and privacy experts—could have considerable influence on the adoption of best practices once they have been identified, so they could help to make privacy protections and IRB/Privacy Board decisions more uniform. For example, Requests for Proposals and other funding mechanisms could be more instructive on the requirements for the protection of privacy.

Many academic researchers depend on their ability to procure funding from a source external to their institutions, and research sponsors have obligations to protect research participants. Thus, major nonfederal funders of health research could be a powerful force for adherence to ethical guidelines even in the absence of strong federal regulations and enforcement. Organizations whose primary missions are focused on promoting responsible and ethical research—such as PRIM&R (Public Responsibility in Medicine and Research) and the Association for the Accreditation of Human Research Protection Programs, Inc., which serve as primary educational vehicles for IRB professionals and offer certification programs—could also contribute much to this dynamic and ongoing process. Increased participation in these

---

[20] Division of Quality Assurance, Health Resources and Services Administration, *National Practitioner Data Bank Guidebook*, Rockville, MD, http://www.npdb-hipdb.hrsa.gov/npdbguidebook.html (accessed August 1, 2008).

organizations by research investigators in particular could extend under-standing of regulatory requirements and foster national discourse about issues of interpretation and application of the HIPAA Privacy Rule.

> **Recommendation II.A.2:** HHS should encourage greater use of par-tially deidentified data called "limited datasets" and develop clear guidance on how to set up and comply with the associated data use agreements more efficiently and effectively, in order to enhance privacy in research by expanding use and usability of data with direct identi-fiers removed.

Rationale

The HIPAA Privacy Rule and the Common Rule both exempt from their provisions research using health data from which personal identifiers have been removed. Because the two rules define personally identifiable information and deidentification differently, however, there is a discrepancy between what research involving existing data is exempt from the Common Rule and what research is exempt from the Privacy Rule.

The standard for deidentification as defined in the Common Rule is that the identity of the subject may not be readily ascertained by the health researcher (e.g., "anonymized" datasets with no direct identifiers included).[21] Thus, health research using information recorded in such a manner that sub-jects cannot be readily identified is exempt from the Common Rule.[22]

Under the HIPAA Privacy Rule, there are two ways to deidentify health information so that it is exempt from the Privacy Rule. One is to remove 18 specified identifiers that identify or could provide a reasonable basis to identify an individual, including both direct identifiers (e.g., name, address, medical records number, Social Security number, health plan beneficiary number) and indirect identifiers (e.g., dates of service and geographic sub-divisions smaller than a state).[23] The second way is to have a qualified stat-istician determine that the risk is very small that any identifiers present on a given data file could be used alone, or in combination with other available information, to identify an individual.[24]

This discrepancy between deidentification standards under the two rules can give rise to situations in which research with anonymized data that is exempt from IRB oversight under the Common Rule may still

---

[21] 45 C.F.R. § 46.102(f)(2) (2006).

[22] 45 C.F.R. § 46.101(b)(4) (2006).

[23] 45 C.F.R. § 164.514(b) (2006). There are no restrictions on the use or disclosure of dei-dentified health information.

[24] *Id.*

require a decision by an IRB or a Privacy Board to determine if a waiver of individuals' authorization of disclosure for the use of their information for research purposes is appropriate under the Privacy Rule. However, IRBs have not had to review these protocols in the past, and they may have difficulty in making appropriate decisions about waivers.

The HIPAA Privacy Rule's restrictions put greater emphasis on the possibility that deidentified health data could be reidentified using publicly available databases. Record linkage technology has advanced rapidly in the past 10 years, making reidentification of data easier now than when the Common Rule was implemented. Yet many researchers maintain that removing all 18 data categories required by the HIPAA Privacy Rule can render a dataset unusable for research. Several organizations—including the Secretary's Advisory Committee on Human Research Protections (SACHRP), NCVHS, and the Association of American Medical Colleges—have recommended changing the HIPAA Privacy Rule to reduce the number of identifiers that must be removed for a dataset to be considered deidentified and thus exempt from IRB and Privacy Board oversight if used in health research. Some elements of the 18 identifiers (e.g., ZIP Codes, geographic subdivisions, and dates of service or tissue collection) do not directly identify individuals, and are essential for some types of health research, such as epidemiology or studies of disease incidence.

In 2002, in response to the concerns that had been raised, HHS modified the HIPAA Privacy Rule to create a category of partially deidentified data called the "limited dataset," in which health information that is stripped of the 16 most direct identifiers can be used and disclosed for research without obtaining individuals' authorization or an IRB/Privacy Board waiver if the covered entity enters into a data use agreement (DUA) with the recipient of the data.[25] Geographic subdivisions (other than street addresses) and dates and other numbers, characteristics, or codes not listed as direct identifiers in the regulation can be included in a limited dataset, making it more useful for research.

Currently, however, there is pervasive confusion regarding the conditions of DUAs and how recipients may meet those conditions. As a result, in some health care settings, the burden of establishing a DUA prevents research from going forward. However, at the other extreme, some covered entities sign DUAs as a matter of course, providing little meaningful privacy protection to the patient. The committee recommends that HHS ameliorate this situation by issuing clear guidance on how to set up and comply with data use agreements more efficiently and effectively, with a goal-oriented focus on the safeguards that researchers should use to protect individuals' privacy.

---

[25] 45 C.F.R. § 164.514(e)(3)(i) (2006).

Recommendation II.A.3: HHS should clarify the distinctions between "research" and "practice" to ensure appropriate IRB and Privacy Board oversight of PHI disclosures for these activities.

• HHS should consult with relevant stakeholders to develop standard criteria for IRBs and Privacy Boards to use when making distinctions between health research and related endeavors such as public health practice and quality improvement practices. These criteria should be evaluated regularly by HHS to ensure that the criteria are helpful and producing the desired outcomes.

Rationale

The HIPAA Privacy Rule makes a somewhat artificial distinction between health research and some closely related activities, such as public health and quality improvement activities, which also may involve collection and analysis of PHI. Under the Privacy Rule (as well as the Common Rule), these activities, which aim to protect the public's health and improve the quality of patient care, are considered health care "practice" rather than health research.

HHS considered public health and quality improvement activities important enough to give them special status under federal regulations by permitting them to be undertaken without authorization or an IRB/Privacy Board waiver of authorization. Yet it can be a challenge for IRBs and Privacy Boards, researchers, health care practitioners, and research participants to distinguish among activities that are or are not subject to the various provisions of the Privacy Rule (and the Common Rule). Inappropriate decisions may prevent important activities from being undertaken or could potentially allow disclosures of PHI that are not permitted under the regulations.

A number of models outlining the criteria IRBs and Privacy Boards should use to distinguish practice and research have been proposed to address these difficulties. One recent model, for example, provides a detailed checklist for IRBs and Privacy Boards to use in determining whether an activity is (1) public health "research" that must comply with the research provisions of the Privacy Rule, or (2) public health "practice" that does not need IRB or Privacy Board review.[26]

The committee believes that standardizing the criteria is essential to support the conduct of these important health care activities. For that reason, the committee recommends that HHS convene the relevant stakeholders to develop standard criteria for IRBs and Privacy Boards to use when making decisions about whether protocols entail research or prac-

---

[26] See Chapter 3 for a complete discussion of this model.

tice, using the available models above as examples. The regulation should have enough flexibility to allow important activities to go forward with appropriate levels of oversight. In addition, it will be important to evaluate whether these criteria are effective in aiding IRB/Privacy Board reviews of proposed protocols and whether they lead to appropriate IRB/Privacy Board decisions.

> **Recommendation II.A.4: HHS guidance documents should simplify the HIPAA Privacy Rule's provisions regarding the use of PHI in activities preparatory to research and harmonize those provisions with the Common Rule, in order to facilitate appropriate IRB and Privacy Board oversight of identification and recruitment of potential research participants.**

Rationale

Many research studies, especially those focused on rare conditions with limited eligible patient populations, rely on large-scale medical chart reviews and searches of patient databases to identify patients who might be eligible for and might benefit from a particular study. Sufficient patient enrollment in a timely fashion is essential to ensure the meaningfulness and reliability of the research results. Researchers may also need to examine medical records in order to develop useful and appropriate research designs and protocols.

The HIPAA Privacy Rule has some specific provisions that allow a covered entity to use or disclose PHI without an individual's authorization if the information is to be used for research. One provision allows a covered entity to use and disclose PHI without an individual's authorization if the covered entity obtains the following representations from the researcher: (1) the use or disclosure of the information is solely to prepare a research protocol or is otherwise preparatory to research; (2) the researcher will not remove any PHI from the covered entity; and (3) the PHI for which access is sought is necessary for the research.[27] However, there is widespread confusion regarding what is permitted under this provision of the Privacy Rule. Surveys and studies also indicate that recruiting patients for research has become more difficult and costly under the HIPAA Privacy Rule.

HHS has issued multiple guidance statements to help address this confusion, but these guidance statements, some of which have been contradictory, have failed to solve the problem.

According to current HHS guidance on the Privacy Rule, researchers (both internal and external to a covered entity) may conduct a review of

---

[27]45 C.F.R. § 164.512(i)(1)(ii) (2006).

medical records under the Privacy Rule's exception that allows the use and disclosure of PHI without an individual's authorization if the information is being used by a researcher for activities preparatory to research. However, HHS guidance also specifies that only internal researchers (an employee or member of the covered entity's workforce) may contact potential research participants about the possibility of enrolling in a study under this provision of the Privacy Rule. External researchers are not allowed to record or remove patient contact information from a covered entity. They must get a partial waiver from an IRB or Privacy Board to perform any recruitment activities. This interpretation of the Privacy Rule creates an artificial distinction between internal and external researchers that actually provides less privacy protection than that afforded by the Common Rule, which requires that any activities preparatory to research involving human subjects, or related to initial recruitment of subjects for research studies, be reviewed and approved by an IRB. Thus, the HIPAA Privacy Rule permits conduct that is prohibited by the Common Rule.

According to SACHRP, HHS statements regarding these provisions for activities preparatory to research have led to "enormous confusion," and many "institutions are hesitant to permit many recruitment activities critical to the continuation of the research enterprise, out of fear that they are in some way misinterpreting the government's current positions on research recruitment." In 2004 SACHRP indicated that it was "very concerned that the bureaucratic complexities here undermine, rather than enhance, the attention that needs to be paid to the welfare and interests of subjects in the research recruitment process."

To address these issues, the committee recommends that all researchers (including those internal to the covered entity) be required to obtain IRB approval (as required under the Common Rule) prior to contacting potential research participants. When making a decision about whether to approve research projects, the IRB should review and consider the investigator's plans for contacting patients, and ensure that the information will be used only for research projects approved by the IRB and will not be disclosed elsewhere. The committee believes that IRBs can protect research participants, including their privacy and confidentiality interests, but as noted in Recommendation II.A.1, educational outreach by HHS is needed to address misunderstandings of these provisions.

Recommendation II.B: HHS should develop guidance materials to facilitate effective use of existing data and materials for health research and public health purposes.

Background

Many institutions create and maintain databases with patient health information or repositories with biological materials collected from patients. These databases and biospecimen banks are used for many types of health research, including studies to understand diseases or to compare patient outcomes following different treatments.

Current interpretations of provisions of the HIPAA Privacy Rule sometimes make it difficult to effectively use these valuable resources for health research. Currently, for example, HHS interprets the Privacy Rule as prohibiting patient authorization for future research use of PHI associated with the individuals' biospecimens collected in the course of a clinical trial or treatment by covered entities.

Such interpretations of the HIPAA Privacy Rule create confusion and unnecessary burdens for patients and researchers alike and lead to lost opportunity by impeding important health research. Furthermore, because such interpretations are inconsistent with the Common Rule, they lead to inequities between covered entities and non-covered entities that hold databases and biospecimen banks.

The committee's four specific recommendations below are intended to facilitate important health research by maximizing the usefulness of patient data associated with biospecimen banks and in research databases, thereby allowing novel hypotheses to be tested with existing data and materials as knowledge and technology improve. The recommendations would align interpretation of the HIPAA Privacy Rule with the Common Rule on several points, simplify or clarify the relevant processes in research, and develop new tools for data aggregation.

> **Recommendation II.B.1: HHS should develop guidance that clearly states that individuals can authorize use of PHI stored in databases or associated with biospecimen banks for specified future research under the HIPAA Privacy Rule with IRB oversight, as is allowed under the Common Rule, to facilitate use of repositories for health research.**

- Future uses should be described in sufficient detail to allow individuals to give informed consent.
- IRBs should determine that the new research is not incompatible with the initial consent.

Rationale

Databases and biospecimen banks, once created, offer a cost-effective resource of information for rapidly addressing new health research questions as technologies and knowledge advance. Collecting the data and biospecimens necessary to address each new research question as it arises would take years, or even decades, at great expense. Thus, the pace and efficiency of medical progress is enhanced significantly by using established resources whenever feasible. When new potential prognostic markers of disease are identified, for example, they must be validated by studying the markers in many patients over the course of the disease. Examining samples stored in biobanks, where disease progression has already been recorded over many years, is a fast and relatively inexpensive way of determining whether the marker has promise for clinical use and warrants further investigation.

The provisions of the HIPAA Privacy Rule, as interpreted by HHS, may impede research with established biospecimen banks and databases. The Privacy Rule requires an individual's authorization for the use or disclosure of protected information to describe, with specificity, the purpose of the proposed use or disclosure of such information.[28] HHS regards all future uses of PHI as nonspecific—and therefore ineligible for inclusion in an authorization for the collection and storage of biological materials and data. In contrast, the Common Rule makes it possible to obtain individuals' consent to future use or disclosure of their health information for health research, with IRB oversight, as long as any intended future use is described in sufficient detail to allow informed consent.

HHS has maintained that allowing individuals to authorize future uses of their PHI could leave decisions about future research projects at the discretion of covered entities, because the HIPAA Privacy Rule, unlike the Common Rule, does not require IRB or Privacy Board review of research uses and disclosures made with individual authorization.[29] For that reason, HHS requires that individuals be recontacted to obtain their authorization for the use or disclosure of their existing data and biospecimens for any additional research studies undertaken unless the researchers obtain a waiver or alteration of individual authorization. Recontacting individuals to obtain their additional authorization is very impractical. Even when another contact is possible, the process can be intrusive and burdensome for patients and their families.

As long as an IRB is overseeing the research, obtaining individuals' authorization for future use of their information in existing databases and biospecimen banks in health research should be adequate for protecting privacy. One way to overcome the discordance between the Privacy Rule and the Common Rule would be for HHS to issue guidance explicitly stating that future research may go forward if the following conditions are

---

[28] 45 C.F.R. § 164.508 (2006).
[29] Id.

met: (1) the individual's authorization describes the types or categories of research that may be conducted with the PHI stored in the database or biobank; and (2) an IRB determines that the proposed new research is not incompatible with the initial consent and authorization, and poses no more than a minimal risk.

Because science is evolving quickly, one cannot adequately anticipate what knowledge will be gained in the future. Significant opportunities for beneficial research could be lost without some revisions in the current interpretation of this portion of the HIPAA Privacy Rule. Databases and biospecimen banks created and maintained with federal funds, in particular, should be used for multiple studies as often as feasible, especially given the high cost of developing such repositories and the high value of investigating and comparing multiple scientific questions from the same pool of data.

> **Recommendation II.B.2: HHS should develop clear guidance for use of a single form that permits individuals to authorize use and disclosure of health information in a clinical trial and to authorize the storage of their biospecimens collected in conjunction with the clinical trial, in order to simplify authorization for interrelated research activities.**

Rationale

Informed consent and authorization are essential for the protection of individuals who volunteer to participate in clinical trials. Thus, it is imperative that the informed consent and authorization documents are easily understood and meaningful to the individuals involved. Ideally, all relevant information should be integrated into one simple document.

The HIPAA Privacy Rule's complex provisions have generated misperceptions about restrictions on individuals' ability to provide compound authorization for the related activities of clinical trial participation and biospecimen donation. Such misperceptions can diminish the informed nature of consent and authorization because they can lead to patient confusion and misunderstanding. HHS has stated that if a covered entity plans to collect and store biospecimens in a research repository in conjunction with a clinical trial, individuals' authorization for storage of the PHI associated with the repository must be separate from authorization for disclosure of the PHI associated with participation in the clinical trial.

HHS arrived at this interpretation through a series of steps. First, it is generally not permissible to condition treatment on an individual's authorization for the use of PHI, although the HIPAA Privacy Rule does permit a covered entity to condition treatment in a clinical trial on signing an authorization.[30] Second, although the HIPAA Privacy Rule generally permits researchers to combine an authorization form with any other type of written permission (including another authorization), it prohibits researchers from combining authorizations where the covered entity conditions the provision of treatment on signing only one of the authorizations, but not the other.[31] Because HHS has concluded that collection of PHI for a clinical trial and for a repository are separate research activities, researchers cannot condition participation in the clinical trial on signing authorization to include PHI in a repository.[32]

Currently, therefore, the two authorizations cannot be combined in one form unless (1) the form has separate signature lines for each authorization, and (2) the text clearly delineates the two activities and states that the participant is not required to sign the portion authorizing the contribution of PHI to the repository in order to receive treatment in a clinical trial.

There is much confusion about these provisions of the HIPAA Privacy Rule, and some institutions require two complete authorization forms with all the attendant language rather than two signature lines on the same form. The excess paperwork that results is burdensome for patients; can reduce the informed nature of authorization by confusing patients; and may reduce patient participation in research. Guidance from HHS to clearly indicate that a single authorization form with two signature lines is permissible in such circumstances would reduce variability and increase the informed nature of authorization.

Recommendation II.B.3: HHS should clarify the circumstances under which DNA samples or sequences are considered PHI, in order to facilitate appropriate use of DNA in health research.

Rationale

With recent technological advances in biomedical research, it is now possible to learn a great deal about disease processes and individual variations in treatment effectiveness or susceptibility to disease from genetic analyses because the DNA sequences that make up a person's genome strongly influence a person's health. In this genomic age of health research, patient blood and tissue samples stored in biospecimen banks can provide a

---

[30] 45 C.F.R. § 164.508(b)(4)(i) (2006).

[31] 45 C.F.R. § 164.508(b)(3) (2006).

[32] National Institutes of Health, *Research Repositories, Databases, and the HIPAA Privacy Rule*, January 2004, http://privacyruleandresearch.nih.gov/pdf/research_repositories_final.pdf (accessed August 1, 2008).

wealth of information for addressing long-standing questions about health and disease.

But HHS has not yet issued clear guidance on how the HIPAA Privacy Rule applies to DNA samples or sequences. HHS guidance documents indicate that blood or tissue samples themselves are not protected under HIPAA unless they contain or are associated with the 18 personal identifiers specified by the HIPAA Privacy Rule. In addition, HHS has stated that the results of an analysis of blood or tissue, if containing or associated with individually identifiable information, would be PHI. Yet the research community remains uncertain about whether genetic information accompanying biospecimens is protected under the HIPAA Privacy Rule because the list of HIPAA identifiers includes vague terms such as "biometric identifiers" and "unique identifying characteristics."[33]

Genetic information does not itself identify an individual in the absence of other identifying information. Even the European Union, which has a more restrictive privacy regime than the United States, does not consider DNA in and of itself to be a direct identifier.[34] In some circumstances, however, a person's genetic code could be construed as a unique identifier in that it could be used to match sequence in another biospecimen bank or databank that does include identifiers. As genetic information becomes more prevalent in research and health care, the latter scenario is more likely to occur. As health care enters the era of personalized medicine, for example, genetic information is more likely to be included in a person's health records. But at the same time, realization of the promises of personalized medicine will require research on DNA from a great many diverse individuals whose medical history is well documented.

The committee believes that establishing consistent standards for the use and protection of genetic information is important. The committee advocates a focus on strong security measures and recommends the adoption of strict prohibitions on the unauthorized reidentification of individuals from DNA sequences, by anyone.

Regardless of how genetic information is regulated under the HIPAA Privacy Rule, a federal prohibition of genetic discrimination is necessary to allay privacy concerns and diminish potential negative consequences of unintended disclosure of genetic information. Many people are concerned about genetic discrimination—the misuse of genetic information by insurance companies, employers, and others to make decisions based on a person's DNA. Thus, in addition to protecting the privacy of individuals'

---

[33] 45 C.F.R. § 164.514 (2006).

[34] Article 29 Data Protection Working Party, European Union, "Opinion 4/2007 on the Concept of Personal Data," WP 136, adopted June 27, 2007, http://ec.europa.eu/justice_home/fsj/privacy/docs/wpdocs/2007/wp136_en.pdf (accessed August 1, 2008).

genetic information, it is important to protect people against genetic discrimination. The hope is that the Genetic Information Nondiscrimination Act of 2008, recently signed into law, will begin to address some of these concerns.

> **Recommendation II.B.4: HHS should develop a mechanism for linking data from multiple sources so that more useful datasets can be made available for research in a manner that protects privacy, confidentiality, and security.**

Rationale

Because a single database may not provide a complete picture of a patient's condition or health history, it is often necessary to combine information about a patient from multiple sources. However, the way in which the HIPAA Privacy Rule has been interpreted and implemented has made linking data from diverse sources for research purposes more difficult. Thus, the Privacy Rule impedes health research and compromises the value and reliability of research that is undertaken.

Under the HIPAA Privacy Rule, it is possible in principle for a researcher to aggregate PHI from multiple covered entities with individual authorization or with an IRB or Privacy Board's waiver of such authorization. Obtaining individuals' authorization for research that entails the review of thousands of medical records is unrealistic, though, and even with a waiver of authorization, covered entities with large datasets are now often reluctant to allow researchers access to PHI. More commonly, covered entities provide data to researchers with direct identifiers removed. Because datasets from multiple sources cannot be linked to generate a more complete record of a patient's health history without a unique identifier, though, datasets with direct identifiers removed are often of minimal value to researchers and are not frequently used. A third party may collect PHI from covered entities and aggregate the data for research by establishing business associate agreements with the various data sources, but in practice, such agreements are used infrequently for this purpose because they are complicated and impractical to set up for individual research projects.

The committee believes a better approach would be to establish secure, trusted intermediaries that could develop a protocol, or key, for routinely linking health data from different sources, and then provide more complete and useful datasets with the identifiers removed to researchers. One way this could be accomplished, for example, might be through data warehouses that are certified for the purpose of linking data from different sources. The organizations responsible for such linking would be required to use strong security measures and would maintain the details about how the linkage was done, should another research team need to recreate the linked dataset. Using such intermediaries would facilitate greater use of health data with direct identifiers removed for research and lead to more meaningful study results while also increasing patient privacy protections and allaying concerns of covered entities.

Some federal agencies are already developing mechanisms for linking information from different sources. The Centers for Medicare & Medicaid Services (CMS), for example, provides a linking service for Medicare and Medicaid data via contractors that create standardized data files tailored for research. CMS also has begun pilot projects to aggregate Medicare claims data with data from commercial health plans and, in some cases, Medicaid, in order to calculate and report quality measures for physician groups.

A broader effort to link data from diverse sources, called the National Health Data Stewardship Entity, has been initiated by the federal Agency for Healthcare Research and Quality (AHRQ). AHRQ is also involved in implementing the Patient Safety and Quality Improvement Act of 2005, which encourages creation of Patient Safety Organizations to receive information from hospitals, doctors, and health care providers on a privileged and confidential basis, for analysis and aggregation. Even though the purpose of these two AHRQ initiatives is to monitor health care quality,[35,36] they could provide a model for data aggregation that is potentially applicable to health research.

The administrative simplification provisions of HIPAA specifically provided for the creation of a unique individual identifier that would permit the linking of data from different sources, but work on developing such an identifier has been halted because there is a great deal of controversy regarding how it could be implemented without compromising individual privacy. In addition, federal agencies are under pressure from the Office of Budget and Management to reduce the use of Social Security numbers as unique identifiers. Nevertheless, it is clear that the development of some type of linking key (not based on Social Security numbers) would make linkages among databases more efficient, standardized, and reliable, and less costly. Moreover, this type of linkage could greatly facilitate many types of information research and improve quality of care.

Recommendation II.C. HHS should revise provisions of the HIPAA Privacy Rule that entail heavy burdens for covered entities and impede

---

[35] National Health Data Stewardship, Request for Information, 72 Fed. Reg. 30803 (June 4, 2007).

[36] Agency for Healthcare Research and Quality, U.S. Department of Health and Human Services, Patient Safety Organizations Website, http://www.pso.ahrq.gov (accessed August 1, 2008); Patient Safety and Quality Improvement Act, Notice of Proposed Rulemaking, 73 Fed. Reg. 8112 (February 12, 2008).

research without providing substantive improvements in patient privacy.

Background

For some provisions of the HIPAA Privacy Rule, the burdens are heavy and the privacy protections are small. Such provisions may need to be reconsidered if society is to derive maximal benefits from health research. The committee recommends revising two components of the HIPAA Privacy Rule that are very burdensome with respect to the level of privacy protection they afford.

Recommendation II.C.1: HHS should reform the requirements for the accounting of disclosures (AOD) of PHI for research.

- The HIPAA Privacy Rule should permit covered entities to inform patients in advance that PHI might be used for health research with IRB/Privacy Board oversight or for public health purposes. Accordingly, the Privacy Rule should be revised to exempt disclosures of PHI made for research and public health purposes from the Privacy Rule's accounting of disclosures requirements. As an alternative to AOD, to ensure transparency, institutions should maintain a list, accessible to the public, of all studies approved by an IRB/Privacy Board.

Rationale

Under the HIPAA Privacy Rule, individuals have a right to receive an accounting of disclosures, a list of all disclosures of their PHI by a covered entity or the covered entity's business associates in the past 6 years. According to HHS, the AOD provision of the HIPAA Privacy Rule was intended "as a means for the individual to find out the nonroutine purposes for which his or her PHI was disclosed by the covered entity, so as to increase the individual's awareness of persons or entities other than the individual's health care provider or health plan in possession of this information." The AOD requirement does not constitute an audit trail, though, because the provision has numerous exceptions—including disclosures of PHI for health care operations, pursuant to an authorization, as part of a limited dataset, for national security or intelligence purposes, and to correctional institutions or law enforcement officials.

Disclosures of PHI by covered entities for research purposes under a waiver of individual authorization approved by an IRB or a Privacy Board, or for public health purposes as required by law, must be included in an AOD report. Furthermore, HHS has noted that "making a set of records available for review by a third party constitutes a disclosure of the PHI in the entire set of records, regardless of whether the third party actually reviews any particular record." The AOD provision of the HIPAA Privacy Rule provides an exception for research involving groups of 50 or more subjects by allowing the covered entity to develop a general list of all protocols for which a person's PHI may have been disclosed. Even then, however, there is a considerable administrative obligation to generate such a list. Furthermore, in many medical facilities, a general list of protocols is extensive and thus relatively meaningless to a particular patient.

The AOD provision of the HIPAA Privacy Rule places a heavy administrative burden on health systems and health services research that achieves little in terms of protecting privacy. Moreover, HHS has provided no guidance to covered entities about practical ways to fulfill this requirement in an efficient manner. On the basis of testimony in 2004, the Secretary's Advisory Committee on Human Research Protections concluded that the cost and burden of compliance with the HIPAA Privacy Rule's AOD requirements were so high that institutions were likely to accept the risk of noncompliance rather than incur the cost of compliance.

Annual surveys of health care privacy officers undertaken by the American Health Information Management Association (AHIMA) since 2004 have similarly found that many facilities report difficulties with the AOD requirement. Such surveys have also found that the demand for AOD reports by individuals is extremely low. Two thirds of health care privacy officers participating in the survey reported receiving no requests at all. Nearly one third of respondents indicated that they would like to see a change to the AOD provision of the HIPAA Privacy Rule—the most frequently cited provision among all respondents and the most frequently cited provision by far among respondents with more than 20,000 admissions/discharges per year. On the basis of these results, AHIMA concluded that "for many, this [AOD] provision is not only burdensome but also significantly inefficient."[37]

Robust safeguards are already in place to protect the privacy of PHI disclosures in health research via IRBs and Privacy Boards. As the health care system moves toward broader implementation of electronic health records, however, automatic tracking of audit trails will be important to incorporate. Technology advances will likely make automatic AOD tracking feasible, affordable, and widely available in the future. Until then, the committee recommends that disclosures of PHI made for health research

---

[37] American Health Information Management Association, 2006, *The State of HIPAA Privacy and Security Compliance*, http://www.ahima.org/emerging_issues/2006StateofHIPAACompliance.pdf (accessed April 20, 2008).

and public health purposes be exempted from the HIPAA Privacy Rule's AOD requirement.

> **Recommendation II.C.2: HHS should simplify the criteria that IRBs and Privacy Boards use in making determinations for when they can waive the requirements to obtain authorization from each patient whose PHI will be used for a research study, in order to facilitate appropriate authorization requirements for responsible research.**

- If HHS decides to retain the current waiver criteria, HHS should provide clear and reasonable definitions of terms used in those criteria, such as "minimal risk" to the privacy of individuals (in the first criterion) and "impracticable" (in the second and third criteria). HHS should also provide specific case examples of what should or should not be considered impracticable or of minimal risk.

Rationale

Under the HIPAA Privacy Rule, researchers seeking to use PHI in medical records for research must obtain authorization from each patient unless an IRB or a Privacy Board makes a determination that a waiver of individual authorization is warranted. For many types of research with medical records, making that determination is a challenge for IRBs and Privacy Boards. Many studies involve thousands of records, making individual authorization unrealistic. But the criteria in the HIPAA Privacy Rule that IRBs and Privacy Boards apply in making these decisions are complex and very subjective.

Currently, IRBs and Privacy Boards must use three criteria in considering whether to approve a waiver of individual authorization for the use of PHI in research.[38] The first criterion is that the use or disclosure of PHI in the research involves no more than a "minimal risk" to the privacy of individuals. The Privacy Rule lists three elements that must be present in making this determination: (1) "an adequate plan to protect the identifiers from improper use and disclosure;" (2) "an adequate plan to destroy the identifiers;" and (3) "adequate written assurances that the PHI will not be reused or disclosed to any other person or entity, except as required by law, for authorized oversight of the research project, or for other research for which the use or disclosure of PHI is otherwise permissible." However, the decision about what is "adequate" is highly subjective, and thus different institutions are likely to set varying thresholds for "minimal risk."

---

[38] 45 C.F.R. § 164.512(i)(2)(ii) (2006).

The other two criteria that IRBs or Privacy Boards currently must use in considering whether to approve a waiver of individual authorization are (1) that "the research could not practicably be conducted without the waiver;" and (2) that the "research could not practicably be conducted without access to and use of PHI"[39] (as opposed to deidentified data or a limited dataset). The concept of practicability is used in both the Common Rule and in the HIPAA authorization criteria, but what is "practicable" or "impracticable" has never been adequately defined by the HHS Office for Human Research Protections or the HHS Office for Civil Rights (e.g., with regard to cost/feasibility). Not surprisingly, therefore, institutions apply varying definitions independently, often too conservatively to allow even low-risk research to proceed. Some institutions interpret the term impracticable to mean not at all possible and even require researchers to demonstrate that a study will fail without a waiver of authorization. The lack of clarity leads to a great deal of variability across institutions and impedes research. Patients have also questioned the meaning of the term.

Simplification or clarification by HHS of the criteria that IRBs or Privacy Boards must use in deciding whether to approve a waiver of individual authorization would be especially helpful for multi-institutional studies, which fall under the jurisdiction of multiple IRBs or Privacy Boards. Covered entities are permitted to rely on a waiver of authorization approved by a single IRB or Privacy Board with jurisdiction. Currently, however, covered entities often decide to require approval from their own IRB or Privacy Board prior to disclosing PHI to the requesting researcher, regardless of whether another IRB or Privacy Board already granted a waiver of authorization. This practice leads to delays and variability in the protocol at different sites.

Simplification of the criteria for approval of waivers by IRBs and Privacy Boards would also be helpful for smaller or community-based institutions that do not have internal counsel or regulatory affairs specialists, and thus are more likely to opt out of research that requires decisions about authorizations. With better guidance, all covered entities would have more confidence in their decisions and might be more willing to rely on a lead IRB or Privacy Board's decision in the case of multi-institutional studies.

If HHS decides to retain the three criteria that IRBs or Privacy Boards currently use in deciding whether to approve a waiver of individual authorization, however, the committee recommends that HHS provide clear and reasonable definitions of the vague terms used in those criteria. Specifically, HHS should define what constitutes "minimal risk" to the privacy of individuals (in the first criterion) and define what constitutes "impracticable" (in the second and third criteria). HHS should also provide specific case

---

[39] *Id.*

examples of what should or should not be considered impracticable or of minimal risk to reduce variability and overly conservative interpretations.

III. Implement Changes Necessary for Both Policy Options Above (Recommendations I and II)

Regardless of whether Recommendation I or II is implemented, the following recommendations, which are independent of the Privacy Rule, should be adopted. Strong security measures are essential to effective privacy protection, willingness to serve in IRBs is important for ensuring appropriate oversight of research, and the public should be provided with more information about health research.

> **Recommendation III.A:** All institutions (both covered entities and non-covered entities) in the health research community that are involved in the collection, use, and disclosure of personally identifiable health information should take strong measures to safeguard the security of health data. For example, institutions could:
>
> - Appoint a security officer responsible for assessing data protection needs and implementing solutions and staff training.
> - Make greater use of encryption and other techniques for data security.
> - Include data security experts on IRBs.
> - Implement a breach notification requirement, so that patients may take steps to protect their identity in the event of a breach.
> - Implement layers of security protection to eliminate single points of vulnerability to security breaches.
>
> In addition, the federal government should support the development and use of:
>
> - Genuine privacy-enhancing techniques that minimize or eliminate the collection of personally identifiable data.
> - Standardized self-evaluations and security audits and certification programs to help institutions achieve the goal of safeguarding the security of personal health data.

Rationale

Effective health privacy protections require effective data security measures. Protecting the privacy of research participants and maintaining the confidentiality of their data have always been imperative to most researchers and a fundamental tenet of clinical research. Recently, however, several highly publicized examples of stolen or misplaced computers containing health data have heightened the public's concerns about privacy. Such events pose problems not only for patient privacy, but also for health research, because public trust is essential for patients to be willing to participate in research. Moreover, data security is a key component of comprehensive privacy protections. Thus, the committee recommends improving the security of personally identifiable health information.

The HIPAA Security Rule (which entails a set of regulatory provisions separate from the Privacy Rule) already sets a floor for data security standards within covered entities, but not all institutions that conduct health research are subject to HIPAA regulations. Moreover, the security protections intended by the HIPAA Security Rule may not be sufficient to prevent breaches.

The committee recommends that all institutions conducting health research undertake measures to strengthen data protections. Given the recent spate of lost or stolen laptops containing patient health information, for example, encryption should be required for all laptops and removable media containing such data. There are differences among the missions and activities of institutions in the health research community, however, so some flexibility in the implementation of specific security measures will be necessary.

Examples of security standards and guidelines already exist in some sectors, but they are not widely applied in academic settings. The National Institute of Standards and Technology (NIST), for example, has developed standards and guidance for the implementation of the Federal Information Security Management Act of 2002, which was meant to bolster computer and network security within the federal government and affiliated parties (e.g., government contractors). The NIST standards include minimum security requirements for information and information systems, as well as guidance for assessing and selecting appropriate security controls for information systems, for determining security control effectiveness, and for certifying and accrediting information systems.[40]

HHS, working through its Office of the National Coordinator for Health Information Technology,[41] could play an important role in developing or adapting standards for health research applications, then encourage and facilitate broader use of such standards in the health research commu-

---

[40]National Institute of Standards and Technology (NIST), Federal Information Security Management Act Implementation Project Website, updated November 1, 2007, http://csrc.nist.gov/groups/SMA/fisma/index.html (accessed August 1, 2008).

[41]Office of the National Coordinator for Health Information Technology, U.S. Department of Health and Human Services, Office of the National Coordinator: Mission, http://www.hhs.gov/healthit/onc/mission/ (accessed August 1, 2008).

nity. The issue of the security of health data will continue to grow in importance as the health care industry moves toward widespread implementation of electronic health records, and Congress has already proposed numerous bills to facilitate and regulate that transition. As noted in the committee's recommendation about the requirements for the accounting of disclosures of PHI for research above (Recommendation II.C.1), advances in information technology will likely make it easier to implement measures such as audit trails and access controls in the future.

Enhancing security could reduce the risk of data theft and reinforce the public's trust in the research community by diminishing anxiety about the potential for unintentional disclosure of information. The publication of best practices and outreach to all stakeholders by HHS, combined with a cooperative approach to compliance with security standards such as self-evaluation and audit programs, would promote progress in this area. As noted in Recommendation II.A.1, research sponsors could also play a role in fostering the adoption of best practices in data security.

Recommendation III.B: HHS—or, as necessary, Congress—should provide reasonable protection against civil suits brought pursuant to federal or state law for members of IRBs and Privacy Boards for decisions made within the scope of their responsibilities under the HIPAA Privacy Rule and the Common Rule, in order to encourage service on Institutional Review Boards and Privacy Boards. The limitation on liability for members of IRBs and Privacy Boards should not include protection for willful and wanton misconduct in reviewing the research, but should instead be reserved for good-faith decisions, backed by minutes or other evidence, in responsibly applying the legal requirements under the HIPAA Privacy Rule or the Common Rule.

Rationale

IRBs, Privacy Boards, and institutions have enormous responsibility in determining whether health research projects are planned and conducted in a way that minimizes or eliminates the potential risk to human research participants, including both direct physical harms and nonphysical harms (e.g., breach of privacy). The workload of IRBs and the complexity of their work have been steadily increasing as a result of new and evolving requirements for research regulation and documentation, including the HIPAA Privacy Rule. Surveys and studies indicate that the IRB review process has become more lengthy and difficult since implementation of the Privacy Rule, which may increase opportunity costs due to delayed or undiscovered research findings that might improve health.

Effective oversight of health research depends on the recruitment of qualified and knowledgeable volunteers to serve on IRBs and Privacy Boards. But the increasing workload and complexity of IRB and Privacy Board service have made it difficult to recruit and retain knowledgeable IRB and Privacy Board members and to ensure time for the ethical reflection necessary to make appropriate decisions about human research projects. Moreover, because of the growth over the past decade of lawsuits naming individual IRB members as defendants, fear of penalties and civil suits can be a significant deterrent in recruiting qualified volunteers to serve on IRBs and Privacy Boards. Such fears could also lead IRB and Privacy Board members to be overly conservative in their decisions about research proposals brought before them.

Members of IRBs and Privacy Boards are generally indemnified by their institutions, but they are not immune from being named in a suit. Therefore, they might still have to devote time and resources to defending themselves for decisions made by an IRB or Privacy Board on which they served. Members of IRBs or Privacy Boards who receive limited protection against lawsuits may be less likely to interpret the HIPAA Privacy Rule too conservatively.

Providing this type of limitation on liability for IRB and Privacy Board members would be similar to the precedent of protection for peer review members under state laws and under the Health Care Quality Improvement Act of 1986. A similar provision was incorporated into the Ontario Personal Health Information Protection Act of 2004, under which members of ethical boards are immune for acts done and omissions made in good faith that are reasonable under the circumstances. In addition to reducing over interpretation of the HIPAA Privacy Rule in health research, such protections might also facilitate multi-institutional research by reducing the variability among local IRBs and Privacy Boards, as they should be more willing to accept the decision of a lead IRB or Privacy Board. Indeed, moving in the direction of national IRBs/Privacy Boards, as is encouraged by the National Cancer Institute for cancer clinical trials, might further reduce overly conservative interpretation of the HIPAA Privacy Rule.

Finally, it should be noted that HHS policy is to seek compliance with the HIPAA Privacy Rule first, rather than penalties, when a concern is brought to its attention. Institutions might be less inclined to interpret the HIPAA Privacy Rule too conservatively if this policy were stated more clearly in guidance materials provided by HHS. Thus, even without the enactment of a new protective statute for IRB and Privacy Board members, simple clarification and clear communication of the way HHS will enforce the HIPAA Privacy Rule and seek penalties would be helpful.

Recommendation III.C: HHS and researchers should take steps to provide the public with more information about health research.

Background

Surveys indicate that the vast majority of Americans believe health research is important, and are interested in the findings of research studies. The majority of patients also appear to be willing to participate in health research, either by volunteering for a study to test a medical intervention or by allowing access to their medical records or stored biospecimens, under certain conditions. Their willingness to participate in research is dependent on trust in researchers to safeguard the rights and well-being of patients, including assurance of privacy and confidentiality, and the belief that the research is a worthwhile endeavor that warrants their involvement. Yet patients often lack information about how health research is conducted and are rarely informed about research results that may have a direct impact on their health. The committee's two recommendations below address the public's desire for more information about health research and are important components in fulfilling two of the committee's overarching goals of the report: (1) improving the privacy and data security of health information, and (2) improving the effectiveness of health research. Both recommendations could be accomplished by HHS and the health research community without any changes to HIPAA or the Privacy Rule by making them a condition of funding from HHS and other research sponsors and by providing additional funds to cover the cost.

Recommendation III.C.1: Health researchers should make greater efforts to inform study participants and the public about the results of research and the relevance and importance of those results.

- Researchers should inform interested research participants (who granted authorization for a particular study) with a simplified summary of the results at the conclusion of a research study.
- HHS should encourage registration of trials and other studies in public databases, particularly when research is conducted with a waiver of authorization.

Rationale

Empirical evidence indicates that people want to be informed about research results, and ethicists have long recommended this kind of feedback and community involvement. In addition, the IOM committee identified transparency—the responsibility to disclose clearly how and why personally identifiable information is being collected—as an important component of comprehensive privacy protections. An IOM report in 2002 titled *Responsible Research: A Systems Approach to Protecting Research Participants* recommended improved communication with the public and research participants to ensure that the protection process is open and accessible to all interested parties, noting that transparency is best achieved by providing graded levels of information and guidance to interested parties.

Effective communication could also build the public's trust in the research community, which is important because trust is necessary for the public's continued participation in research under both the HIPAA Privacy Rule and the committee's new framework. Learning about clinically relevant findings from a study in which a patient has participated could make patients feel more integrated into the process and could encourage more patients to participate in future studies. Moreover, if the study results indicate that an altered course of care is warranted, direct feedback about these results could lead to improved health care for study participants.

Thus, the committee recommends that when patients grant authorization for their medical records to be used in a particular study, health researchers should make greater efforts at the conclusion of the study to inform study participants about the results, and the relevance and importance of those results. Broader adoption of electronic medical records may be helpful in accomplishing this goal, but multiple impediments, beyond cost and technology, may prevent delivery of meaningful feedback to participants. Although some guidelines for providing and explaining study results to research participants have been proposed, they differ in details because limited data are available on this subject, and thus standards are lacking. A summary of the results alone, while necessary and reasonable, can be seen as a token, and also raises questions about issues such as how best to write summaries and how to present research with uninformative outcomes.

HHS should also encourage registration of trials and other studies in public databases, particularly when research is conducted with a waiver of authorization as a way to make information about research studies more broadly available to the public. Numerous clinical trial registries already exist, and registration has increased in recent years. The National Library of Medicine established a clinical trials registry[42] in 2000, which has expanded to serve as the FDA's required site for submissions about clinical trials subject to the FDA databank requirement and now also includes information from several other trial registries. The FDA Amendments Act of 2007 expanded the scope of required registrations and provided the first federally funded trials results database. In fall 2005, the International Committee of Medical Journal Editors adopted a policy requiring prospective trial registration as a precondition for publication.

The development of clinical trial registries is an important first step toward providing high-quality clinical trial information to the public. Cur-

---

[42] See http://clinicaltrials.gov (accessed August 6, 2008).

rently, however, there is no centralized system for disseminating information about clinical trials of drugs or other interventions. Thus, patients and their health care providers have difficulty identifying ongoing studies. Moreover, some trials are still exempt from registration and data reporting. An additional limitation of clinical trial databases is that noninterventional studies (including observational studies that play an increasingly critical role in biomedical research) are not generally included. Because many noninterventional studies are conducted with a waiver of authorization, including those studies in a registry could be an important method for increasing public knowledge of those studies.

Recommendation III.C.2: HHS and the health research community should work to educate the public about how health research is done, and what value it provides.

Rationale

Health research provides a community benefit by determining the most effective treatments and by developing new therapies. Interventional clinical trials are the most visible of the various types of health research, but a great deal of informative health research entails analysis of thousands of patient records to better understand human diseases, to determine treatment effectiveness, and to identify adverse side effects of therapies. This form of research is likely to increase in frequency as the availability of electronic health records continues to expand. As medicine moves toward the goal of personalized medicine, research results will be even more likely to be directly relevant to patients, but more study participants will be needed to derive meaningful results.

However, many patients probably are not aware that their medical records are being used in database research. Moreover, surveys show that many patients desire not only notice, but also the opportunity to decide about whether to consent to such research with medical records. As noted in Recommendation III.A, strengthening security protections of health data should reduce the risk of security breaches and their potential negative consequences, and thus should help to alleviate patient concerns in this regard. But educating patients about how health research is conducted, monitored, and reported could also help to increase patients trust in the research community, which is important for the public's continued participation under both the HIPAA Privacy Rule and the committee's new framework.

In addition, an educated public could also decrease the potential for biased research samples. A universal requirement to obtain authorization for medical records research can lead to a biased study sample, and thus inaccurate conclusions, because those who decline to participate may be more or less likely than average to have a particular health problem. A study sample may also be biased if certain members are underrepresented or overrepresented relative to others in the population. A biased sample is problematic, because any statistic computed from that sample has the potential to be consistently erroneous, and thus, conclusions drawn from a biased sample are likely to be invalid. Conveying to the public the importance of health care improvements derived from medical records research and stressing the negative impact of incomplete datasets on research findings may increase the public's participation in research and their willingness to support information-based research that is conducted with IRB or Privacy Board oversight and a waiver of patient authorization.

There are numerous examples of important research findings from medical records research that would not have been possible if direct patient consent and authorization were always required, including the finding that infants exposed to diethylstilbestrol (DES) during the first trimester of pregnancy had an increased risk of breast, vaginal, and cervical cancer and reproductive anomalies as adults. Studies of medical records also led to the discovery that folic acid supplementation during pregnancy can prevent neural tube defects.

Thus, HHS and the health research community should work to educate the public about how research is done, and what value it provides. All stakeholders, including professional organizations, nonprofit funders, and patient organizations, have different interests and responsibilities to make sure their constituencies are well informed, but coordination and identification of best practices by HHS would be helpful. For example, the American Society of Clinical Oncology and the American Heart Association already have some online resources to help patients gather information about research that may be relevant to their conditions. Research is needed to identify which segments of the population would be receptive to and benefit from various types of information about how research is done and its value in order to create and implement an effective education plan.

Greater use of community-based participatory research, in which community-based organizations or groups bring community members into the research process as partners to help design studies and disseminate the knowledge gained,[43] would also help achieve this goal. These groups help researchers to design activities that the community is likely to value and to recruit research participants, by using the knowledge of the community to understand health problems. They also inform community members about how the research is done and what comes out of it, with the goal of providing immediate community benefits from the results when possible.

---

[43] Agency for Healthcare Research and Quality, U.S. Department of Health and Human Services, *Creating Partnerships, Improving Health: The Role of Community-Based Participatory Research*, June 2003, http://www.ahrq.gov/research/cbprrole.htm (accessed August 1, 2008).

1

Introduction

BRIEF HISTORY OF HIPAA AND THE PRIVACY RULE

The Health Insurance Portability and Accountability Act (HIPAA) was passed on August 21, 1996, with the dual goals of making health care delivery more efficient and increasing the number of Americans with health insurance coverage. These objectives were pursued through three main provisions of the Act: (1) the portability provisions, (2) the tax provisions, and (3) the administrative simplification provisions. The focus of this report, the HIPAA Privacy Rule, was promulgated under the third provision. The administrative simplification provisions of HIPAA instructed the Secretary of the U.S. Department of Health and Human Services (HHS) to issue several regulations concerning electronic transmission of health information, which was expanding greatly in the early 1990s. The primary purpose of these provisions was to standardize the use of electronic health information, but Congress also recognized that advances in electronic technology could endanger the privacy of health information. Thus, HIPAA mandated the development of nationwide security standards and safeguards for the use of electronic health care information as well as the creation of privacy standards for protected health information.[1]

---

[1] Protected health information is personally identifiable health information transmitted by electronic media, maintained in electronic media, or transmitted or maintained in any other form or medium. Protected health information excludes education records covered by the Family Educational Rights and Privacy Act, as amended, 20 U.S.C. 1232(g), records described at 20 U.S.C. 1232(g)(a)(4)(B)(iv), and employment records held by a covered entity in its role as employer.

Although the Common Rule[2] imposed some requirements on the use of health information in research, federal regulations specifically targeting health information privacy were lacking. In accordance with the administrative simplification provisions, HHS developed the HIPAA Privacy Rule, which set out detailed regulations regarding the types of uses and disclosures of personally identifiable health information that are permitted by the covered entities.[3] HHS first issued a proposed version of the HIPAA Privacy Rule for public comment in 1999, but because of the enormous volume of comments received regarding the regulations, as well as a change in executive branch leadership following the 2000 Presidential election, the HIPAA Privacy Rule evolved through several iterations before the final version was issued in 2002 (45 C.F.R. parts 160 and 164). Most health care providers and health plans were required to be in compliance with this version of the HIPAA Privacy Rule by April 14, 2003. Small health plans were given until April 14, 2004, to be in compliance.

The primary targets of the HIPAA Privacy Rule were information uses and transactions necessary for the provision of health care, but the final regulations also apply to a great deal of health research. Congress recognized the important role that health records play in conducting health research, and wanted to ensure that implementation of the HIPAA Privacy Rule would not impede researchers' continued access to such data. This is reflected in two House reports on HIPAA with identical language, stating: "The conferees recognize that certain uses of individually identifiable information are appropriate, and do not compromise the privacy of an individual. Examples of such use of information include . . . the transfer of information from a health plan to an organization for the sole purpose of conducting health care–related research. As health plans and providers continue to focus on outcomes research and innovation, it is important that the exchange and aggregated use of health care data be allowed" (U.S. Congress, 1996a,b).

In response, HHS attempted to create a system that mandated privacy protection for individually identifiable health information while allowing important uses of the information in health care and research. Thus, researchers must now follow the provisions of the HIPAA Privacy Rule when obtaining data from a covered entity.

---

[2] The "Common Rule" is the term used by 18 federal agencies who have adopted the same regulations governing the protection of human subjects of research.

[3] 45 C.F.R. § 160.103 (2006), a health plan, a health care clearinghouse, or a health care provider that transmits health information in electronic form in connection with a transaction for which HHS has adopted a standard.

PRIVACY AND HEALTH RESEARCH

Health research and privacy protections both provide valuable benefits to society, and the two topics are interrelated. Researchers know that trust is essential for patients to be willing to participate in research, and many patients value research and are willing to share their health information in the hope of reaping some benefit from scientific advances for themselves or their families. Collection and analysis of health information is necessary to attain the full benefits of health research for the individual, the family, and the community. The challenge is to identify the most essential components of both privacy protection and research, to ensure maximal benefit and minimal risk.

Some health research projects with important implications for health care improvements and public health protections entail the analysis of information that many would consider sensitive. For example, some research examines information regarding individuals' sexuality, or smoking, alcohol, and drug use habits. Also, it may be necessary to collect information on an individual's social, racial, or economic status to study the influence of poverty, nutrition, and social relationships on health. Many research projects now also study a person's genetic profile to gain insight into predispositions for diseases. Epidemiology and public health research may trace disease incidence and characteristics, or response to treatments.

Research participants are more willing to share personal information and more likely to truthfully answer research questions when they believe the privacy of their personal information is protected against inadvertent or unwanted disclosure. This helps to assure individuals that their risk of harm in participating, including economic, social, or psychological harm, is minimal (Hodge et al., 1999). Furthermore, when researchers have access to accurate and comprehensive medical datasets, the results are more likely to be valid and meaningful to broad populations.

PRIVACY CONCERNS

Since the HIPAA Privacy Rule was implemented, privacy advocates and others have argued that the United States needs stronger privacy protections than are provided in the HIPAA Privacy Rule (Friedman, 2006; Gellman, 2006; Sobel, 2007). These demands have generally focused on health care rather than health research, and are based to a large extent on theory, opinions, and anecdotal experiences. As noted in the methods section below, a Harris Poll undertaken during the course of this study provided new and current insight into the experiences and expectations of the U.S. public with regard to privacy in health research. A review of the relevant literature, including surveys and focus group studies, can be found in Chapter 2.

After reviewing the available evidence, the committee concluded that the public is deeply concerned about the privacy and security of personal health information, and that the HIPAA Privacy Rule has reduced, but not eliminated, those concerns. In some surveys, the majority of respondents were not comfortable with their health information being provided for health research except with notice and express consent. But in others, a majority of respondents were willing to forgo notice and consent if various safeguards and specific types of research were specified. As noted in Chapter 3, surveys also indicate that the majority of Americans are supportive of health research, but they lack information about how research is conducted and are rarely informed about research results that may have a direct impact on their health.

THE CONCERNS OF HEALTH RESEARCHERS

Researchers began raising concerns about the potential impact of the HIPAA Privacy Rule on health research when the regulations were first proposed. However, researchers did not play a large role in shaping the final version of the HIPAA Privacy Rule published by HHS. Most of the comments that HHS received from the research community during the notice of proposed rulemaking period were focused on urging HHS not to include research within the HIPAA Privacy Rule regulations at all. Few comments suggested alternatives to the regulatory scheme proposed by HHS, or gave HHS constructive comments on how to incorporate the research provisions into the rule (IOM, 2006).

After the date of compliance for the HIPAA Privacy Rule, the concerns of researchers escalated. Numerous anecdotal reports and expert opinions, along with a number of surveys, indicate that the HIPAA Privacy Rule has had a negative effect on the ability of researchers to conduct valid research due to new restrictions on access to health data, and has not produced a measurable increase in the protection of data used in research (NCVHS, 2003; Ramirez and Niederhuber, 2003; Tovino, 2004; Walker, 2005) (see also Chapter 5). Because of the reported concerns about the HIPAA Privacy Rule's effect on research, several organizations have provided HHS with recommendations on how to improve the way the HIPAA Privacy Rule regulates research. The past recommendations of the National Committee on Vital and Health Statistics, the Association of American Medical Colleges, and the HHS Secretary's Advisory Committee on Human Research Protections are listed in Appendix A. As noted in the methods section below, several new surveys were also undertaken during the course of this study to provide more current, systematic data for the committee's deliberations. The committee also reviewed a number of studies that attempted to assess the impact of the HIPAA

Privacy Rule on health research. A complete review of the literature can be found in Chapter 5.

ORIGINS OF THE STUDY

The 2003 Annual Report of the President's Cancer Panel, which made a number of recommendations regarding issues affecting cancer survivors, also included a recommendation that "The Institute of Medicine (IOM) should be commissioned to evaluate the impact of HIPAA provisions and provide guidance to legislators on amendments needed to make this law serve the interests of cancer survivors and others" after concluding that the HIPAA Privacy Rule slowed research on cancer survivors in a variety of ways (President's Cancer Panel, 2004). The Panel's 2005–2006 report again called for an evaluation of the HIPAA Privacy Rule provisions that were thought to inhibit the ability to track and collect data for research on cancer survivors (President's Cancer Panel, 2006). Based on those recommendations, the IOM's National Cancer Policy Forum held a workshop on the topic, inviting a diverse group of speakers representing many relevant stakeholders from academia, industry, and the public. The proceedings of that workshop, held June 16, 2006, were then reported in a summary published by the IOM (IOM, 2006).

At that workshop, speakers reiterated many of the challenges described above in applying the HIPAA Privacy Rule to health research, noting that despite having several years to learn and adapt to the new rules, as well as new guidance from HHS and the Office for Civil Rights (OCR), researchers are still facing difficulty in working under the HIPAA Privacy Rule. Although the goal of the HIPAA Privacy Rule was to establish a uniform set of federal standards to be applied nationwide, many speakers testified that there is enormous variation among institutions and oversight boards in the way the regulations are interpreted and applied, with many adopting exceptionally conservative interpretations. Moreover, it was reported that many smaller institutions lacked the staff and infrastructure to implement the regulations on research and ensure compliance, and were opting out of research entirely to avoid the risk of penalties for HIPAA noncompliance (IOM, 2006). However, many speakers also stressed the need to maintain or strengthen the privacy protections for personal health information.

Following the publication of the IOM's National Cancer Policy Forum's workshop summary, the governing board of the National Academies determined that a consensus study to examine the effects of the HIPAA Privacy Rule on health research would be of value, and funding for the study was obtained from diverse sources, including the National Institutes of Health, the National Cancer Institute, the Burroughs Wellcome Fund, the Robert Wood Johnson Foundation, the American Heart Association (AHA)/

American Stroke Association, the American Cancer Society, the American Society for Clinical Oncology (ASCO), and C-Change.

COMMITTEE APPOINTMENT AND CHARGE

The funders of the study asked the IOM to examine the available evidence to determine whether the HIPAA Privacy Rule was impacting the conduct of health research. As a major funder of the study, HHS had a particular interest in distinguishing direct effects of mandates in the HIPAA Privacy Rule on the conduct of research from the variable influence of interpretation and implementation of the regulations by various institutions and oversight boards.

To examine the question, the IOM appointed a 15-member committee with a broad range of expertise and experience covering various fields of health research; privacy of health information; health law, regulation, and ethics; human research protections and IRBs; health center administration; use and protection of electronic health information; and patient advocacy. The IOM committee was charged with the task of proposing recommendations that would facilitate the efficient and effective conduct of responsible health research while maintaining or strengthening the privacy protections of identifiable health information (Box 1-1).

METHODS

The committee reviewed the available published literature and obtained input from experts in the field and interested individuals and institutions. The literature review, as well as the proceedings of the IOM workshop described above, demonstrated there was a dearth of systematic data to determine whether the HIPAA Privacy Rule was having an impact on health research. Because many published reports were based on isolated anecdotes or small surveys, the IOM committee sought larger surveys with national coverage. As a result, the IOM, in consultation with committee members, took the unusual step of commissioning[4] several surveys to assess current perceptions among health researchers of the effect of the HIPAA Privacy Rule on research, and to gauge the public's perception of and expectations for privacy in health research. The first survey entailed a national web-based survey of U.S. epidemiologists overseen by Dr. Roberta Ness at the University of Pittsburgh. A second project, undertaken by Sarah Greene and Dr. Ed Wagner at the Group Health Center for Health Studies in Seattle, involved a survey of HMO Research Network (HMORN) investigators and

---

[4] The surveys were commissioned with private funding. No federal funds were used to support collection of survey data.

BOX 1-1
Committee Statement of Task

An Institute of Medicine committee will investigate the effects on health research of the Privacy Rule regulations implementing the Health Insurance Portability and Accountability Act of 1996 (HIPAA) section on Administrative Simplification and prepare a report. In conducting the study, the committee will:

1. Consider the range of study types, such as clinical trials, epidemiologic designs, research using tissue repositories and databases, public health research, and health services research, to the extent that available data and evidence allow;
2. Consider research carried out by the full range of sponsors: government, public and private academic, and for-profit sectors, including the pharmaceutical, biotechnology, and medical device industries;
3. Review provisions of the Privacy Rule relevant to health research, including those dealing with authorizations and accounting of disclosures of personal health information, deidentification of data, reviews preparatory to research, and others, and on reviewing them, may identify provisions that merit priority attention and analysis;
4. Consider issues of interpretation and implementation of the Privacy Rule, as well as of harmonization with overlapping provisions of the Common Rule and Food and Drug Administration regulations, which have existed much longer;
5. Examine the potential impact of the Rule on public health research, on the recruitment of research subjects for studies, on carrying out research internationally, and on research using data and biomaterials in databases and tissue repositories; and
6. Consider the needs for privacy of identifiable personal health information and the value of such privacy to patients and the public. As data and evidence allow, the needs and benefits of patient privacy will be balanced against the needs, risks, and benefits of identifiable health information for various kinds of health research. The committee will formulate recommendations for alterations or retention of the status quo accordingly.

---

a survey of HMORN Institutional Review Boards. A Harris Interactive Poll of the public, developed by Alan Westin of the Privacy Consulting Group, served as the third survey. Detailed descriptions of the methodologies and analysis for each of the surveys can be found in Appendix B. Several additional surveys and focus groups were undertaken independently by organizations, with the intent of providing input to the IOM committee. Those organizations include AcademyHealth, AHA, ASCO, the American Association of Central Cancer Registries, and the Association of Academic Health Centers.

Surveys are useful in identifying the main issues surrounding the HIPAA Privacy Rule's regulation of research, but it is important to recognize the limitations of opinion surveys. As noted briefly in Chapters 2, 3, and 5, designing quality surveys presents many challenges. These challenges include ensuring that the respondents are truly representative of the population being surveyed, developing the wording of questions, framing the responses provided, analyzing the relationship and potential influence of questions to each other in the survey process, and applying statistical analyses to the data acquired. Although they are helpful in gaining the perspective of populations of interest, such as current members of the health research community or of the public, survey methods are also prone to subject bias and error. Motivational factors may influence the results of surveys that address sensitive subjects, and respondents may be unwilling to provide accurate information for reasons of self-protection or personal gain (Wentland and Smith, 1993). In addition, experiments in social psychology suggest that responses to survey questions regarding attitude are influenced by environment, survey type, and the context in which the question is presented (Tourangeau et al., 2000). The committee's intention in presenting findings from opinion surveys, including those commissioned by the IOM, is to shed light on opinions regarding the influence of the HIPAA Privacy Rule on health research and patient privacy; it is not an attempt to definitively determine cause and effect.

THE COMMITTEE'S CONCLUSIONS AND RECOMMENDATIONS

The recommendations put forth in this report represent committee consensus that was developed through review and discussion of the above information sources. There are three general methods for improving the current system: (1) HHS and its OCR could provide more guidance to IRBs, Privacy Boards, institutions, and other participants and stakeholders, which is the simplest and most direct way to achieve change; (2) regulatory changes to the HIPAA Privacy Rule provisions may be necessary in some cases, but are more difficult to undertake; and (3) statutory change of HIPAA or other legislation at the federal or state level, which is the most difficult to accomplish. The committee tried to be as modest as possible in proposing recommendations to achieve its goals, with the aim of making it easier to effect change if policy makers agree with our proposals.

After reviewing the available evidence, the committee concluded that covered entities, Institutional Review Boards (IRBs), Privacy Boards, and researchers alike have faced difficulty in interpreting and implementing the complex regulation. There is a great deal of variation in how these stakeholders have responded to the HIPAA Privacy Rule, with many covered entities, IRBs, and Privacy Boards interpreting the HIPAA Privacy

Rule very conservatively. These interpretations impede some important research activities, and can also limit the validity and generalizability of some research results. The variation in interpretation is especially problematic for multi-institutional research projects. Gaining IRB or Privacy Board approval from multiple institutions for a particular project is challenging and can lead to significant delays or even abandoned studies, and also can result in protocol variations at different research sites. The committee also found that for some provisions of the HIPAA Privacy Rule, the burdens are heavy and the privacy protections in research are small.

Therefore, the committee concluded that the HIPAA Privacy Rule, as currently interpreted and implemented, impedes research without protecting privacy as well as it should. The committee's approach to its task evolved as the study progressed and the group began thinking about potential recommendations. The committee decided to approach the problem in two ways. First, the committee proposes a bold, innovative, and more uniform approach to the dual challenge of protecting privacy and supporting beneficial and responsible research.[5] Although this new approach may be harder to implement in the short term, it should help stimulate fresh ideas about the best ways to protect privacy and improve research as the nation thinks about these two interrelated values over the next several years. Second, the committee makes a series of detailed proposals to improve the HIPAA Privacy Rule and associated guidance. These recommendations aim to reduce variability in the interpretation of the HIPAA Privacy Rule as applied to research, and to facilitate important health research within the scope of the HIPAA Privacy Rule through revised and expanded guidance, or by altering some provisions that pose a hindrance to research but do not provide significant privacy protections. The committee's last set of recommendations do not directly relate to the HIPAA Privacy Rule, but should be adopted regardless of which of the committee's approaches is implemented (the new framework or revisions to the HIPAA Privacy Rule and associated guidance). These include improving the security of identifiable health information, encouraging service on Institutional Review Boards and Privacy Boards, and providing more information to the public about research results, how health research is conducted, and how it contributes to the welfare of individuals and society as a whole.

---

[5] Responsible health research is methodologically sound, scientifically valid, protects the rights and interests of study subjects, and addresses a question or problem relevant to improving human health.

FRAMEWORK OF THE REPORT

Chapter 2 describes the value and importance of health information privacy with an overview of how informational privacy has been protected by law; a review of survey data on public opinions, expectations, and experiences; and a discussion on the security of health data.

Chapter 3 describes the value and importance of responsible health research, and includes an overview of how health information is used in research and how federal regulations govern the conduct of research.

Chapter 4 provides an overview of the HIPAA Privacy Rule and how privacy regulations apply to health research, including a discussion of the HIPAA Privacy Rule's relation to other regulations that govern the privacy of health information in research.

Chapter 5 reviews the available evidence, including results from recent surveys, on the impact of the HIPAA Privacy Rule on the conduct of health research.

Chapter 6 describes the limitations of the HIPAA Privacy Rule, and proposes a new and broader framework for the protection of privacy in health research.

The **Appendixes** provide a summary of previous recommendations to HHS about the HIPAA Privacy Rule and health research, as well as a description of the surveys commissioned by the committee (survey methods and analysis).

REFERENCES

Friedman, D. S. 2006. HIPAA and research: How have the first two years gone? *American Journal of Ophthalmology* 141(3):543–546.

Gellman, R. 2006. Crimes and sanctions. *Journal of AHIMA* 77(9):96–97.

Hodge, J. G., Jr., L. O. Gostin, and P. D. Jacobson. 1999. Legal issues concerning electronic health information: Privacy, quality, and liability. *Journal of the American Medical Association* 282(15):1466–1471.

IOM (Institute of Medicine). 2006. *Effect of the HIPAA Privacy Rule on health research: Proceedings of a workshop presented to the National Cancer Policy Forum.* Washington, DC: The National Academies Press.

National Committee on Vital and Health Statistics, Subcommittee on Privacy and Confidentiality. *Susan Ehringhaus's testimony on behalf of the Association of American Medical Colleges.* November 19, 2003.

President's Cancer Panel. 2004. *Living beyond cancer: Finding a new balance.* http://deainfo.nci.nih.gov/ADVISORY/pcp/pcp03-04rpt/Survivorship.pdf (accessed May 1, 2008).

President's Cancer Panel. 2006. *Assessing progress, advancing change.* http://deainfo.nci.nih.gov/ADVISORY/pcp/pcp07rpt/pcp07rpt.pdf (accessed June 15, 2008).

Ramirez, A. G., and J. E. Niederhuber. 2003 (November 5). Letter to The Honorable Tommy G. Thompson, Secretary of Department of Health and Human Services. Washington, DC.

Sobel, R. 2007. The HIPAA paradox: The Privacy Rule that's not. *Hastings Center Report* 37(4):40–50.

Tourangeau, R., L. Rips, and K. Rasinski. 2000. *The psychology of survey response.* Cambridge, UK: Cambridge University Press.

Tovino, S. A. 2004. The use and disclosure of protected health information for research under the HIPAA Privacy Rule: Unrealized patient autonomy and burdensome government regulation. *South Dakota Law Review* 49(3):447–502.

U.S. Congress, House of Representatives, Committee on Ways and Means. 1996a. *Health Coverage Availability and Affordability Act of 1996.* 104th Cong., 2d Sess. March 25, 1996.

U.S. Congress, House of Representatives, Committee of Conference. 1996b. *Health Insurance Portability and Accountability Act of 1996.* 104th Cong., 2d Sess. July 31, 1996.

Walker, D. K. 2005. *Impact of the HIPAA Privacy Rule on health services research.* Philadelphia, PA: Abt Associates, Inc.

Wentland, E. J., and K. W. Smith. 1993. *Survey responses: An evaluation of their validity.* San Diego, CA: Academic Press.

2

The Value and Importance of Health Information Privacy

Ethical health research and privacy protections both provide valuable benefits to society. Health research is vital to improving human health and health care. Protecting patients involved in research from harm and preserving their rights is essential to ethical research. The primary justification for protecting personal privacy is to protect the interests of individuals. In contrast, the primary justification for collecting personally identifiable health information for health research is to benefit society. But it is important to stress that privacy also has value at the societal level, because it permits complex activities, including research and public health activities to be carried out in ways that protect individuals' dignity. At the same time, health research can benefit individuals, for example, when it facilitates access to new therapies, improved diagnostics, and more effective ways to prevent illness and deliver care.

The intent of this chapter[1] is to define privacy and to delineate its importance to individuals and society as a whole. The value and importance of health research will be addressed in Chapter 3.

CONCEPTS AND VALUE OF PRIVACY

Definitions

Privacy has deep historical roots (reviewed by Pritts, 2008; Westin, 1967), but because of its complexity, privacy has proven difficult to

---

[1] Sections of this chapter were adapted from a background paper by Pritts (2008).

define and has been the subject of extensive, and often heated, debate by philosophers, sociologists, and legal scholars. The term "privacy" is used frequently, yet there is no universally accepted definition of the term, and confusion persists over the meaning, value, and scope of the concept of privacy. At its core, privacy is experienced on a personal level and often means different things to different people (reviewed by Lowrance, 1997; Pritts, 2008). In modern society, the term is used to denote different, but overlapping, concepts such as the right to bodily integrity or to be free from intrusive searches or surveillance. The concept of privacy is also context specific, and acquires a different meaning depending on the stated reasons for the information being gathered, the intentions of the parties involved, as well as the politics, convention and cultural expectations (Nissenbaum, 2004; NRC, 2007b).

Our report, and the Privacy Rule itself, are concerned with health informational privacy. In the context of personal information, concepts of privacy are closely intertwined with those of confidentiality and security. However, although privacy is often used interchangeably with the terms "confidentiality" and "security," they have distinct meanings. *Privacy* addresses the question of who has access to personal information and under what conditions. Privacy is concerned with the collection, storage, and use of personal information, and examines whether data can be collected in the first place, as well as the justifications, if any, under which data collected for one purpose can be used for another (secondary)[2] purpose. An important issue in privacy analysis is whether the individual has authorized particular uses of his or her personal information (Westin, 1967).

Confidentiality safeguards information that is gathered in the context of an intimate relationship. It addresses the issue of how to keep information exchanged in that relationship from being disclosed to third parties (Westin, 1976). Confidentiality, for example, prevents physicians from disclosing information shared with them by a patient in the course of a physician–patient relationship. Unauthorized or inadvertent disclosures of data gained as part of an intimate relationship are breaches of confidentiality (Gostin and Hodge, 2002; NBAC, 2001).

Security can be defined as "the procedural and technical measures required (a) to prevent unauthorized access, modification, use, and dissemination of data stored or processed in a computer system, (b) to prevent any deliberate denial of service, and (c) to protect the system in its entirety from physical harm" (Turn and Ware, 1976). Security helps keep health

---

[2]The National Committee on Vital and Health Statistics has noted that the term "secondary uses" of health data is ill defined and therefore urged abandoning it in favor of precise description of each use. Consequently, the IOM committee has chosen to minimize use of the term in this report.

records safe from unauthorized use. When someone hacks into a computer system, there is a breach of security (and also potentially, a breach of confidentiality). No security measure, however, can prevent invasion of privacy by those who have authority to access the record (Gostin, 1995).

The Importance of Privacy

There are a variety of reasons for placing a high value on protecting the privacy, confidentiality, and security of health information (reviewed by Pritts, 2008). Some theorists depict privacy as a basic human good or right with intrinsic value (Fried, 1968; Moore, 2005; NRC, 2007a; Terry and Francis, 2007). They see privacy as being objectively valuable in itself, as an essential component of human well-being. They believe that respecting privacy (and autonomy) is a form of recognition of the attributes that give humans their moral uniqueness.

The more common view is that privacy is valuable because it facilitates or promotes other fundamental values, including ideals of personhood (Bloustein, 1967; Gavison, 1980; Post, 2001; Solove, 2006; Taylor, 1989; Westin, 1966) such as:

- Personal autonomy (the ability to make personal decisions)
- Individuality
- Respect
- Dignity and worth as human beings

The bioethics principle nonmaleficence[3] requires safeguarding personal privacy. Breaches of privacy and confidentiality not only may affect a person's dignity, but can cause harm. When personally identifiable health information, for example, is disclosed to an employer, insurer, or family member, it can result in stigma, embarrassment, and discrimination. Thus, without some assurance of privacy, people may be reluctant to provide candid and complete disclosures of sensitive information even to their physicians. Ensuring privacy can promote more effective communication between physician and patient, which is essential for quality of care, enhanced autonomy, and preventing economic harm, embarrassment, and discrimination (Gostin, 2001; NBAC, 1999; Pritts, 2002). However, it should also be noted that perceptions of privacy vary among individuals and various groups. Data that are considered intensely private by one person may not be by others (Lowrance, 2002).

But privacy has value even in the absence of any embarrassment or

---

[3]The ethical principle of doing no harm, based on the Hippocratic maxim, primum non nocere, first do no harm.

tangible harm. Privacy is also required for developing interpersonal relationships with others. Although some emphasize the need for privacy to establish intimate relationships (Allen, 1997), others take a broader view of privacy as being necessary to maintain a variety of social relationships (Rachels, 1975). By giving us the ability to control who knows what about us and who has access to us, privacy allows us to alter our behavior with different people so that we may maintain and control our various social relationships (Rachels, 1975). For example, people may share different information with their boss than they would with their doctor.

Most discussions on the value of privacy focus on its importance to the individual. Privacy can be seen, however, as also having value to society as a whole (Regan, 1995). Privacy furthers the existence of a free society (Gavison, 1980). For example, preserving privacy from widespread surveillance can be seen as protecting not only the individual's private sphere, but also society as a whole: Privacy contributes to the maintenance of the type of society in which we want to live (Gavison, 1980; Regan, 1995).

Privacy can foster socially beneficial activities like health research. Individuals are more likely to participate in and support research if they believe their privacy is being protected. Protecting privacy is also seen by some as enhancing data quality for research and quality improvement initiatives. When individuals avoid health care or engage in other privacy-protective behaviors, such as withholding information, inaccurate and incomplete data are entered into the health care system. These data, which are subsequently used for research, public health reporting, and outcomes analysis, carry with them the same vulnerabilities (Goldman, 1998).

The bioethics principle of respect for persons also places importance on individual autonomy, which allows individuals to make decisions for themselves, free from coercion, about matters that are important to their own well-being. U.S. society also places a high value on individual autonomy, and one way to respect persons and enhance individual autonomy is to ensure that people can make the choice about when, and whether, personal information (particularly sensitive information) can be shared with others.

Public Views of Health Information Privacy

American society places a high value on individual rights, personal choice, and a private sphere protected from intrusion. Medical records can include some of the most intimate details about a person's life. They document a patient's physical and mental health, and can include information on social behaviors, personal relationships, and financial status (Gostin and Hodge, 2002). Accordingly, surveys show that medical privacy is a major concern for many Americans, as outlined below (reviewed by Pritts, 2008;

Westin, 2007). As noted in Chapter 1, however, there are some limits to what can be learned from surveys (Tourangeau et al., 2000; Wentland, 1993; Westin, 2007). For example, how the questions and responses are worded and framed can significantly influence the results and their interpretation. Also, responses are biased when respondents self-report measures of attitudes, behavior, and feelings in such a way as to represent themselves favorably.

In a 1999 survey of consumer attitudes toward health privacy, three out of four people reported that they had significant concerns about the privacy and confidentiality of their medical records (Forrester Research, 1999). In a more recent survey, conducted in 2005 after the implementation of the Health Insurance Portability and Accountability Act (HIPAA) Privacy Rule, 67 percent of respondents still said they were concerned about the privacy of their medical records, suggesting that the Privacy Rule had not effectively alleviated public concern about health privacy. Ethnic and racial minorities showed the greatest concern among the respondents. Moreover, the survey showed that many consumers were unfamiliar with the HIPAA privacy protections. Only 59 percent of respondents recalled receiving a HIPAA privacy notice, and only 27 percent believed they had more rights than they had before receiving the notice (Forrester Research, 2005). One out of eight respondents also admitted to engaging in behaviors intended to protect their privacy, even at the expense of risking dangerous health effects. These behaviors included lying to their doctors about symptoms or behaviors, refusing to provide information or providing inaccurate information, paying out of pocket for care that is covered by insurance, and avoiding care altogether (Forrester Research, 2005).

A series of polls conducted by Harris Interactive suggest, however, that the privacy of health information has improved since implementation of the Privacy Rule. Prior to its creation, a 1993 survey by Harris Interactive showed that 27 percent of Americans believed their personal medical information had been released improperly in the past 3 years. In contrast, 14 percent and 12 percent of respondents believed this had happened to them in 2005 and 2007, respectively (Harris Interactive, 2005, 2007). In the 2005 survey, about two-thirds of respondents reported having received a HIPAA privacy notice, and of these people, 67 percent said the privacy notice increased their confidence that their medical information is being handled properly (Harris Interactive, 2005).

Responses to other questions on recent public opinion polls conducted by Harris Interactive only partially corroborate these findings. In one survey, 70 percent of respondents indicated that they are generally satisfied with how their personal health information is handled with regard to privacy protections and security. Nearly 60 percent of the respondents reported that they believe the existing federal and state health privacy protection laws provide a reasonable level of privacy protection for their health information (Harris Interactive, 2005). Nonetheless, half of the respondents also believed that "[P]atients have lost all control today over how their medical records are obtained and used by organizations outside the direct patient health care such as life insurers, employers, and government health agencies." In another survey, 83 percent of respondents reported that they trust health care providers to protect the privacy and confidentiality of their personal medical records and health information (Westin, 2007). However, in that survey, 58 percent of respondents believed the privacy of personal medical records and health information is not protected well enough today by federal and state laws and organizational practices.

A number of studies suggest that the relative strength of privacy, confidentiality, and security protections can play an important role in people's concerns about privacy (reviewed by Pritts, 2008). When presented with the possibility that there would be a nationwide system of electronic medical records, one survey found 70 percent of respondents were concerned that sensitive personal medical record information might be leaked because of weak data security, 69 percent expressed concern that there could be more sharing of medical information without the patient's knowledge, and 69 percent were concerned that strong enough data security will not be installed in the new computer system.

Confidentiality is particularly important to adolescents who seek health care. When adolescents perceive that health services are not confidential, they report that they are less likely to seek care, particularly for reproductive health matters or substance abuse (Weddle and Kokotailo, 2005). In addition, the willingness of a person to make self-disclosures necessary to mental health and substance abuse treatment may decrease as the perceived negative consequences of a breach of confidentiality increase (Petrila, 1999; Roback and Shelton, 1995; Taube and Elwork, 1990). These studies show that protecting the privacy of health information is important for ensuring that individuals seek and obtain quality care.

The potential for economic harm resulting from discrimination in health insurance and employment is also a concern for many people (reviewed by Pritts, 2008). Polls consistently show that people are most concerned about insurers and employers accessing their health information without their permission (Forrester Research, 2005; PSRA, 1999). This concern arises from fears about employer and insurer discrimination. Concerns about employer discrimination based on health information, in particular, increased 16 percent between 1999 and 2005, with 52 percent of respondents in the later survey expressing concern that their information might be seen by an employer and used to limit job opportunities (Forrester Research, 2005; PSRA, 1999). Reports alleging that major employers such as Wal-Mart base some of their hiring decisions on the health of applicants suggest that these concerns may be justified (Greenhouse and Barbaro, 2005).

Studies show that individuals are especially concerned about genetic information being used inappropriately by their insurers and employers (reviewed by Pritts, 2008). Even health care providers appear to be affected by these concerns. In a survey of cancer-genetics specialists, more than half indicated that they would pay out of pocket rather than bill their insurance companies for genetic testing, for fear of genetic discrimination (Hudson, 2007). Although surveys do not reveal a significant percentage of individuals who have experienced such discrimination, geneticists have reported that approximately 550 individuals were refused employment, fired, or denied life insurance based on their genetic constitution (NBAC, 1999). In addition, a study in the United Kingdom suggested that life insurers in that country do not have a full grasp on the meaning of genetic information and do not assess or act in accord with the actuarial risks presented by the information (Low et al., 1998). There is, therefore, some legitimate basis to individuals' concerns about potential economic harm and the need to protect the privacy of their genetic information. Recent passage of the Genetic Information Nondiscrimination Act in the United States will hopefully begin to address some of these concerns.[4]

Patient Attitudes About Privacy in Health Research

Ideally, there would be empirical evidence regarding the privacy value of all the specific Privacy Rule provisions that impact researchers, but there are only limited data on this topic from the consumer/patient perspective. A few studies have attempted to examine the public's attitudes about the use of health information in research. However, few have attempted to do so with respect to the intricacies of the protections afforded by the Privacy Rule or the Common Rule,[5] which are likely not well known to the public.

A review by Westin of 43 national surveys with health privacy questions fielded between 1993 and September 2007 identified 9 surveys[6] with one or more questions about health research and privacy (Westin, 2007). In some, the majority of respondents were not comfortable with their health

---

[4] The Genetic Information Nondiscrimination Act of 2008 establishes some protections to prevent discrimination based on a patient's genetic background.

[5] The "Common Rule" is the term used by 18 federal agencies who have adopted the same regulations governing the protection of human subjects of research. See Chapter 3 for a detailed description of the rule.

[6] These surveys were undertaken by a wide range of sponsors (Markle Foundation, Equifax, Institute for Health Freedom, Geneforum, Privacy Consulting Group) and a wide range of surveyors (Harris Interactive, Public Opinion Strategies, Genetics and Public Policy Center).

information being provided for health research except with notice and express consent. But in others, a majority of respondents were willing to forgo notice and consent if various safeguards and specific types of research were offered. For example, a recent Harris Poll found that 63 percent of respondents would give general consent to the use of their medical records for research, as long as there were guarantees that no personally identifiable health information would be released from such studies (Harris Interactive, 2007). This is similar to the percentage of people willing to participate in a "clinical research study" (Research!America, 2007; Woolley and Propst, 2005) (see also Chapter 3). A 2006 British survey also found strong support for the use of personally identifiable information without consent for public health research and surveillance, via the National Cancer Registry (Barrett et al., 2007).

Westin noted that opinions varied in the surveys according to developments on the health care scene and with consumer privacy trends. He concluded from this review that the majority of consumers are positive about health research, and if asked in general terms, support their medical information being made available for research. However, he also noted that most of these surveys presented the choice in ways that did not articulate the key permission process, and that there was much ambiguity in who "researchers" are, what kind of "health research" is involved, and how the promised protection of personal identities would be ensured (Westin, 2007).

Reviewing the handful of detailed studies examining patient views of the use of their medical information in research through surveys, structured interviews, or focus groups, Pritts determined that a number of common themes emerge (reviewed by Pritts, 2008):

- Patients were generally very supportive of research provided safeguards are established to protect the privacy and security of their medical information (Damschroder et al., 2007; Kass et al., 2003; Robling et al., 2004; Westin, 2007; Willison et al., 2007).
- Patients were much more comfortable with the use of anonymized data (e.g., where obvious identifiers have been removed) than fully identifiable data for research (Damschroder et al., 2007; Kass et al., 2003; Robling et al., 2004; Whiddett et al., 2006).
- Patients were less comfortable with sharing information about "sensitive" conditions such as mental health with researchers (Damschroder et al., 2007; Robling et al., 2004).

In studies where patients were able to provide unstructured comments, they expressed concern about the potential that anonymized data would be reidentified. They were also concerned that insurers or employers or others who could discriminate against subjects could potentially access information maintained by researchers (Damschroder et al., 2007; Kass et al., 2003; Robling et al., 2004). Some feared that researchers would sell information to drug companies or other third parties (Damschroder et al., 2007).

Although supportive of research, the majority of patients in these studies expressed a desire to be consulted before their information was released for research (Damschroder et al., 2007; Kass et al., 2003; Robling et al., 2004; Westin, 2007; Whiddett et al., 2006; Willison et al., 2007). Some surveys also show that even if researchers would receive no directly identifying information (e.g., name, address, and health insurance number), the majority of respondents still wanted to have some input before their medical records were disclosed (Damschroder et al., 2007; Robling et al., 2004; Willison et al., 2007). For example, in a 2005 Australian survey, 67 percent of respondents indicated they would be willing to allow their deidentified health records to be used for medical research purposes, but 81 percent wanted to be asked first (Flannery and Tokley, 2005).

Studies indicate that public support for research and willingness to share health information can vary with the purpose or type of activity being conducted (reviewed by Pritts, 2008). Studies have found there was less support for activities that were primarily for a commercial purpose, or that might be used in a manner that would not help patients (Damschroder et al., 2007; Willison et al., 2007). Some participants expressed concern that some researchers were motivated by monetary rewards and that decision makers would act out of self-interest (Damschroder et al., 2007).

One recent study suggests that the biggest predictor of whether patients are willing to share their medical records with researchers is the patients' trust that their information will be kept private and confidential (Damschroder et al., 2007). In this study, the patients who most trusted the Veterans Affairs system to keep their medical records private were more likely to accept less stringent requirements for informed consent. Thirty-four percent of veterans who participated in intensive focus groups using deliberative democracy were willing to allow researchers associated with the Veterans Health Administration to use their medical records without any procedures for patient input, subject to Institutional Review Board (IRB) approval, and another 17 percent reported that patients should have to ask for their medical records to be *excluded* from research studies (opt-out).

But participants in focus groups also have expressed a desire to be informed of how their health information was used for research. This desire was tied to a sense of altruism—they wanted to know that their information was useful and that they may have contributed to helping others by allowing their medical records to be used for research (Damschroder et al., 2007; Robling et al., 2004). The veterans also recommended methods to give research participants more control over how their medical records are used in research. These recommendations included requiring that participants are fully informed about how their medical records are being used in research; providing assurances that the research being conducted will benefit fellow veterans; updating research participants about findings and ongoing research; and setting out clear and consistent consequences for anyone who violates a patient's privacy (Damschroder et al., 2007).

The recent Harris poll[7] commissioned by the Institute of Medicine (IOM) committee for this study found that 8 percent of respondents had been asked to have their medical information used in research, but declined. When asked why, 30 percent indicated they were concerned about the privacy and confidentiality of their personal information, but many other reasons were also commonly cited (ranging from 5 to 24 percent of respondents), including worry that participation would be risky, painful, or unpleasant; lack of trust in the researchers; or belief that it would not help their condition or their family (Westin, 2007).

Some studies also suggest that individuals' attitudes toward the use of their medical records in research may be influenced by a person's state of health. Although the commissioned Harris Poll found that people who are in only fair health, who have a disability, or who had taken a genetic test were slightly more concerned than the public about health researchers seeing their medical records (55 percent versus 50 percent), other data suggest that people with health concerns may be more supportive of using medical records in research. For example, qualitative market research by the National Health Council showed that individuals with chronic conditions have a very favorable attitude toward the implementation of electronic personal health records (EPHRs). During the focus group discussions, participants noted that EPHRs could be very advantageous in medical research and were supportive of this use even though many had expressed concern about the privacy and confidentiality of EPHRs (Balch et al., 2005, 2006). Although the Council did not specifically ask about attitudes toward health research and privacy, these results suggest that individuals with chronic conditions may be more likely to grant researchers access to their medical records, and to place less emphasis on protecting privacy than members of the general population.

Also, a Johns Hopkins University survey of patients having, or at risk for, serious medical conditions examined these patients' attitudes about the use of their medical records in research, and compared those results to polls from the general population. Thirty-one percent of respondents stated that medical researchers should have access to their medical records without their permission if it would help to advance medical knowledge.

In contrast, the recent Harris poll of the public found that 19 percent of respondents would be willing to forgo consent to use personal medical and health information, as long as the study never revealed their identity

---

[7]The survey was conducted online by Harris Interactive between September 11 and 18, 2007, with 2,392 respondents. The methodology for the survey is described in Appendix B.

and it was supervised by an IRB (Westin, 2007). An additional 8 percent indicated they would be willing to give general consent in advance to have personally identifiable medical or health information used in future research projects without the researchers having to contact them, and 1 percent said researchers should be free to use their personal medical and health information without their consent at all. Thus, 28 percent of respondents would be willing to grant researchers access to their medical records without giving specific consent for each research project. Thirty-eight percent believed they should be asked to consent to each research study seeking to use their personally identifiable medical or health information, and 13 percent did not want researchers to contact them or to use their personal or health information under any circumstances. However, those who preferred not to be contacted at all were actually less likely than those who would grant conditional permission to have declined participating in a research study. Notably, 20 percent of respondents were unsure how to respond to the question about notice and consent for research.

Among the 38 percent who said they wanted notice and consent, 80 percent indicated that they would want to know the purpose of the research, and 46 percent wanted to know specifically whether the research could help their health condition or those of family members. Sixty-two percent indicated that knowing about the specific research study and who would be running it would allow the respondent to decide whether to trust the researchers. A little more than half of the respondents (54 percent) said they would be worried that their personally identifiable information may be disclosed outside the study. Among those 54 percent, three-quarters agreed with the statement "I would feel violated and my trust in the researchers betrayed." Between 39 and 67 percent were concerned about discrimination in a government program, by an employer, or in obtaining life or health insurance (Westin, 2007).

However, about 70 percent of all respondents indicated that they trusted health researchers to protect the privacy and confidentiality of the medical records and health information they obtain about research participants. Furthermore, among respondents who had participated in health research, only 2 percent reported that any of their personally identifiable medical information used in a study was given to anyone outside the research staff, and half of those disclosures were actually made to other researchers or research institutions (Westin, 2007).

In summary, very limited data are available to assess the privacy value of the Privacy Rule provisions that impact researchers. Surveys indicate that the public is deeply concerned about the privacy and security of personal health information, and that the HIPAA Privacy Rule has perhaps reduced—but not eliminated—those concerns. Patients were generally very supportive of research, provided safeguards were established to protect the privacy and security of their medical information, although some surveys indicate that a significant portion of the public would still prefer to control access to their medical records via consent, even if the information is anonymized. Studies indicate that public support for research and willingness to share health information varies with health status and the type of research conducted, and depends on the patients' trust that their information will be kept private and confidential. An understanding the public's attitude toward privacy is important throughout the rest of this report, because many of the IOM committee's recommendations affect the nature of the privacy protections afforded by the federal health research regulations.

HISTORICAL DEVELOPMENT OF LEGAL PROTECTIONS OF HEALTH INFORMATION PRIVACY

The medical community has long recognized the importance of protecting privacy in maintaining public trust in doctors and researchers, and codes of medical ethics reflect a desire to increase this public trust. Since the time of Hippocrates, physicians have pledged to keep information about their patients private and confidential (Feld and Feld, 2005). The Hippocratic Oath states, "What I may see or hear in the course of the treatment or even outside of the treatment in regard to the life of men, which on no account one must spread abroad, I will keep to myself. . . ." This pledge to privacy has been included in the code of ethics of nearly all health care professionals in the United States. For example, the first Code of Ethics of the American Medical Association in 1847 included the concept of confidentiality (OTA, 1993).

The value of health information privacy has also been recognized by affording it protection under the law (reviewed by Pritts, 2008). The rules for protecting the privacy of health information in the clinical care and health research contexts developed along fairly distinct paths until the promulgation of the federal privacy regulations under HIPAA.[8] Prior to HIPAA, health information in the clinical setting was protected primarily under a combination of federal and state constitutional law, as well as state common law and statutory protections (Box 2-1).

In contrast, research practices have been governed largely by federal regulations called the Common Rule, which have historically focused on protecting individuals from physical and mental harm in clinical trials (see subsequent sections of this chapter). Although the standards apply to research that uses personally identifiable health information, the protection of information is not their primary focus.

---

[8] Health Insurance Portability and Accountability Act, Public Law 104–191 (1996) (most relevant sections codified at 42 U.S.C. §§ 1320(d)–1320(d)(8).

BOX 2-1
Overview of Privacy Protections in the Law

Constitutional Protections

Both federal and state constitutions generally afford citizens some protection for the privacy of their health information. However, with limited exceptions, individuals are only protected against governmental intrusions into their personal health information and may not raise constitutional concerns about private action. Even when state action is involved, individuals rarely prevail on claims premised on constitutional rights to informational privacy because state interests generally outweigh the individual's privacy interest.

The U.S. Constitution does not expressly provide a right to privacy, but the courts have determined that various constitutional provisions implicitly create zones of privacy that are protected by the Constitution. The privacy interests recognized include both the individual's interest in making certain kinds of important decisions, and the individual's interest in avoiding disclosure of personal matters. With respect to informational privacy, the courts have afforded limited constitutional protections, although the right is not absolute, with the courts weighing factors such as the type of record and information that it contains, the potential for harm in an unauthorized disclosure and the injury from disclosure to the relationship in which the record was generated against the public interest or need for the disclosure, and the adequacy of safeguards to prevent unauthorized access or disclosure. Several federal courts have expressly recognized the constitutional right of privacy in connection with medical and prescription records.

All states have constitutional provisions similar to those in the U.S. Constitution, which give rise to an implied right of privacy. Unlike the U.S. Constitution, however, constitutions in 10 states grant individuals an express right to privacy. Courts have consistently determined that health or medical information is an area of privacy that is protected by state constitutions.

Common Law Protections

State common law generally recognizes that some health care relationships are based on maintaining the confidentiality of information obtained in the course of care and affords a remedy when that confidentiality is breached. Traditionally, the law's regulation of "privacy" consisted essentially of the protection of confidentiality within the doctor–patient relationship. Courts have found that actions may be maintained against private parties for unauthorized disclosures of health information under a number of legal theories, including invasion of privacy, implied breach of contract, breach of confidentiality, and breach of fiduciary relationship. Obtaining a remedy for disclosure of health information under any of these theories, however, is difficult.

In the health care context, the promise of confidentiality is intended to encourage patients to fully disclose their most personal information to assist in accurate

continued

BOX 2-1 Continued

diagnosis and treatment. Courts have thus found the duty of confidentiality applies to physicians, hospitals, psychiatrists, and social workers. The underlying duty of confidentiality is not absolute, and the courts have indicated that there is no breach of confidentiality when a disclosure is made as required by statute (e.g., mandatory reporting to state officials of infectious or contagious diseases) or common law (e.g., a duty to disclose information concerning the safety of third persons). The extent to which state common law protects the confidentiality of health information in the evolving health care paradigm, where many people and organizations that receive and maintain health information do not have a direct relationship with the patient, is unclear. In most states, common law protections, particularly in tort, have been codified in statute.

Statutory and Regulatory Protections

Since the 1970s, the trend has been to augment existing constitutional and common law rights with statutory protections specifically designed to protect the privacy and confidentiality of health information (see Table 2-1). Although the common law continues to be important, the federal and state governments have increasingly focused on promulgating distinct standards for the protection of health information.

The shift to statutory and regulatory protections for health information was largely a response to the changing nature of recordkeeping in general, and of the nature of the provision of health care. As noted by the 1977 Privacy Protection Study Commission, "The emergence of third-party payment plans; the use of health care information for non-healthcare purposes; the growing involvement of government agencies in virtually all aspects of health care; and the exponential increase in the use of computers and automated information systems for health-care record information have combined to put substantial pressure on traditional confidentiality protections."

SOURCES: Bodger (2006); Gostin (1995); Magnussen (2004); NCSL (2008); Pritts (2002, 2008); Privacy Protection Study Commission (1977); Richards and Solove (2007); Terry and Francis (2007).

TABLE 2-1 Federal Health Privacy Statutes and Executive Orders That Regulate the Collection and Disclosure of Information

Statute	Year	Privacy Protection
Freedom of Information Act (FOIA)	1966	Prevents personally identifiable health information from being included in the release of information as part of a FOIA request
Privacy Act	1974	Protects the privacy of health, research, and other records held by federal agencies
Family Educational Rights and Privacy Act	1974	Requires schools to have written permission from a parent or student prior to releasing information from a student's education record
Veterans Omnibus Health Care Act	1976	Protects the privacy of medical records relating to the treatment of drug abuse, alcohol abuse, infection with AIDS or sickle cell anemia, in the Department of Veterans Affairs
Protection of Pupil Rights Amendment	1978	Protects the rights of pupils and the parents of pupils in programs funded by the Department of Education
Social Security Act, Section 1106	1986	Prohibits unauthorized disclosure of individually identifiable records held by the Department of Health and Human Services, the Social Security Administration, and their contractors
Clinical Laboratory Improvement Amendments	1988	Requires clinical laboratories to protect the confidentiality of test results and reports, including information on patient and clinical study subjects; medical information may only be disclosed to authorized persons as defined by state or federal law
Public Health Service Act, Health Omnibus Program Extension	1988	Provides for Certificates of Confidentiality that protect personally identifiable research information

continued

BOX 2-1 Continued

TABLE 2-1 Continued

Statute	Year	Privacy Protection
Americans with Disabilities Act	1990	Employers must treat employees' and applicants' medical information and medical conditions confidentially
Public Health Service Act, Section 543, Federal Confidentiality Requirements for Substance Abuse Patient Records	1992	Federally assisted alcohol or substance abuse programs must keep patient alcohol and drug abuse treatment records confidential, absent patient consent or a court order
Health Insurance Portability and Accountability Act (HIPAA), Privacy Rule	1996	Protects the privacy of individually identifiable information held by covered entities
Balanced Budget Act	1997	Added language to the Social Security Act to require Medicare+Choice organizations to establish safeguards for the privacy of individually identifiable patient information
Clinton's Executive Order 13145	2000	Bans the use of genetic information in federal hiring and promotion decisions
Confidential Information Protection and Statistical Efficiency Act	2002	Ensures that information supplied by individuals or organizations to a federal agency for statistical purposes under a pledge of confidentiality is used exclusively for statistical purposes
Medicare Prescription Drug, Improvement and Modernization Act	2003	Requires prescription drug plan sponsors to comply with the HIPAA Privacy Rule and the Security Rule requirements
Genetic Information Nondiscrimination Act	2008	Prohibits discrimination against individuals based on their genetic information in health insurance and employment

Principles of Fair Information Practice

The framework in which detailed statutory and regulatory protections of privacy originated was in the 1973 report of an advisory committee to the U.S. Department of Health, Education and Welfare (HEW), "designed to call attention to issues of recordkeeping practice in the computer age that may have profound significance for us all" (HEW, 1973). The principles were intended to "provide a basis for establishing procedures that assure the individual a right to participate in a meaningful way in decisions about what goes into records about him and how that information shall be used" (HEW, 1973). In addition to affording individuals the meaningful right to control the collection, use, and disclosure of their information, the fair information practices also impose affirmative responsibilities to safeguard information on those who collect it (reviewed by Pritts, 2008).

The fundamental principles of fair information practice articulated in the report have since been amplified and adopted in various forms at the international, federal, and state levels (Gelman, 2008). The fair information practices endorsed by the Organisation for Economic Co-operation and Development (OECD), which have been widely cited, include the following principles (OECD, 1980):

- *Collection Limitation*
  There should be limits to the collection of personal data, and any such data should be obtained by lawful and fair means and, where appropriate, with the knowledge or consent of the data subject.
- *Data Quality*
  Personal data should be relevant to the purposes for which they are to be used, and to the extent necessary for those purposes, should be accurate, complete, and kept updated.
- *Purpose Specification*
  The purposes for which personal data are collected should be specified not later than at the time of data collection, and the subsequent use limited to the fulfillment of those purposes or such others as are not incompatible with those purposes, and as are specified on each occasion of change of purpose.
- *Use Limitation*
  Personal data should not be disclosed, made available, or otherwise used for purposes other than those specified in accordance with [the Purpose Specification] except:
    (a) with the consent of the data subject; or
    (b) by the authority of law.

- *Security Safeguards*
  Personal data should be protected by reasonable security safeguards against such risks as loss or unauthorized access, destruction, use, modification, or disclosure of data.
- *Openness*
  There should be a general policy of openness about developments, practices, and policies with respect to personal data. Means should be readily available of establishing the existence and nature of personal data, and the main purposes of their use, as well as the identity and usual residence of the data controller.
- *Individual Participation*
  An individual should have the right to know whether a data controller has data relating to him/her, to obtain a copy of the data within a reasonable time in a form that is intelligible to him/her, to obtain a reason if the request for access is denied, to challenge such a denial, to challenge data relating to him/her, and, if the challenge is successful, to have the data erased, rectified, completed, or amended.
- *Accountability*
  A data controller should be accountable for complying with measures, which give effect to the principles stated above.

These principles have been adopted at the federal and state levels to varying degrees. The United States has taken a sector-driven approach toward adopting the principles of fair information practices, with the federal and state governments promulgating statutes and regulations that apply only to specific classes of record keepers or categories of records.[9,10]

At the federal level, the fair information practices were first incorporated into the Privacy Act of 1974, which governs the collection, use, and disclosure of personally identifiable data held by the federal government and some of its contractors. Hospitals operated by the federal government and health care or research institutions operated under federal contract are subject to the Privacy Act, while other health care entities remained outside its scope (Gostin, 1995). Nevertheless, the Privacy Act afforded perhaps the broadest

---

[9]The original 1973 HEW Advisory Committee contemplated and rejected the creation of a centralized, federal approach to regulating the use of all automated personal data systems (see HEW, 1973).

[10]Europe, in contrast, has adopted fair information practices in a broad, more uniform fashion by incorporating them into the European Union (EU) Directive, which protects individuals with regard to the processing of any personal data and on the free movement of such data. The EU Directive applies to personal data of many types, including medical and financial, and widely applies to all who process such data, resulting in protections (Gelman, 2008).

protection for health information at the federal level until the promulgation of the HIPAA Privacy Rule.

For their part, states have adopted (and continue to adopt) laws that not only mirror the Privacy Act in protecting government-held records, but also that afford broader protections for personally identifiable health information held by private parties. However, these principles have not been adopted uniformly among states, resulting in a patchwork of state health privacy laws that provide little consistency from entity to entity or from state to state.

For example, the states have enacted the fair information practice restriction on use and disclosure of information in varying ways (reviewed by Pritts, 2008). Some allow the disclosure of health information for research without the individual's permission and others require such permission. Others only require such permission to release only certain types of information for research. Similarly, state statutes vary widely in how they have applied the accountability principle, both in the way they provide remedies for breaches in confidentiality and security and with respect to the standard imposed for initiating a suit. Also, only a few states have statutorily required providers to undertake security measures to ensure that health information is used and disclosed properly.

SECURITY OF HEALTH DATA

Protecting the security of data in health research is important because health research requires the collection, storage, and use of large amounts of personally identifiable health information, much of which may be sensitive and potentially embarrassing. If security is breached, the individuals whose health information was inappropriately accessed face a number of potential harms. The disclosure of personal information may cause intrinsic harm simply because that private information is known by others (Saver, 2006). Another potential danger is economic harm. Individuals could lose their job, health insurance, or housing if the wrong type of information becomes public knowledge. Individuals could also experience social or psychological harm. For example, the disclosure that an individual is infected with HIV or another type of sexually transmitted infection can cause social isolation and/or other psychologically harmful results (Gostin, 2008). Finally, security breaches could put individuals in danger of identity theft (Pritts, 2008).

Protecting the privacy of research participants and maintaining the confidentiality of their data have always been paramount in research and a fundamental tenet of clinical research. However, several highly publicized examples of stolen or misplaced computers containing health data have heightened the public's concerns about the security of health data (for a list of security breaches in health research, see Table 2-2). The extent to which these breaches have caused tangible harm to the individuals involved is difficult to quantify (Pritts, 2008). A Government Accountability Office (GAO) report studying major security breaches involving nonmedical personal information concluded that most security breaches do not result in identity theft (GAO, 2007). However, the lack of identity theft resulting from past breaches is no guarantee that future breaches will not result in more serious harm. A recent report from the Identity Theft Resources Center found that identity theft is up by 69 percent for the first half of 2008, compared to the same time period in 2007 (ITRC, 2008). Also, regardless of actual harm, security breaches are problematic for health research because they undermine public trust, which is essential for patients to be willing to participate in research (Hodge et al., 1999). A recent study found patients believe that requiring researchers to have security plans encourages researchers to take additional precautions to protect data (Damschroder et al., 2007). Moreover, data security is important to protect because it is a key component of comprehensive privacy practices.

The HIPAA Security Rule and Its Limitations

The goals of security are threefold: to ensure that (1) only authorized individuals see stored data; (2) they only see the data when they need to use it for an authorized purpose; and (3) what they see is accurate. Traditionally, these goals have been pursued through protections intended to make data processing safe from unauthorized access, alteration, deletion, or transmission. The HIPAA Security Rule employs this traditional solution to protecting security, and sets a floor for data security standards within covered entities (Box 2-2).[11]

The HIPAA Security Rule has several major gaps in security protection. First, like the HIPAA Privacy Rule, the HIPAA Security Rule only applies to covered entities. Many researchers who rely on protected health information (PHI)[12] to conduct health research are not covered entities, and thus are not required to implement any of the security requirements outlined in the Security Rule. Although federal research regulations include protections of privacy, there are no other laws that specifically require researchers to implement security protections for research data. Second, the HIPAA Security Rule only protects electronic medical records; it does not require covered entities

---

[11] Security Standards, 45 C.F.R. parts 160, 162, and 164 (2003). The final standards were adopted on February 20, 2003. Covered entities were required to be in compliance with the regulation on April 21, 2005 (and April 21, 2006, for small health plans).

[12] Protected health information (PHI) refers to all personally identifiable health information maintained by a HIPAA covered entity. 45 C.F.R. § 160.103 (2002).

TABLE 2-2 Research Security Breaches: 2006–2008

Date	Organization	Event	No. of Records Affected	Consequence
3/3/06	Georgetown University	A cyber attack on a server exposed the personal information of elderly District of Columbia (DC) residents. The compromised server was used by researchers to monitor services provided to the elderly for the DC Office on Aging.	41,000	The person making the attack came from outside the University and was not authorized to access the data. However, there is no evidence that personal data have been misused.
6/20/06	University of Alabama School of Medicine	A computer containing the personal information on donors, recipients, and potential recipients from the university's kidney transplant program was stolen.	9,800	The computer was stolen in February, but individuals were not notified until June, because it took months for the University to reconstruct the missing data.
9/29/06	University of Iowa, Department of Psychology	A computer was attacked that stored the personal information of research subjects participating in a study on maternal and child health from 1995 to the present.	14,500	There is no evidence that any personal information on the computer was accessed.
10/24/06	Jacobs Neurological Institute (Buffalo, NY)	A laptop containing patient records and research data was stolen from a researcher's locked office.	Unknown	The chief technology officer reported that no personally identifiable information was stored on the laptop.
1/4/07	SickKids (Ontario)	A laptop containing personal health information on research participants from 10 research studies was stolen.	Unknown	The computer was password protected, so it is unlikely that any data were accessed.

continued

TABLE 2-2 Continued

Date	Organization	Event	No. of Records Affected	Consequence
2/16/07	U.S. Department of Veterans Affairs (VA)	An unencrypted computer hard drive disappeared from a VA research center in Alabama.	Unknown	The Secretary of the VA shut down the Research Enhancement Award Programs until proper security standards are in place.
3/30/07	University of California–San Francisco	A computer that contained the personal information on cancer research subjects was stolen from a locked research office.	+3,000	There is no evidence that any information on the computer was used by unauthorized persons.
6/7/07	U.S. Marines/Pennsylvania State University	A researcher posted the personal information of many U.S. Marines online. This information then turned up in a cache on Google's search engine.	10,554	During the time period that the information was online, the website was only accessed by one individual—a Marine whose information was released.
8/17/07	Walter Reed Army Institute of Research	Boxes of documents containing personal information were found in the dumpster at an apartment building. The documents should have been shredded.	Unknown	The boxes were intact when discovered, so it is unlikely that any of the personal information was accessed.
2/23/08	National Institutes of Health	A laptop computer that contained sensitive medical information on patients enrolled in a clinical trial was stolen. The information was not encrypted, in violation of the government's data-security policy.	2,500	Because the information was not encrypted, it is possible that private health information was accessed on the computer.

SOURCES: ITRC (2006, 2007); PRC (2008).

BOX 2-2
The HIPAA Security Rule

The final HIPAA Security Standards were adopted on February 20, 2003. Covered entities were required to be in compliance with the regulation on April 21, 2005 (and April 21, 2006, for small health plans). In designing the HIPAA Security Rule, the Department of Health and Human Services (HHS) recognized that covered entities affected by this Rule were varied in terms of size, sophistication in technology use, and relative risks. Rather than dictate specific technological solutions, HHS deliberately made the rule flexible and usable by all covered entities regardless of size and purpose. HHS also specifically stayed away from requiring any particular technology solutions to protect security. The Rule was intended to encourage covered entities to use future technology as it developed.

Unlike the HIPAA Privacy Rule, the HIPAA Security Rule only protects electronic protected health information (EPHI). The Security Rule requires covered entities that process EPHI to maintain sufficient security measures to ensure the confidentiality, integrity, and availability of all EPHI. The Rule enumerates specific administrative, technical, and physical security safeguards for covered entities to implement. Each safeguard is either classified as "addressable" or "required." For the former, a "covered entity must conduct a risk analysis to determine whether each specification is reasonable and appropriate for its unique situation," and only those safeguards that are "reasonable and appropriate" must be implemented. Required security safeguards are those mandated by the Rule.

The Rule gives covered entities the responsibility for training their workforces to comply with the security regulation and for having written security policies and procedures in place. However, covered entities are only required to protect against reasonably anticipated threats or hazards to the security of the data, and reasonably anticipated uses or disclosures of such information that are not permitted under the Privacy Rule.

SOURCES: 68 Fed. Reg. 8333, 8334 (2003); 45 C.F.R. § 164.306; 45 C.F.R. § 164.316 (2007).

---

to implement any security protections for health information stored in paper records. There is an ongoing effort to implement electronic health records. However, many health records now exist only in paper form and may not be securely protected.

Third, many covered entities apparently are not yet in full compliance with all the requirements of the HIPAA Security Rule, based on surveys[13] of

---

[13]Since 2004, the American Health Information Management Association has annually surveyed health care privacy officers and others whose jobs related to the HIPAA privacy function to gain an understanding of where health care organizations stand with regard to implementing the Privacy and Security Rules required by HIPAA (AHIMA, 2006).

health care privacy officers and other individuals responsible for implementing the HIPAA regulations conducted by the American Health Information Management Association (AHIMA). The surveys found that although the percentage of respondents who believe their facilities are in full compliance with the HIPAA Security Rule is increasing yearly, the number is still not 100 percent. In 2006, 1 year after implementation of the HIPAA security regulations, 25 percent of respondents described themselves as fully compliant with the Security Rule, and 50 percent described themselves as 85 to 95 percent compliant (compared to 17 percent of respondents in 2005 reporting they were fully compliant, and 43 percent describing themselves as 85 to 95 percent compliant). More than half—54 percent—of respondents reported that their covered entity had upgraded its electronic software system to comply with the HIPAA Security Rule. All the respondents reported that their covered entity has an individual responsible for assessing data protection needs and implementing solutions and staff training (compared to 89 percent in 2005), but the number of facilities reporting that they have an entire committee or task related to security decreased from 2005 (59 percent versus 78 percent) (AHIMA, 2006).

The Centers for Medicare & Medicaid Services (CMS) has the authority to enforce the HIPAA Security Rule, and has received 378 security complaints as of 2008 without issuing any fines or penalties. A recent report issued by the HHS Office of Inspector General evaluated CMS's oversight and enforcement of the HIPAA Security Rule and "found that CMS had taken limited steps to ensure that covered entities adequately implement security protections" (OIG, 2008). However, a 2008 Resolution Agreement entered into by the U.S. Department of Health and Human Services (HHS) and CMS with Seattle-based Providence Health & Services for breaches of the HIPAA Privacy and Security Rules may indicate that CMS is starting to take a more affirmative approach to enforcement. The agreement requires Providence Health & Services to pay $100,000 and to implement a corrective action plan to ensure electronic patient information is appropriately safeguarded against future security breaches (OCR, 2008). In addition, CMS has recently partnered with PricewaterhouseCoopers to conduct security audits of covered entities to examine how well they are implementing the requirements of the HIPAA Security Rule. Ten to 20 assessments are planned for 2008 (Conn, 2008). Together these actions may have a positive effect on the percentage of covered entities fully compliant with the HIPAA Security Rule.

Regardless of whether the HIPAA Security Rule is actively enforced, the other gaps in the HIPAA Security Rule's protection of personal health information are problematic because enhanced security is necessary to reduce the risk of data theft and to reinforce the public's trust in the research community by diminishing anxiety about the potential for unintentional disclosure of information. **Thus, the IOM committee recommends that all institutions (both covered entities and non-covered entities) in the health research community that are involved in the collection, use, and disclosure of personally identifiable health information take strong measures to safeguard the security of health data.** Given the differences among the missions and activities of institutions in the health research community, some flexibility in the implementation of specific security measures will be necessary.

Examples of measures that institutions should implement include appointment of a security officer on IRBs and Privacy Boards to be responsible for assessing data protection needs and implementing solutions and staff training; use of encryption and encoding techniques, especially for laptops and removable media containing personally identifiable health information; and implementation of a breach notification requirement, so that patients may take steps to protect their identity in the event of a breach (IOM, 2000). More generally, institutions should implement layers of security protections, so that if security fails at one layer the breach will likely be stopped by another layer of security protection. The publication of best practices combined with a cooperative approach to compliance with security standards—such as self-evaluation, security audits, and certification programs—would also promote progress in this area. Research sponsors could play a role in the adoption of best practices in data security, by requiring researchers to implement appropriate security measures prior to providing funding. In addition, the federal government should support the development of technologies to enhance the security of health information.

Examples of security standards and guidelines already exist in some sectors, but they are not widely applied in health research. For instance, the National Institute of Standards and Technology has developed standards and guidance for the implementation of the Federal Information Security Management Act of 2002, which was meant to bolster computer and network security within the federal government and affiliated parties (e.g., government contractors). These include standards for minimum security requirements for information and information systems, as well as guidance for assessing and selecting appropriate security controls for information systems, for determining security control effectiveness, and for certifying and accrediting information systems (NIST, 2007). However, two recent GAO reports found that although the federal government is improving information security performance, a number of significant information security control deficiencies remain (GAO, 2008a,b). HHS, working through its Office of the National Coordinator for Health Information Technology,[14] could play an important role in developing or adapting standards for health

---

[14] See http://www.hhs.gov/healthit/onc/mission/.

research applications, and then encourage and facilitate broader use of such standards in the health research community.

POTENTIAL TECHNICAL APPROACHES TO HEALTH DATA PRIVACY AND SECURITY

The security of data will continue to grow in importance as the health care industry moves toward greater implementation of electronic health records, and Congress has already proposed numerous bills to facilitate and regulate that transition (see also Chapter 6). Advances in information technology will likely make it easier to implement such measures as audit trails and access controls in the future. Although the committee does not recommend a specific technology solution, there are at least four technological approaches to enhancing data privacy and security that have been proposed by others as having the potential to be particularly influential in health research: (1) Privacy-preserving data mining and statistical disclosure limitation, (2) personal electronic health record devices, (3) independent consent management tools, and (4) pseudonymisation. Each seeks to minimize or eliminate the transfer of personally identifiable data (Burkert, 2001). The advantages, limitations, and current feasibility of each are described briefly below.

Privacy-preserving data mining and statistical disclosure limitation. In recent years, a number of techniques have been proposed for modifying or transforming data in such a way so as to preserve privacy while statistically analyzing the data (reviewed in Aggarwal and Yu, 2008; NRC, 2000, 2005, 2007b,c). Typically, such methods reduce the granularity of representation in order to protect confidentiality. There is, however, a natural trade-off between information loss and the confidentiality protection because this reduction in granularity results in diminished accuracy and utility of the data, and methods used in their analysis. Thus, a key issue is to maintain maximum utility of the data without compromising the underlying privacy constraints. In addition, there are a very large number of definitions of privacy and its protection in the statistical disclosure limitation and the privacy-preserving data mining literatures, in part because of the varying goals.

Examples of statistical disclosure limitation and privacy-preserving data mining methods include perturbation methods such as noise addition, which attempts to mask the identifiable attributes of individual records, aggregation methods such as k-anonymity, which attempts to reduce the granularity of representation of the data in such a way that a given record cannot be distinguished from at least $(k - 1)$ other records, the release of summary statistics that can be used for actual statistical analyses such as marginal totals from contingency tables, and various approaches to the generation of synthetic data. Several of these are reviewed in Aggarwal and Yu (2008).

Other technologies include cryptographic methods for distributive privacy protection, which operate by allowing researchers to query various databases online using cryptographic algorithms (Brands, 2007; reviewed in Aggarwal and Yu, 2008), query auditing techniques, and output perturbation using methodology known as differential privacy (many of these techniques are reviewed in Aggarwal and Yu, 2008, and Dwork, 2008). These technologies aim to protect privacy by minimizing the outflow of information to researchers, as the providers of the databases do not make any of the actual data available to the researchers. The principal drawback of many of these methods relates to the potentially limited utility of the released information, especially for secondary analyses not planned in advance.

Each of the methods referred to above have strengths and weaknesses for specific kinds of statistical analyses. Precisely how this body of developing methodologies may be effectively used in the types of health research of the sort envisioned in this report remains an open question and this is an area of active research. Thus, alternative mechanisms for data protection going beyond the removal of obvious identifiers and the application of limited modifications of data elements are required. These mechanisms need to be backed up by legal penalties and sanctions.

Personal electronic health record devices. The use of personal electronic health record devices requires that all individuals possess a personal electronic device, such as a personal digital assistant (PDA) or personal computer, to manage their health information. The electronic device is intended to be used by individuals to aggregate all of their health information into one location (i.e., the electronic device). The infrastructure for implementing this privacy-enhancing technology exists, but there are several serious problems with relying on this technology in health research. First, it is unclear who would provide individuals with the devices, how they would be maintained, and who would bear the cost of the maintenance. Second, it is impossible for researchers to query every single individual for permission to access his/her personal electronic health record device in order to determine if he/she meets the criteria for the relevant study. Only individuals who are on the Internet and are involved in health research could easily be queried. Third, the use of personal electronic devices would make it almost impossible to aggregate data because of the difficulty of accessing data from multiple sources. These problems are sufficiently serious that the use of this technology is unlikely to offer a satisfactory solution to the privacy and security concerns in health research (Brands, 2007).

Independent consent management tools. The independent consent management tool (or infomediary) relies on a health trust to store all of an individual's health data. When researchers are interested in accessing an individual's health information for a study, the researchers must contact the health trust. The health trust will then approach the individual and asks whether he/she is willing to give consent for the research. Examples of this technology include Microsoft's HealthVault, Google Health, and Revolution Health.

Independent consent management tools allow individuals to make blanket consents for their health information to be released for certain types of researchers. For example, an individual can have a standing consent that his/her information can be released to all researchers at the Mayo Clinic, or for all research on cancer, etc. Thus, the use of a health trust allows an individual to have the power of consent for all uses of his/her health information, but does not require a specific consent in all instances (Brands, 2007). Some privacy advocates are very favorable about the use of this technology because they see it as a way to give patients complete control over who can see and use their health information (PPR, 2008).

However, the use of this technology in health research has several major problems. The first problem is that the health trust in this system becomes a "honey pot" (i.e., the health trust holds ALL of an individual's data). This creates serious trust and security issues because a person's entire health record is stored in a single entity (Brands, 2007). A 2006 survey of global financial services institutions found that respondents reported that nearly 50 percent of all security breaches were a result of an internal failure (e.g., a virus or worm originating inside the organization, insider fraud, or inadvertent leakage of consumer data) (Melek and MacKinnon, 2006). Many security breaches in health care are likely also a result of internal failures. In addition, these organizations are currently not regulated by the HIPAA Privacy Rule, so there are no legal federal privacy restrictions preventing these entities from releasing individuals' data to the government, marketing companies, or others, and no mandatory data security requirements. New legislation or regulation making health trusts liable for security breaches may be necessary before the public is willing to trust these organizations to store personal health data (Metz, 2008).

The second major impediment to the widespread adoption of independent consent management tools is the difficulty of providing individuals with secure online access to view their health information. The companies marketing this technology need to develop a mechanism where individuals can access their medical information held by the health trust without endangering its security and privacy. The current methods for individual authentication online do not work well (NRC, 2003), but the use of a strong authentication system in a single domain may solve this problem. The companies will also need to address the fact that a significant portion of the population does not have online access at all (Brands, 2007).

The final problem with using independent consent management systems in health research is the inability to ensure the authenticity and integrity of responses. There is no existing method for the health trusts to provide the researchers with a guarantee that the information contained in their database is accurate. If data are authenticated using existing methods, such as through the use of digital signing, then it is impossible to truly protect the privacy of the individuals' information being disclosed (NRC, 2003). Cryptographic selective disclosure techniques may be able to solve this problem, but the technology does not exist yet (Brands, 2007).

Pseudonymization. Pseudonymization is a method "used to replace the true identities (nominative) of individuals or organizations in databases by pseudo-identities (pseudo-IDs) that cannot be linked directly to their corresponding nominative identities" (Claerhout and De Moor, 2005). The benefit of using pseudonymization in health research is that it protects individuals' identities while allowing researchers to link personal data across time and place by relying on the pseudo-IDs.

Most pseudonymization methods use a trusted third party to perform the pseudonymization process. This results in at least three entities being involved in the creation of each database. There is the data source that has access to nominative personal data (e.g., PHI), the trusted third party, and the data register that uses the pseudonymized data for research.

Two methods of pseudonymization are the batch data collection and the interactive data collection. In the batch data collection, the data supplier splits the data into two parts: (1) the identifiers that relate to a specific person (e.g., Social Security number, name), and (2) the payload data, which includes all the nonidentifiable data associated with each individual. The data are prepseudonymized at the data source and transferred to the trusted third party, which converts the prepseudonyms data into a final pseudo-ID. Both the final pseudo-ID and payload data are transferred to the data register, where they are stored and used for research; no data are stored with the trusted third party. Privacy concerns are minimized because the only version of the data that is available to researchers is pseudonymized data.

The interactive data collection is used in situations where neither the data supplier nor the data register has a need for local storage of the data. All the data is stored by a trusted third party in pseudonymous form. Both the data supplier and the data register must query the trusted third party to access the data (Claerhout and De Moor, 2005; De Moor et al., 2003).

It is unclear how technologies relying on pseudonymization would be implemented under the requirements of the HIPAA Privacy Rule. In order for information to be considered deidentified, the HIPAA Privacy Rule specifically states that covered entities can assign a code or other means of record identification (such as a pseudo-ID), but the code cannot be derived from, or related to, information about the subject of the information.[15] This means that any pseudo-IDs created using this technology must be based entirely on nonpersonal information. Alternatively, any researchers using the pseudonymized data must go through the normal IRB/Privacy Board review process.

CONCLUSIONS AND RECOMMENDATIONS

Based on its review of the information described in this chapter, the committee agreed on an overarching principle to guide the formation of recommendations. The committee affirms the importance of maintaining and improving the privacy of health information. In the context of health research, privacy includes the commitment to handle personal information of patients and research participants with meaningful privacy protections, including strong security measures, transparency, and accountability.[16] These commitments extend to everyone who collects, uses, or has access to personally identifiable health information of patients and research participants. Practices of security, transparency, and accountability take on extraordinary importance in the health research setting: Researchers and other data users should disclose clearly how and why personal information is being collected, used, and secured, and should be subject to legally enforceable obligations to ensure that personally identifiable information is used appropriately and securely. In this manner, privacy protection will help to ensure research participation and public trust and confidence in medical research.

As part of the process of implementing this principle into the federal oversight regime of health research, **the committee recommends that all institutions in the health research community that are involved in the collection, use, and disclosure of personally identifiable health information should take strong measures to safeguard the security of health data.** For example, institutions could:

- Appoint a security officer responsible for assessing data protection needs and implementing solutions and staff training.
- Make greater use of encryption and other techniques for data security.
- Include data security experts on IRBs.

---

[15] Standards for Privacy of Individually Identifiable Health Information: Final Rule, 67 Fed. Reg. 53182, 53232 (2002).

[16] This is derived from the principles of fair information practices (see Chapter 2 for more detail).

- Implement a breach notification requirement, so that patients may take steps to protect their identity in the event of a breach.
- Implement layers of security protection to eliminate single points of vulnerability to security breaches.

In addition, the federal government should support the development and use of:

- Genuine privacy-enhancing techniques that minimize or eliminate the collection of personally identifiable data.
- Standardized self-evaluations and security audits and certification programs to help institutions achieve the goal of safeguarding the security of personal health data.

Effective health privacy protections require effective data security measures. The HIPAA Security Rule (which entails a set of regulatory provisions separate from the Privacy Rule) already sets a floor for data security standards within covered entities, but not all institutions that conduct health research are subject to HIPAA regulations. Also, the survey data presented in this chapter show that neither the HIPAA Privacy Rule nor the HIPAA Security Rule have directly improved public confidence that personal health information will be kept confidential. Therefore, all institutions conducting health research should undertake measures to strengthen data protections. For example, given the recent spate of lost or stolen laptops containing patient health information, encryption should be required for all laptops and removable media containing such data. However, in general, given the differences among the missions and activities of institutions in the health research community, some flexibility in the implementation of specific security measures will be necessary.

Enhanced security would reduce the risk of data theft and reinforce the public's trust in the research community by diminishing anxiety about the potential for unintentional disclosure of information. The publication of best practices and outreach to all stakeholders by HHS, combined with a cooperative approach to compliance with security standards, such as self-evaluation and audit programs, would promote progress in this area. Research sponsors could also play a roll in fostering the adoption of best practices in data security.

REFERENCES

Aggarwal, C. C., and P. S. Yu, eds. 2008. *Privacy-preserving data mining: Models and algorithms.* Boston, MA: Kluwer Academic Publishers.

AHIMA (American Health Information Management Association). 2006. *The state of HIPAA privacy and security compliance.* http://www.ahima.org/emerging_issues/2006StateofHIPAACompliance.pdf (accessed April 20, 2008).

Allen, A. 1997. Genetic privacy: Emerging concepts and values. In *Genetic secrets: Protecting privacy and confidentiality in the genetic era*, edited by M. Rothstein. New Haven, CT: Yale University Press. Pp. 31–59.

Balch, G. I., L. Doner, M. K. Hoffman, and E. Macario. 2005. *An exploration of how patients and family caregivers think about counterfeit drugs and the safety of prescription drug retail outlets for the National Health Council.* Oak Park, IL: Balch Associates.

Balch, G. I., L. M. A. Doner, M. K. Hoffman, M. P. Merriman, E. Monroe-Cook, and G. Rathjen. 2006. *Concept and message development research on engaging communities to promote electronic personal health records for the National Health Council.* Oak Park, IL: Balch Associates.

Barrett, G., J. A. Cassell, J. L. Peacock, and M. P. Coleman. 2007. National survey of British public's view on use of identifiable medical data by the National Cancer Registry. *British Medical Journal* 332(7549):1068–1072.

Bloustein, E. 1967. Privacy as an aspect of human dignity: An answer to Dean Prosser. *New York Law Review* 39:34.

Bodger, J. A. 2006. Note, taking the sting out of reporting requirements: Reproductive health clinics and the constitutional right to informational privacy. *Duke Law Journal* 56:583–609.

Burkert, H. 2001. Privacy-enhancing technologies: Typology, critique, vision. In *Technology and privacy: The new landscape*, edited by P. E. Agre and M. Rotenberg. Cambridge, MA: The MIT Press. Pp. 125–142.

Claerhout, B., and G. J. E. De Moor. 2005. Privacy protection for clinical and genomic data: The use of privacy-enhancing techniques in medicine. *Journal of Medical Informatics* 74:257–265.

Conn, J. 2008. CMS' HIPAA watchdog presents potential conflict. *Modern Healthcare*. http://www.modernhealthcare.com (accessed July 28, 2008).

Damschroder, L. J., J. L. Pritts, M. A. Neblo, R. J. Kalarickal, J. W. Creswell, and R. A. Hayward. 2007. Patients, privacy and trust: Patients' willingness to allow researchers to access their medical records. *Social Science & Medicine* 64(1):223–235.

De Moor, G. J. E., B. Claerhout, and F. De Meyer. 2003. Privacy enhancing techniques: The key to secure communication and management of clinical and genomic data. *Methods of Information in Medicine* 42:148–153.

Dwork, C. S., 2008. An ad omnia approach to defining and achieving private data analysis, proceedings of the first sigkdd international workshop on privacy, security, and trust in kdd (invited). *Lecture Notes in Computer Science* 4890.

Feld, A. D., and A. D. Feld. 2005. The Health Insurance Portability and Accountability Act (HIPAA): Its broad effect on practice. *American Journal of Gastroenterology* 100(7):1440–1443.

Flannery, J., and J. Tokley. 2005. *AMA poll shows patients are concerned about the privacy and security of their medical records.* Australian Medical Association. http://www.ama.com.au/web.nsf/doc/WEEN-6EG7LY (accessed December 10, 2007).

Forrester Research. 1999. *National survey: Confidentiality of medical records.* http://www.chcf.org (accessed February 12, 2007).

Forrester Research. 2005. *National consumer health privacy survey 2005.* http://www.chcf.org/topics/view.cfm?itemID=115694 (accessed February 12, 2007).

Fried, C. 1968. Privacy. *Yale Law Journal* 77:475–493.

GAO (Government Accountability Office). 2007. *Personal information: Data breaches are frequent, but evidence of resulting identity theft is limited.* Washington, DC: GAO.

GAO. 2008a. *Although progress reported, federal agencies need to resolve significant deficiencies: Statement of Gregory C. Wilshusen, Director, Information Security Issues.* Washington, DC: GAO.

GAO. 2008b. *Information security: Progress reported, but weaknesses at federal agencies persist: Statement of Gregory C. Wilshusen, Director, Information Security Issues.* Washington, DC: GAO.

Gavison, R. 1980. Privacy and the limits of the law. *Yale Law Journal* 89:421–471.

Gelman, R. 2008. *Fair information practices: A basic history.* http://bobgellman.com/rg-docs/rg-FIPshistory.pdf (accessed April 15, 2008).

Goldman, J. 1998. Protecting privacy to improve health care. *Health Affairs* 17(6):47–60.

Gostin, L. O. 1995. Health information privacy. *Cornell Law Review* 80:101–184.

Gostin, L. 2001. Health information: Reconciling personal privacy with the public good of human health. *Health Care Analysis* 9:321.

Gostin, L. 2008. Surveillance and public health research: Personal privacy and the "right to know." In *Public health law: Power, duty, restraint.* 2nd ed. Berkeley, CA: University of California Press.

Gostin, L. O., and J. G. Hodge. 2002. Personal privacy and common goods: A framework for balancing under the national health information Privacy Rule. *Minnesota Law Review* 86:1439.

Greenhouse, S., and M. Barbaro. 2005. Walmart memo suggests ways to cut employee benefit costs. *The New York Times.* http://www.nytimes.com/2005/10/26/business/26walmart.ready.html?pagewanted=1&_r=1 (accessed April 14, 2008).

Harris Interactive. 2005. *Health Information Privacy (HIPAA) notices have improved public's confidence that their medical information is being handled properly.* http://www.harrisinteractive.com/news/printerfriend/index.asp?NewsID=849 (accessed April 3, 2007).

Harris Interactive. 2007. *Many U.S. adults are satisfied with use of their personal health information.* http://www.harrisinteractive.com/harris_poll/index.asp?PID=743 (accessed May 15, 2007).

HEW (Department of Health, Education and Welfare). 1973. *Records, computers and the rights of citizens: Report of the Secretary's Advisory Committee on Automated Personal Data Systems.* http://aspe.hhs.gov/datacncl/1973privacy/tocprefacemembers.htm (accessed July 12, 2008)

Hodge, J. G., Jr., L. O. Gostin, and P. D. Jacobson. 1999. Legal issues concerning electronic health information: Privacy, quality, and liability. *JAMA* 282(15):1466–1471.

Hudson, K. L. 2007. Prohibiting genetic discrimination. *New England Journal of Medicine* 356:2021.

IOM (Institute of Medicine). 2000. *Protecting data privacy in health services research.* Washington, DC: National Academy Press.

ITRC (Identity Theft Resource Center). 2006. *2006 disclosures of U.S. Data incidents.* http://idtheftmostwanted.org/ITRC%20Breach%20Report%202006.pdf (accessed July 7, 2008).

ITRC. 2007. *2007 breach list.* http://idtheftmostwanted.org/ITRC%20Breach%20Report%202007.pdf (accessed July 7, 2008).

ITRC. 2008. *Security breaches.* http://www.idtheftcenter.org/artman2/publish/lib_survey/ITRC_2008_Breach_List_printer.shtml (accessed July 22, 2008).

Kass, N. E., M. R. Natowicz, S. C. Hull, R. R. Faden, L. Plantinga, L. O. Gostin, and J. Slutsman. 2003. The use of medical records in research: What do patients want? *Journal of Law, Medicine & Ethics* 31:429–433.

Low, L., S. King, and T. Wilkie. 1998. Genetic discrimination in life insurance: Empirical evidence from a cross sectional survey of genetic support groups in the United Kingdom. *British Medical Journal* 317:1632–1635.

Lowrance, W. W. 1997. *Privacy and health research: A report to the U.S. Secretary of Health and Human Services.* http://aspe.hhs.gov/DATACNCL/PHR.htm (accessed May 10, 2008).

Lowrance, W. W. 2002. *Learning from experience, privacy and the secondary use of data in health research.* London: The Nuffield Trust.

Magnussen, R. 2004. The changing legal and conceptual shape of health care privacy. *The Journal of Law, Medicine & Ethics* 32:681.

Melek, A., and M. MacKinnon. 2006. *Deloitte global security survey.* http://www.deloitte.com/dtt/cda/doc/content/us_fsi_150606globalsecuritysurvey(1).pdf (accessed July 23, 2008).

Metz, R. 2008. *Google makes health service publicly available.* Associated Press. http://biz.yahoo.com/ap/080519/google_health.html (accessed August 13, 2008).

Moore, A. 2005. Intangible property: Privacy, power and information control. In *Information ethics: Privacy, property, and power,* edited by A. Moore. Seattle, WA: University of Washington Press.

NBAC (National Bioethics Advisory Commission). 1999. *Research involving human biological materials: Ethical issues and policy guidance, report and recommendations.* Vol. 1. Rockville, MD: NBAC.

NBAC. 2001. *Ethical and policy issues in research involving human participants.* Rockville, MD: NBAC.

NCSL (National Conference of State Legislatures). 2008. *Privacy protections in state constitutions.* http://www.ncsl.org/programs/lis/privacy/stateconstpriv03.htm (accessed June 10, 2008).

Nissenbaum, H. 2004. Privacy as Contextual Integrity. *Washington Law Review* 79:101–139.

NRC (National Research Council). 2000. *Improving access to and confidentiality of research data: Report of a workshop.* Washington, DC: National Academy Press.

NRC. 2003. *Who goes there?: Authentication through the lens of privacy.* Washington, DC: The National Academies Press.

NRC. 2005. *Expanding access to research data: Reconciling risks and opportunities.* Washington, DC: The National Academies Press.

NRC. 2007a. *Engaging privacy and information technology in a digital age.* Washington, DC: The National Academies Press.

NRC. 2007b. *Privacy and information technology in a digital age.* Washington, DC: The National Academies Press.

NRC. 2007c. *Putting people on the map: Protecting confidentiality with linked social-spatial data.* Washington, DC: The National Academies Press.

OCR (Office for Civil Rights). 2008. *HIPAA compliance and enforcement.* http://www.hhs.gov/ocr/privacy/enforcement/ (accessed August 13, 2008).

OECD. 1980. *Guidelines on the protection of privacy and transborder flows of personal data.* http://www.oecd.org/document/0,2340,en_2649_34255_1815186_1_1_1_1,00.html (accessed August 13, 2008).

OIG (Office of Inspector General). 2008. *Nationwide review of the Centers for Medicare & Medicaid Services Health Insurance Portability and Accountability Act of 1996 oversight.* Washington, DC: Department of Health and Human Services.

OTA (Office of Technology Assessment). 1993. *Protecting privacy in computerized medical information.* Washington, DC: OTA.

Petrila, J. 1999. Medical records confidentiality: Issues affecting the mental health and substance abuse systems. *Drug Benefit Trends* 11:6–10.

Post, R. 2001. Three concepts of privacy. *Georgetown Law Journal* 89:2087–2089.

PPR (Patient Privacy Rights). 2008 (October 4). Press release: *Microsoft raises the bar for privacy in electronic health record solutions.* http://www.patientprivacyrights.org/site/PageServer?pagename=HealthVault_PressRelease/ (accessed August 13, 2008).

PRC (Privacy Rights Clearinghouse). 2008. *A chronology of data breaches.* http://www.privacyrights.org/ar/ChronDataBreaches.htm (accessed July 8, 2008).

Pritts, J. L. 2002. Altered states: State health privacy laws and the impact of the federal health Privacy Rule. *Yale Journal of Health Policy, Law & Ethics* 2(2):327–364.

Pritts, J. 2008. *The importance and value of protecting the privacy of health information: Roles of HIPAA Privacy Rule and the Common Rule in health research.* http://www.iom.edu/CMS/3740/43729/53160.aspx (accessed March 15, 2008).

Privacy Protection Study Commission. 1977. *Personal privacy in an information society.* http://epic.org/privacy/ppsc1977report/ (accessed April 21, 2008).

PSRA (Princeton Survey Research Associates). 1999. *Medical privacy and confidentiality survey.* http://www.chcf.org/topics/view.cfm?itemID=12500 (accessed August 11, 2008).

Rachels, J. 1975. Why privacy is important. *Philosophy and Public Affairs* 4:323–333.

Regan, P. 1995. *Legislating privacy: Technology, social values, and public policy.* Chapel Hill, NC: University of North Carolina Press.

Research!America. 2007. *America speaks: Poll summary.* Vol. 7. Alexandria, VA: United Health Foundation.

Richards, N. M., and D. J. Solove. 2007. Privacy's other path: Recovering the law of confidentiality. *Georgetown Law Journal* 96:124.

Roback, H., and M. Shelton. 1995. Effects of confidentiality limitations on the psychotherapeutic process. *Journal of Psychotherapy Practice and Research* 4:185–193.

Robling, M. R., K. Hood, H. Houston, R. Pill, J. Fay, and H. M. Evans. 2004. Public attitudes towards the use of primary care patient record data in medical research without consent: A qualitative study. *Journal of Medical Ethics* 30:104–109.

Saver, R. 2006. Medical research and intangible harm. *University of Cincinnati Law Review* 74:941–1012.

Solove, D. J. 2006. A taxonomy of privacy. *University of Pennsylvania Law Review* 154:516–518.

Taube, D. O., and A. Elwork. 1990. Researching the effects of confidentiality law on patients' self-disclosures. *Professional Psychology: Research and Practice* 21:72–75.

Taylor, C. 1989. *Sources of the self: The making of modern identity.* Cambridge, MA: Harvard University Press.

Terry, N. P., and L. P. Francis. 2007. Ensuring the privacy and confidentiality of electronic health records. *University of Illinois Law Review* 2007(2):681–736.

Tourangeau, R., L. J. Rips, and K. Rasinski. 2000. *The psychology of survey response.* Cambridge, UK: Cambridge University Press.

Turn, R., and W. H. Ware. 1976. Privacy and security issues in information systems. *The RAND Paper Series.* Santa Monica, CA: The RAND Corporation.

Weddle, M., and P. Kokotailo. 2005. *Confidentiality and consent in adolescent substance abuse: An update.* Virtual Mentor, American Medical Association Journal of Ethics. http://virtualmentor.ama-assn.org/2005/03/pdf/pfor1-0503.pdf (accessed August 1, 2008).

Wentland, E. J. 1993. Survey responses: An evaluation of their validity. San Diego, CA: Academic Press.

Westin, A. 1966. Science, privacy and freedom. *Columbia Law Review* 66(7):1205–1253.

Westin, A. 1967. *Privacy and freedom.* New York: Atheneum.

Westin, A. 1976. *Computers, health records, and citizen rights.* http://eric.ed.gov/ERICWebPortal/custom/portlets/recordDetails/detailmini.jsp?_nfpb=true&_&ERICExtSearch_SearchValue_0=ED143358&ERICExtSearch_SearchType_0=no&accno=ED143358 (accessed July 30, 2008).

Westin, A. 2007. *How the public views privacy and health research.* Institute of Medicine. http://www.iom.edu/Object.File/Master/48/528/%20Westin%20IOM%20Srvy%20Rept%2011-1107.pdf (accessed November 11, 2007).

Whiddett, R., I. Hunter, J. Engelbrecht, and J. Handy. 2006. Patients' attitudes towards sharing their health information. *International Journal of Medical Informatics* 75(7):530–541.

Willison, D. J., L. Schwartz, J. Abelson, C. Charles, M. Swinton, D. Northrup, and L. Thabane. 2007 (September 25–28). *Alternatives to project-specific consent for access to personal information for health research. What do Canadians think?* Paper presented at 29th International Conference of Data Protection and Privacy Commissioners, Montreal, Canada.

Woolley, M., and S. M. Propst. 2005. Public attitudes and perceptions about health related research. *JAMA* 294:1380–1384.

3

The Value, Importance, and Oversight of Health Research

The previous chapter reviewed the value of privacy, while this chapter examines the value and importance of health research. As noted in the introduction to Chapter 2, the committee views privacy and health research as complementary values. Ideally, society should strive to facilitate both for the benefit of individuals as well as the public.

In addition to defining health research and delineating its value to individuals and society, this chapter provides an overview and historical perspective of federal research regulations that were in place long before the Privacy Rule was implemented. Because a great deal of medical research falls under the purview of multiple federal regulations, it is important to understand how the various rules overlap or diverge. The chapter also explains how the definition of research has become quite complex under the various federal regulations, which make a distinction between research and some closely related health practice activities that also use health data, such as quality improvement initiatives.

The chapter also reviews the available survey data regarding public perceptions of health research and describes the importance of effective communication about health research with patients and the public.

CONCEPTS AND VALUE OF HEALTH RESEARCH

Definitions

Under both the Health Insurance Portability and Accountability Act (HIPAA) Privacy Rule and the Common Rule, "research" is defined as "a systematic investigation, including research development, testing and evaluation, designed to develop or contribute to generalizable knowledge." This is a broad definition that may include biomedical research, epidemiological studies,[1] and health services research,[2] as well as studies of behavioral, social, and economic factors that affect health.

Perhaps the most familiar form of health research is the clinical trial, in which patients volunteer to participate in studies to test the efficacy and safety of new medical interventions. But an increasingly large portion of health research is now information based. A great deal of research entails the analysis of data and biological samples that were initially collected for diagnostic, treatment, or billing purposes, or that were collected as part of other research projects, and are now being used for new research purposes. This secondary[3] use of data is a common research approach in fields such as epidemiology, health services research, and public health research, and includes analysis of patterns of occurrences, determinants, and natural history of disease; evaluation of health care interventions and services; drug safety surveillance; and some genetic and social studies (Lowrance, 2002; Lowrance and Collins, 2007).

The Importance of Health Research

Like privacy, health research has high value to society. It can provide important information about disease trends and risk factors, outcomes of treatment or public health interventions, functional abilities, patterns of care, and health care costs and use. The different approaches to research provide complementary insights. Clinical trials can provide important information about the efficacy and adverse effects of medical interventions by controlling the variables that could impact the results of the study, but feedback from real-world clinical experience is also crucial for comparing and improving the use of drugs, vaccines, medical devices, and diagnostics. For example, Food and Drug Administration (FDA) approval of a drug for a particular indication is based on a series of controlled clinical trials, often

---

[1] Epidemiology is the study of the occurrence, distribution, and control of diseases in populations.

[2] Health services research has been defined as a multidisciplinary field of inquiry, both basic and applied, that examines the use, costs, quality, accessibility, delivery, organization, financing, and outcomes of health care services to increase knowledge and understanding of the structure, processes, and effects of health services for individuals and populations (IOM, 1995).

[3] The National Committee on Vital and Health Statistics has noted that "secondary uses" of health data is an ill-defined term, and urges abandoning it in favor of precise description of each use (NCVHS, 2007a). Thus, the committee chose to minimize use of the term in this report.

with a few hundred to a few thousand patients, but after approval it may be used by millions of people in many different contexts. Therefore, tracking clinical experience with the drug is important for identifying relatively rare adverse effects and for determining the effectiveness in different populations or in various circumstances. It is also vital to record and assess experience in clinical practice in order to develop guidelines for best practices and to ensure high-quality patient care.

Collectively, these forms of health research have led to significant discoveries, the development of new therapies, and a remarkable improvement in health care and public health.[4] Economists have found that medical research can have an enormous impact on human health and longevity, and that the resulting increased productivity of the population contributes greatly to the national economy (Hatfield et al., 2001; Murphy and Topel, 1999) in addition to the individual benefits of improved health. If the research enterprise is impeded, or if it is less robust, important societal interests are affected.

The development of Herceptin as a treatment for breast cancer is a prime example of the benefits of research using biological samples and patient records (Box 3-1) (Slamon et al., 1987). Many other examples of findings from medical records research have changed the practice of medicine as well. Such research underlies the estimate that tens of thousands of Americans die each year from medical errors in the hospital, and research has provided valuable information for reducing these medical errors by implementing health information technology, such as e-prescribing (Bates et al., 1998; IOM, 2000b). This type of research also has documented that disparities in health care and lack of access to care in inner cities and rural areas result in poorer health outcomes (Mick et al., 1994). Furthermore, medical records research has demonstrated that preventive services (e.g., mammography) substantially reduce mortality and morbidity at reasonable costs (Mandelblatt et al., 2003), and has established a causal link between the nursing shortage and patient health outcomes by documenting that patients in hospitals with fewer registered nurses are hospitalized longer and are more likely to suffer complications, such as urinary tract infections and upper gastrointestinal bleeding (Needleman et al., 2002). These findings have all informed and influenced policy decisions at the national level. As the use of electronic medical records increases, the pace of this form of research is accelerating, and the opportunities to generate new knowledge about what works in health care are expanding (CHSR, 2008).

---

[4] See Standards for Privacy of Individually Identifiable Health Information, 64 Fed. Reg. 59918, 59967 (preamble to rule proposed November 3, 1999) for a discussion on the benefits of health records research.

BOX 3-1
Examples of Important Findings from
Medical Database Research

Herceptin and breast cancer: Data were collected from a cohort of more than 9,000 breast cancer patients whose tumor specimens were consecutively received at the University of San Antonio (1974–1992, from across the United States). Data were collected prospectively with audits for verification, and recurrences were recorded through systematic patient follow-up. This database was analyzed to identify prognostic factors, and the results showed that amplification of the HER-2 oncogene was a significant predictor of both overall survival and time to relapse in patients with breast cancer. This information subsequently led to the development of Herceptin (trastuzumab), a targeted therapy that is effective for many women with HER-2–positive breast cancer.

Folic acid and birth defects: Medical records research led to the discovery that supplementing folic acid during pregnancy can prevent neural tube birth defects (NTDs). Studies in the 1970s found that vitamin (folate) deficiency and use of anticonvulsive drugs that deplete folate were associated with higher rates of NTDs, and studies in the 1980s found that use of folate supplements was associated with decreased rates. Population-based surveillance systems showed that the number of NTDs decreased 31 percent after mandatory fortification of cereal grain products.

Effects of intrauterine DES exposure: Starting in the 1940s, diethylstilbestrol (DES) was used by millions of pregnant women to prevent miscarriages and other disorders in pregnancy. In the 1970s, retrospective studies of medical records began to show that infants exposed to DES during the first trimester of pregnancy had an increased risk as adults of breast, vaginal, and cervical cancer as well as reproductive anomalies. In November 1971, the FDA sent a *FDA Drug Bulletin* to all U.S. physicians advising them to stop prescribing DES to pregnant women and ordered that prevention of miscarriage be removed from Indications and pregnancy be added to Contraindications in the physician-prescribing information for DES.

Patient safety: Health services research estimated that tens of thousands of Americans die each year from medical errors in the hospital. A 1998 study led by David Bates (Brigham & Women's Hospital) found that computerized order entry of prescriptions at Brigham & Women's Hospital reduced medical error rates by 55 percent; rates of serious errors fell by 86 percent. In response to this groundbreaking work, hospitals around the country are installing their own computerized physician order entry systems. For example, The Leapfrog Group—a large national coalition of more than 100 public and private organizations that provide health care benefits—includes computerized physician order entry as one of the safety standards it encourages hospitals to adopt.

Mortality risks of antipsychotic drugs in the elderly: In 2005, the FDA issued a public health advisory stating that the atypical (second generation) antipsychotic medications increase mortality among elderly patients. This decision was based on the results of 17 placebo-controlled trials with such drugs that enrolled a total of 5,106 elderly patients with dementia who had behavioral disorders. Fifteen of the studies showed numerical increases in mortality in the drug-treated group compared to the placebo-treated patients (approximately 1.6-1.7–fold increase in mortality), most often due to heart-related events (e.g., heart failure, sudden death) or infections (mostly pneumonia). However, the risk of death with older, conventional agents was not known. Results from two subsequent retrospective reviews of 27,000 and 37,000 medical records of elderly patients who had been treated with either conventional or atypical antipsychotic drugs indicated that conventional antipsychotic medications are at least as likely as atypical agents to increase the risk of death among those patients. As a result, the FDA now requires that the prescribing information for all antipsychotic drugs includes the same information about this risk in a boxed warning and a warnings section.

Child safety: Using the Partners for Child Passenger Safety (PCPS)—an ongoing child-focused, real-time, crash surveillance system established with the State Farm Insurance Companies in 1997—Flaura Winston (Children's Hospital of Pennsylvania) found that only 25 percent of children between 3 and 7 years of age were appropriately restrained in crashes; children in seat belts alone were at a 3.5-fold increased risk of serious injury. Winston's analysis of PCPS data led to the rapid adoption of belt-positioning boosters as the appropriate form of restraint for children once they have outgrown car seats. Appropriate restraint by children in this age group has doubled, and child fatality from crashes is at its lowest level ever.

Obesity: Eric Finkelstein (RTI International) used data from the late 1990s to find that obesity is responsible for up to $92.6 billion in medical expenditures each year; approximately half of obesity-related health care costs are borne by Medicare and Medicaid. A 2002 study by Roland Sturm (RAND) found that the effects of obesity on a number of chronic conditions were larger than those of smoking or problem drinking. Since then, obesity has been escalated to the top of the list of health care priorities, and policy makers have appropriated funds for federal agencies to fund health services research that encourages people to understand the effects of diet and exercise on their health.

Rural health: Stephen Mick (Virginia Commonwealth University) and colleagues examined rural hospital performance in the late 1980s and early 1990s and found that activity typical of urban hospitals is beyond the capacity of most rural facilities and recommended that a new federal approach would be required to preserve rural acute-care services. This work helped form the intellectual basis for Medicare's highly successful Critical Access Hospital program, which was designed to improve rural health care access and reduce closures of hospitals that provide essential community services.

continued

BOX 3-1 Continued

Workforce and health outcomes: In 1997, Jack Needleman (University of California–Los Angeles) and Peter Buerhaus (Vanderbilt University) analyzed more than 6 million patient discharge records from 799 hospitals in 11 states. They found that patients in hospitals with fewer registered nurses stay hospitalized longer and are more likely to suffer complications, such as urinary tract infections and upper gastrointestinal bleeding. This research established a causal link between the nursing shortage and outcomes, and helped move the nursing shortage into the public's eye and onto policy makers' radar. In 2002, Congress passed the Nurse Reinvestment Act to increase the domestic supply of nurses.

SOURCES: Bates et al. (1998); FDA (1971, 2005, 2008); Finkelstein et al. (2003); Gill et al. (2007); Herbst et al. (1971); IOM (2000b); Mick et al. (1994); Needleman et al. (2002); Pitkin (2007); Schneeweiss et al. (2007); Slamon et al. (1987); Thorpe et al. (2004); Veurink et al. (2005); Winston et al. (2000).

Advances in health information technology are enabling a transformation in health research that could facilitate studies that were not feasible in the past, and thus lead to new insights regarding health and disease. As noted by the National Committee on Vital and Health Statistics, "Clinically rich information is now more readily available, in a more structured format, and able to be electronically exchanged throughout the health and health care continuum. As a result, the information can be better used for quality improvement, public health, and research, and can significantly contribute to improvements in health and health care for individuals and populations" (NCVHS, 2007a). The informatics grid recently developed with support from the National Cancer Institute (Cancer Biomedical Informatics Grid, or caBIG) is an example of a how information technologies can facilitate health research by enabling broader sharing of health data while still ensuring regulatory compliance and protecting patient privacy (Box 3-2).

Science today is also changing rapidly and becoming more complex, so no single researcher or single site can bring all the expertise to develop and validate medical innovations or to ensure their safety. Thus, efficient sharing of information between institutions has become even more important than in previous eras, when there were fewer new therapies introduced. The expansion of treatment options, as well as the escalating expense of new therapies, mandates greater scrutiny of true effectiveness,[5] once efficacy

---

[5] Effectiveness can be defined as the extent to which a specific test or intervention, when used under *ordinary* circumstances, does what it is intended to do. Efficacy refers to the extent to which a specific test or intervention produces a beneficial result under *ideal* conditions (e.g., in a clinical trial).

BOX 3-2
caBIG (Cancer Biomedical Informatics Grid)

The National Cancer Institute's caBIG Data Sharing and Intellectual Capital Workspace's mission is to enable all constituencies in the cancer community—including researchers, physicians, and patients—to share data and knowledge through an informatics grid "by addressing the legal, regulatory, ethical, policy, academic, proprietary, and contractual barriers."

The caBIG strives to achieve this objective through a number of different initiatives. First, caBIG provides decision support tools for institutions that share data through the informatics grid. This analytic framework is intended to encourage institutions to make consistent analysis of legal, regulatory, and ethical constraints on data sharing. The program has identified four sets of considerations for institutions to analyze: (1) intellectual property considerations, (2) privacy and confidentiality considerations, (3) IRB and ethical considerations, and (4) sponsor considerations.

Second, caBIG has identified a number of best practices and processes for facilitating the approval of data sharing agreements via the caBIG infrastructure. Currently identified best practices include suggestions for conducting the patient informed consent process in a manner that permits data to be shared via caBIG, standardizing expectations for sharing unpublished data, creating recommendations for developing contract clauses for sponsored research projects that permit broad data sharing, and providing information documents for IRBs and Privacy Boards to use in reviewing proposals for data sharing via caBIG.

Third, caBIG has created model documents intended to facilitate and expedite the arrangements between institutions to share data. These include model informed consent provisions, model researcher questionnaires and data sharing checklists, and security-related agreements. Finally, caBIG has developed security policies and requirements for systems that are attached to or access the caBIG infrastructure.

Under caBIG, each institution retains legal responsibility for the research data it generates; this includes responsibility for complying with the HIPAA Privacy Rule, the Common Rule, as well as any applicable state laws. The institutions also retain the right to determine who they will share their data with, what type of data (deidentified versus identifiable) they will share and under what terms and conditions. The advantage to conducting research within the caBIG technical infrastructure is that the program has identified the common legal and ethical considerations that apply to all researchers across the country, and has simplified the process for sharing data. In addition, the caBIG infrastructure has increased institutions' trust in one another because "everyone is playing by the same rules" and a common set of expectations exist. Recently, the BIG Health Consortium was developed to extend the concept of caBIG beyond cancer research, and to link all stakeholders in biomedicine through a new biomedical configuration.

SOURCES: Big Health (2008); NCI (2008); NCVHS (2007b).

has been demonstrated. This requires registries of patient characteristics, outcomes, and adverse events. Large populations are required to facilitate comparison of patient populations and to calculate risk/benefit estimates. For example, INTERMACS[6] (Interagency Registry for Mechanically Assisted Circulatory Support) is a national registry for patients who are receiving mechanical circulatory support device therapy to treat advanced heart failure. This registry was devised as a joint effort of the National Heart, Lung and Blood Institute, Centers for Medicare & Medicaid Services, FDA, clinicians, scientists and industry representatives. Analysis of the data collected is expected to facilitate improved patient evaluation and management while aiding in better device development. Registry results are also expected to influence future research and facilitate appropriate regulation and reimbursement of such devices. Similarly, the Extracorporeal Life Support Organization (ELSO),[7] an international consortium of health care professionals and scientists who focus on the development and evaluation of novel therapies for support of failing organ systems, maintains a registry of extracorporeal membrane oxygenation and other novel forms of organ system support. Registry data are used to support clinical practice and research, as well as regulatory agencies. Another example is the database developed by the United Network for Organ Sharing (UNOS) for the collection, storage, analysis and publication of data pertaining to the patient waiting list, organ matching, and transplants.[8] Launched in 1999, this secure Internet-based system contains data regarding every organ donation and transplant event occurring in the United States since 1986.

Information-based research, such as research using health information databases has many advantages (reviewed by Lowrance, 2002). It is often faster and less expensive than experimental studies; it can analyze very large sets of data and may detect unexpected phenomena or differences among subpopulations that might not be included in a controlled experimental study; it can often be undertaken when controlled trials are simply not possible for ethical, technical, or other reasons, and it can be used to study effectiveness of a specific test or intervention in clinical practice, rather than just the efficacy as determined by a controlled experimental study. It can also reexamine data accrued in other research studies, such as clinical trials, to answer new questions quickly and inexpensively. However, information-based research does have limitations. Often it has less statistical rigor than controlled clinical studies because it lacks scientific control over the original data collection, quality, and format that prospective experimental research can dictate from the start. In addition to these scientific limitations, because

---

[6] See http://www.intermacs.org.
[7] See http://www.elso.med.umich.edu.
[8] See http://www.unos.org/Data.

of its relational and often distant physical separation from the data subjects, and the sheer volume of the records involved, obtaining individual consent for the research can be difficult or impossible.

Advances in information-based medical research could also facilitate the movement toward personalized medicine, which will make health research more meaningful to individuals. The goal of personalized medicine is to tailor prevention strategies and treatments to each individual based on his/her genetic composition and health history. In spite of the strides made in improving health through new treatments, it is widely known that most drugs are effective in only a fraction of patients who have the condition for which the drug is indicated. Moreover, a small percentage of patients are likely to have adverse reactions to drugs that are found to be safe for the majority of the population at the recommended dose. Both of these phenomena are due to variability in the patient population. Revolutionary advances in the study of genetics and other markers of health and disease are now making it possible to identify and study these variations, and are leading to more personalized approaches to health care—that is, the ability to give "the appropriate drug, at the appropriate dose, to the appropriate patient, at the appropriate time." Achieving the goals of personalized medicine will lead to improvements in both the effectiveness and the safety of medical therapies.

Public Perceptions of Health Research

A number of studies have been undertaken to gauge the public's attitude toward research and the factors that influence individuals' willingness to participate in research. The surveys reviewed in this chapter focus on interventional clinical trials. A review of survey questions to gauge the public willingness to allow their medical records to be used in research can be found in Chapter 2.

The Public Values Health Research

A number of studies suggest that most Americans have a positive view of medical research and believe that research is beneficial to society. A recent Harris poll found that nearly 80 percent of respondents were interested in health research findings, consistent with previous survey results (Westin, 2007). A study in 2005 compiled data from 70 state surveys and 18 national surveys and found that the majority of Americans believe maintaining world leadership in health-related research is important. Seventy-eight percent of respondents said that it is very important, and 17 percent said that it is somewhat important. Only 4 percent of Americans reported that maintaining world leadership in health-related research is not important (Woolley and Propst, 2005). Similar results were found in a 2007 survey—76 percent of respondents reported that science plays a very important role in our health, and 78 percent reported that science plays a very important role in our competitiveness (Research!America, 2007).

The Virginia Commonwealth University 2004 Life Sciences Survey also found that most Americans have a positive view of research. In this study, 90 percent of respondents agreed that developments in science have made society better; 92 percent reported that "scientific research is essential for improving the quality of human lives"; and 84 percent agreed that "the benefits of scientific research outweigh the harmful results" (NSF, 2006).

Overall Experience When Participating in Research

Little is known about the attitudes of individuals who have actually participated in medical research. However, the available evidence suggests that most research participants have positive experiences. A recent Harris Poll found that 13 percent of respondents had participated in some form of health research, and 87 percent of those felt comfortable about their experience (Westin, 2007). In a study focused on cancer, 93 percent of respondents who participated in research reported it as a very positive experience; 76 percent said they would recommend participation in a clinical trial to someone with cancer. Most physicians surveyed in this study stated that they believe clinical trial participants receive the best possible care, and have outcomes at least as good as patients receiving standard cancer treatment (Comis et al., 2000). Another study found that 55 percent of individuals who participated in a research study would be willing to participate again in a future research study (Trauth et al., 2000).

Willingness to Participate in Research

Public opinion surveys indicate that a majority of Americans are willing to participate in clinical research studies. In 2001, a compilation of studies commissioned by Research!America found that 63 percent of Americans would be willing to participate in a clinical research study (Woolley and Propst, 2005). This percentage has remained stable over time. A 2007 Research!America survey also found that 63 percent of Americans would be very likely to participate in a clinical research study if asked (Research!America, 2007); 68 percent of respondents reported that their desire to improve their own health or the health of others was a major factor in deciding whether to participate in a clinical research project (Research!America, 2007).

Other surveys also suggest that willingness to participate in research focused on specific diseases is quite high. In one survey, the percentage of respondents indicating a willingness to participate in a medical research study was 88 percent for cancer, 86 percent for heart disease, 83 percent for a noncurable fatal disease, 79 percent for addiction, 78 percent for depression, and 76 percent for schizophrenia (Trauth et al., 2000). Respondents with greater knowledge of how research is conducted were more willing to participate (Trauth et al., 2000). Another study found that 8 of 10 Americans would consider participating in a clinical trial if faced with cancer. More than two-thirds of respondents said they would be willing to participate in a clinical trial designed to prevent cancer (Comis et al., 2000).

Americans also seem to be very supportive of medical research that relies on genetic data. A 2007 survey found that 93 percent of Americans supported the use of genetic testing if the information collected is used by researchers to find new ways to diagnose, prevent, or treat disease (Genetics & Public Policy Center, 2007). Two separate surveys found that 66 percent of Americans would be willing to donate their genetic material for medical research (Genetics & Public Policy Center, 2007; Research!America, 2007). However, despite this apparent positive view of genetic research, 92 percent of Americans reported they were concerned about their genetic information being used in a "harmful way" (Genetics & Public Policy Center, 2007).

Many factors, in addition to concerns about privacy and confidentiality (Genetics & Public Policy Center, 2007; Research!America, 2007), may influence an individual's willingness to participate in a medical research study. The Trauth survey found that individuals with higher income levels, with a college or graduate degree, or with children were more likely to participate in research. Age affected willingness to participate: 57 percent of respondents ages 18–34 were willing to participate in research, but only 31 percent of respondents ages 65 or older were willing (Trauth et al., 2000).

Other factors that potentially influence an individual's willingness to participate in research are race and ethnicity. It is well documented that minorities participate in health research at a much lower percentage than white Americans. Many cultural, linguistic, and socioeconomic barriers could be responsible for this difference (Giuliano et al., 2000), and study results have been variable on this issue. Several studies suggest that the low participation rates by racial and ethnic minority groups are due to their strong distrust of the medical research community compared to the general population (Braunstein et al., 2008; Corbie-Smith et al., 1999; Farmer et al., 2007; Grady et al., 2006; Shavers et al., 2002).

However, other evidence suggests that the low percentage of minorities participating in research is related to minority groups' lack of access to the research community (Brown et al., 2000; Wendler et al., 2006; Williams and Corbie-Smith, 2006). Thus, it is likely that the low number of minority individuals participating in medical research is at least partly due to recruitment techniques that are ineffective for minority populations.

The survey that focused on cancer research suggests that one of the main reasons why individuals do not participate in research is lack of knowledge about the availability of clinical trials. In a survey of nearly 6,000 cancer patients, 85 percent said they were unaware of the opportunity to participate in a clinical trial. Respondents who did participate said they did so because of one of the following beliefs: (1) trials provide access to the best quality of care (76 percent), (2) their participation would benefit future cancer patients (72 percent), (3) they would receive newer and better treatment (63 percent), and (4) participation would get them more care and attention (40 percent) (Comis et al., 2000).

A recommendation from a physician can also impact participation. In the United States, 48 percent of respondents to one survey reported that a physicians' recommendation would be a major factor in deciding whether to take part in a research study. Nearly three-fourths of respondents also cited an institution's reputation as a key factor to consider when deciding whether to participate in a study (Research!America, 2007). Twenty percent of respondents in an Italian public survey indicated that the presence of a physician as a reference during a research study influenced their willingness to participate (Mosconi et al., 2005).

In sum, surveys indicate that the vast majority of Americans have a positive view of medical research, believe that research is beneficial to society, and are interested in health research findings. Although little is known about the attitudes of individuals who have actually participated in medical research, the available evidence suggests that most research participants have positive experiences. Surveys also suggest that a majority of Americans are willing to participate in clinical research studies. Similar to the findings in Chapter 2, surveys indicate that many factors, in addition to concerns about privacy and confidentiality, can potentially influence an individual's willingness to participate in medical research, including the type of research and personal characteristics such as health status, age, education, and race. Notably, respondents with greater knowledge of how research is conducted were more willing to participate in research.

OVERSIGHT OF HEALTH RESEARCH

Historical Development of Federal Protections of Health Information in Research

The development of international codes, federal legislation, and federal regulation of human subjects often occurred in response to past abuses in biomedical experiments (reviewed by Pritts, 2008) (Box 3-3). The most well-known examples included (1) reported abuses of concentration camp prisoners in Nazi experiments during World War II, and (2) the Tuskegee syphilis study begun in 1932, in which researchers withheld effective treatment from affected African American men long after a cure for syphilis was found. Most of the current principles and standards for conducting human subjects research were developed primarily to protect against the physical and mental harms that can result from these types of biomedical experiments. Therefore, they focus on the principles of autonomy and consent. Although the standards apply to research that uses identifiable health information, research based solely on information is not their primary focus.

In the United States, perhaps the most influential inquiry into the protection of human subjects in research was the Belmont Report. The Belmont principles have been elaborated on in many settings, and served as the basis for formal regulation of human subjects research in the United States. In general, states do not directly regulate the activity of most researchers (Burris et al., 2003). However, the Belmont Commission's recommendations were reflected in the Department of Health and Human Services' (HHS's) Policy for Protection of Human Subjects Research, Subpart A of 45 C.F.R. 46 ("Subpart A") in 1979.[9] These protections were considered a benchmark policy for federal agencies, and in December 1981, the President's Commission for the Study of Ethical Problems in Medicine and Biomedical and Behavioral Research recommended[10] that all federal departments and agencies adopt the HHS regulations.[11]

In 1982, the President's Office of Science and Technology Policy appointed a Committee for the Protection of Human Research Subjects to respond to the recommendations of the President's commission. The committee agreed that uniformity of federal regulations on human subjects protection is desirable to eliminate unnecessary regulations and to promote increased understanding by institutions that conduct federally supported or regulated research. As a result, in 1991, other federal departments and agencies joined HHS in adopting a uniform set of rules for the protection of human subjects of research, identical to Subpart A of 45 C.F.R. 46, which is now informally known as the "Common Rule." Eighteen federal agencies have now adopted the Common Rule as their own respective regulations.

Overview of the Common Rule

The Common Rule governs most federally funded research conducted on human beings and aims to ensure that the rights of human subjects

---

[9] The Department of Health, Education and Welfare (now HHS) had previously issued policy and guidance on the protection of human subjects. See Williams (2005).

[10] In its report "First Biennial Report on the Adequacy and Uniformity of Federal Rules and Policies, and their Implementation, for the Protection of Human Subjects in Biomedical and Behavioral Research, Protecting Human Subjects."

[11] 45 C.F.R. part 46 (2005).

BOX 3-3
The Basis for Human Subjects Protections
in Biomedical Research

Nuremberg Code

The Nuremberg Code, created by the international community after the Nazi War Crimes Trials, is generally seen as the first codification of ethical norms governing experimentation on humans. Although it did not carry the force of law, the Nuremberg Code was the first international document to advocate voluntary participation and informed consent, which is partially based on autonomy. The Code established a set of ethical standards for physical experiments on humans emphasizing the following principles:

- The need to obtain the informed consent of the research subject;
- The duty to avoid all unnecessary physical and mental suffering and injury; and
- The requirement that any and all risks associated with the research must be outweighed by associated benefits.

Declaration of Helsinki

In 1964, The World Medical Association adopted the "Ethical Principles for Medical Research Involving Human Subjects," also known as the "Declaration of Helsinki," noting that all "[m]edical research is subject to ethical standards that promote respect for all human beings and protect their health and rights." The Declaration, which sets forth ethical principles to provide guidance to investigators and participants in human subjects research, made expressly clear that ethical standards on medical research encompass the protection of research on identifiable human material or identifiable data. The Declaration reiterated the principles of informed consent found in the Nuremberg Code and amplified them by, among other things, requiring that all experimental research be reviewed by an independent body. The principles are based on the general concept that it is the duty of medical researchers "to protect the life, health, privacy, and dignity of the human subject." The principles also require that "[e]very precaution [is made] . . . to respect the privacy of the subject, the confidentiality of the patient's information and to minimize the impact of the study on the subject's physical and mental integrity and on the personality of the subject." Thus, the Helsinki Declaration promotes the concepts of respect, autonomy, privacy, and confidentiality.

---

are protected during the course of a research project. The Common Rule stresses the importance of individual autonomy and consent; requires independent review of research by an Institutional Review Board (IRB); and seeks to minimize physical and mental harm. Privacy and confidentiality

Belmont Report

In 1979, the National Commission for the Protection of Human Subjects of Biomedical and Behavioral Research, created largely in response to the ethical breaches of the Tuskegee Syphilis Study, issued the "Belmont Report" to guide the resolution of ethical problems arising from research involving human subjects. The report first distinguished between practice (interventions designed solely to enhance the well-being of a patient) and research (activities intended to test a hypothesis and gain generalizable knowledge) and concluded that when elements of research are present in an activity, that activity should undergo review for the protection of human subjects. The Commission then identified and defined three overarching principles applicable to research involving human subjects: respect for persons, beneficence, and justice. Two of these principles, respect for persons and beneficence, are particularly relevant to privacy. The principle of respect for persons encompasses the requirement to treat competent adults as autonomous individuals capable of making their own choices. In application, this requires that subjects, to the degree that they are capable, be given the opportunity to choose what will or will not happen to them. Informed consent is closely tied to the principle of respect for persons because it provides information about potential benefits and risks, including how personal data will be protected, and requires comprehension of those risks and voluntariness to participate. The principle of respect for persons also seeks to protect persons with diminished autonomy, such as children and persons with serious mental disabilities. The principle of beneficence consists of the obligations to not harm the subject and to maximize possible benefits and minimize possible harms. Such an assessment should consider not only physical and psychological harms, but also social and economic harms, including breach of privacy. These harms are to be weighed against the anticipated benefit to the subject (if any) and the anticipated benefit to society. Although not as salient to questions of privacy and research, the third Belmont principle of justice is also worth emphasizing. Justice requires that the benefits and burdens of human subjects research be fairly allocated. It therefore protects the least advantaged in society.

SOURCES: Furrow et al. (2004); HEW (1979); Pritts (2008); Williams (2005); WMA (1964).

protections, although not defined in a detailed and prescriptive manner, are included as important components of risk in research.

The framework for achieving the goal of protecting human subjects is based on two foundational requirements: the informed consent of the research participant and the review of proposed research by an IRB. This section describes some of the basic parameters of the Common Rule (reviewed by Pritts, 2008). Particular provisions that interact with the HIPAA Privacy Rule are described in more detail in Chapter 4.

Scope of the Common Rule

In general, the Common Rule applies only to research on human subjects that is supported by the federal government.[12] As noted previously, research is defined as "a systematic investigation, including research development, testing, and evaluation, designed to develop or contribute to generalizable knowledge."[13]

Under the Common Rule, a "human subject" is defined as "a living individual about whom an investigator . . . conducting research obtains (1) Data through intervention or interaction with the individual, or (2) Identifiable private information." Private information is considered to be personally identifiable if the identity of the subject is or may readily be ascertained by the investigator or associated with the information.

The Common Rule applies to most human subjects research conducted using federal funds, but its influence is broader because most institutions that accept federal funds sign an agreement (a Federalwide Assurance or FWA) with HHS to abide by the Common Rule requirements in all research, regardless of funding source. Nonetheless, some privately funded human subjects research is conducted outside the purview of federal regulation (Goldman and Choy, 2001; Williams, 2005). Companies and other organizations may voluntarily choose to apply the Common Rule to their research projects, and many do. However, research projects in which compliance is voluntary are not subject to oversight or disciplinary action by HHS (Goldman and Choy, 2001; Williams, 2005).

Informed Consent[14]

The Common Rule requires that a researcher obtain informed consent (usually in writing) from a person before he/she can be admitted to a study (Williams, 2005). Informed consent is sought through a process in which a person learns key facts about a research study, including the potential risks and benefits, so that he/she can then agree voluntarily to take part or decide against it.

---

[12] See 45 C.F.R. § 46.101 (2005).

[13] See 45 C.F.R. § 46.102(d) (2005).

[14] This section on informed consent is based largely on a Congressional Research Service report (Williams, 2005), as adapted by Pritts (2008).

The Common Rule informed consent regulations focus primarily on the elements and documentation of informed consent rather than on the process used to obtain it. As to the process, the regulations require that informed consent be sought only under circumstances that provide the prospective subject with adequate opportunity to consider whether to participate. The Common Rule requires that information pertaining to informed consent be given in language understandable to the subject, and that the consent does not imply that the subject is giving up his/her legal rights or that the investigator is released from liability for negligence during the conduct of the study.[15]

The Common Rule also specifies a number of elements that must be provided when informed consent is sought. These elements include:

- an explanation of the purposes of the research,
- the expected duration of the subject's participation,
- the potential risks and benefits of the research,
- how confidentiality will be maintained,
- the fact that participation is strictly voluntary, and
- who the subject can contact to answer questions about the study or about his/her rights as a research participant.

In certain limited circumstances, the Common Rule allows an informed consent to be for unspecified future research. For example, under the Common Rule an informed consent can be used to obtain a person's permission to study personally identifiable information maintained in a repository for future, unspecified research purposes (HHS, 2003).

For the most part, the required elements of an informed consent address all types of research, although some are more relevant to biomedical research (e.g., the consent must include a disclosure of appropriate alternative procedures or courses of treatment, if any, that might be advantageous to the subject). One required element of informed consent is particularly relevant to research involving personally identifiable health information. The Common Rule requires an informed consent to include a statement describing the extent, if any, to which confidentiality of records identifying the subject will be maintained.[16]

Institutional Review Boards

Adopting the principles of the Belmont Report, the Common Rule requires that protocols for human subjects research be reviewed by an IRB

---

[15] See 45 C.F.R. § 46.116 (2005).
[16] See 45 C.F.R. § 46.116(b) (2005).

(Box 3-4) before research may begin.[17] The IRB must meet certain membership requirements, including having members with different expertise and at least one member who is not affiliated with the investigator's institution. The Common Rule specifies which level of IRB review is needed for various types of research and provides criteria for the IRB to consider during the review. Although the Common Rule does not specify the procedures an IRB must follow in its review of protocols, it does require the IRB to have written procedures for how it will review protocols and document IRB decisions.

The Common Rule requires that an IRB determine the following factors are satisfied to approve proposed research:

- Risks to subjects are minimized;
- Risks to subjects are reasonable in relation to anticipated benefits, if any, to subjects, and the importance of the knowledge that may reasonably be expected to result;
- The selection of subjects is equitable;
- Informed consent will be sought in accordance with the rules and will be documented;
- When appropriate, the research plan makes adequate provision for monitoring the data collected to ensure the safety of subjects; and
- When appropriate, adequate provisions are in place to protect the privacy of subjects and to maintain the confidentiality of data.[18]

An IRB may waive the requirement to obtain informed consent or approve an alteration of the consent form for some minimal risk research. The IRB may also waive the requirement for signed consent in certain circumstances.[19]

Anonymized Data

As noted above, the Common Rule considers use of "private identifiable information" to be human subjects research. Data are considered personally identifiable if the identity of the subject is or may be readily ascertained by the investigator or associated with the information accessed by the researcher.[20] However, the Common Rule exempts from its requirements research that involves:

---

[17] See 45 C.F.R. § 46.103 (2005).
[18] See 45 C.F.R. § 46.111 (2005). There are additional factors if the study includes subjects who are likely to be vulnerable to coercion or undue influence.
[19] See 45 C.F.R. § 46.116(d); 46.117(c) (2005).
[20] See 45 C.F.R. § 46.102(f) (2005).

BOX 3-4
Institutional Review Boards

According to the Department of Health and Human Services (HHS) Institutional Review Board (IRB) guidebook, "the IRB is an administrative body established to protect the rights and welfare of human research subjects recruited to participate in research activities conducted under the auspices of the institution with which it is affiliated. The IRB has the authority to approve, require modifications in, or disapprove all research activities that fall within its jurisdiction as specified by both the federal regulations and local institutional policy."

Therefore, IRBs have enormous responsibility in determining whether health research projects are planned and orchestrated in a way that minimizes or eliminates the potential risk to human research participants, including direct physical harms as well as nonphysical harms such as breach of privacy.

An IRB must be made up of at least five members with varying backgrounds who are sufficiently qualified through experience and expertise, and the diversity of the members must be sufficient to analyze the proposed research project. The IRB cannot consist entirely of members from one profession. At least one member must be unaffiliated with the institution conducting the research, and must not be part of the immediate family of someone affiliated with the institution. Members cannot have conflicts of interest with regard to the proposed research project. Also, there must be one member whose primary concerns are scientific, and one member whose primary concerns are nonscientific on each IRB.

SOURCE: OHRP (2008a).

[T]he collection or study of existing data, documents, records, pathological specimens, or diagnostic specimens, if these sources are publicly available or if the information is recorded by the investigator in such a manner that subjects cannot be identified, directly or through identifiers linked to the subjects.[21]

Otherwise identifiable data may be deidentified or "anonymized" for purposes of the Common Rule if it is coded and certain other conditions are met (HHS, 2004). Under Guidance issued by the Office for Human Research Protection, information is "coded" if identifying information (such as name or Social Security number) that would enable the investigator to readily ascertain the identity of the individual to whom the private information or specimens pertain has been replaced with a number, letter, symbol, or combination thereof (the code), and a key to decipher the code

---

[21] See 45 C.F.R. § 46.101(b)(4) (2005).

exists, enabling linkage of the identifying information to the private information or specimen.

Research involving only coded private information or specimens is not considered to involve human subjects under the Common Rule if the following conditions are met:

- The private information or specimens were not collected specifically for the currently proposed research project through an interaction or intervention with living individuals; and
- The investigator(s) cannot readily ascertain the identify of the individual(s) to whom the coded private information or specimens pertain because, for example:
  — The key to decipher the code is destroyed before the research begins;
  — The investigators and the holder of the key enter into an agreement prohibiting the release of the key to the investigators under any circumstances, until the individuals are deceased;
  — IRB-approved written policies and operating procedures for a repository or data management center prohibit the release of the key to investigators under any circumstances, until the individuals are deceased; or
  — Other legal requirements prohibit the release of the key to the investigators, until the individuals are deceased.

Under this standard, when a researcher accesses or receives data that have been coded and does not have access to the identifying key, the research is not considered human subjects research and is not subject to the Common Rule's requirements of informed consent or IRB review and approval of protocol.

Enforcement of the Common Rule

The Common Rule requirements for informed consent do not preempt any applicable federal, state, or local laws that require additional information to be disclosed to a subject in order for informed consent to be legally effective.[22]

Federal funding can be suspended or withdrawn from an institution when it is found to be in material violation of the Common Rule.[23] There is no authority to impose penalties directly on individual researchers for violations. Neither does the Common Rule expressly provide a research

---

[22] See 45 C.F.R. § 46.116(e) (2005).
[23] See 45 C.F.R. § 46.123 (2005).

participant with a private right of action. It should be noted, however, that recent cases indicate that courts may be willing to hold an institution liable under common law negligence theories where the approved informed consent form is determined to be less than adequate (Shaul et al., 2005).[24]

FDA Protection of Human Research Subjects

Some health research is also subject to FDA regulations. The FDA is charged by statute with ensuring the protection of the rights, safety, and welfare of human subjects who participate in clinical investigations[25] involving articles subject to the Federal Food, Drug, and Cosmetic Act[26] (the Act), as well as clinical investigations that support applications for research or marketing permits for products regulated by the FDA, including drugs, medical devices, and biological products for human use (Box 3-5).

In January 1981, the FDA adopted regulations governing informed consent of human subjects[27] and regulations establishing standards for the composition, operation, and responsibilities of IRBs that review clinical investigations involving human subjects.[28] At the same time, HHS adopted the Common Rule regulations on the protection of human research subjects.[29] The FDA's regulations were harmonized with the Common Rule in 1991 to the extent permitted by statute. Key differences between FDA and HHS regulations include that the FDA does not allow for waiver or alteration of informed consent and requires that subjects be informed that the FDA may inspect their medical records. In addition, studies of efficacy based solely on medical records research are not permitted to support registration. Remaining differences in the rules are due to differences in the statutory scope or requirements (Lee, 2000).

DISTINGUISHING HEALTH RESEARCH FROM PRACTICE

The Common Rule and Privacy Rule make a somewhat artificial distinction between health research and some closely related health care practices, such as public health practice, quality improvement activities, program

---

[24]See also *Grimes v. Kennedy Krieger Institute*, 782 A. 2d 807 (Md. Ct. App. 2001); *Gelsinger v. University of Pennsylvania* (Philadelphia County Court of Common Pleas filed September 18, 2000), available at http://www.sskrplaw.com/links/healthcare2.html.

[25]The FDA has defined "clinical investigation" to be synonymous with "research."

[26]The Food, Drug, and Cosmetic Act Section 505(i), 507(d), or 520(g) of 21 U.S.C. 355(i), 357(d), or 360j(g) (1972).

[27]See 21 C.F.R. part 50 (2008); 46 Fed. Reg. 8942 (1981).

[28]See 21 C.F.R. part 56 (2008); 46 Fed. Reg. 8958 (1981).

[29]See 45 C.F.R. part 46 (2005); 46 Fed. Reg. 8366 (1981).

BOX 3-5
FDA Protection of Human Subjects Regulations

The Food and Drug Administration (FDA) Protection of Human Subjects Regulations aim to protect the rights of human subjects enrolled in research involving products that the FDA regulates (i.e., drugs, medical devices, biologicals, foods, and cosmetics). For example, the regulations set out a number of steps researchers must go through before conducting drug research on human subjects. Researchers must submit a brief statement to the FDA promising that they will uphold ethical research standards, and identifying the Institutional Review Board (IRB) that will review the study prior to its start date. Sponsors of the study are required to submit to the FDA the results of any chemical and animal studies conducted on the new drug, provide the proposed study procedures for using human subjects, and ensure that the researchers' designated IRB will review the proposed study. The FDA will then review this information to ensure that there are no unacceptable risks to human subjects, that the project is ethically sound, and that the research is likely to achieve the study's objectives. The regulations give the FDA the right to request modifications to the proposed study, or the right to reject the proposal as presenting an unacceptable risk to human subjects.

Additionally, the FDA Protection of Human Subjects Regulations allow the FDA to conduct onsite inspections of IRBs to determine whether they are adhering to the requirements of the regulation. This portion of the regulation provides the FDA with the ability to examine IRB minutes, IRB written operating procedures, and other documents that substantiate the IRB's review of the research project. The FDA can also ensure that the IRB reviewing the study meets the membership requirements stipulated in the regulations, and that the consent forms contain all the required elements and are signed by all the subjects.

SOURCE: GAO (1996).

---

evaluations,[30] and utilization reviews,[31] all of which may involve collection and analysis of personally identifiable health information. However, determining which activities meet the definition of "research" is a major

---

[30] The Centers for Disease Control and Prevention defines program evaluation as the "systematic investigation of the merit, worth, or significance of organized public health action," noting that such evaluations are "systematic ways to improve and account for public health actions by involving procedures that are useful, feasible, ethical, and accurate." They can be based on goals, processes, outcomes, or value (http://www.cdc.gov/mmwr/preview/mmwrhtml/rr4811a1.htm).

[31] The Utilization Review Accreditation Commission defines utilization review as "the evaluation of the medical necessity, appropriateness, and efficiency of the use of health care services, procedures, and facilities under the provisions of the applicable health benefits plans" (http://www.urac.org/about/).

challenge for IRBs, Privacy Boards,[32] investigators, and health care practitioners because neither the regulations nor their interpretations by HHS provide clear guidance on how to distinguish research from activities that use similar techniques to analyze health information (IOM, 2000a).

It is important for IRBs and Privacy Boards to correctly distinguish among activities that are or are not subject to the various provisions of the Privacy Rule and the Common Rule. Only research requires formal IRB or Privacy Board review and informed consent.[33] Inappropriate classification of an activity as research can make it difficult or impossible for important health care activities, such as public health practice and quality improvement, to be undertaken. On the other hand, failure to correctly identify an activity as research could potentially allow improper disclosure of personally identifiable health information without sufficient oversight.

Thus, standard criteria are urgently needed for IRBs and Privacy Boards to use when making distinctions between health research and related activities, and the committee recommends that HHS consult with relevant stakeholders to develop such standard criteria. HHS is aware of this need, and created a working document titled "What Is Research?" However, the work on this project apparently has been delayed for unknown reasons (NCURA, 2007).[34] As described below, a number of other models have already been proposed to help determine whether activities should be classified as research in the fields of public health and quality improvement, and these could be instructive for developing HHS guidance. Any criteria adopted by HHS should be regularly evaluated to ensure that they are helpful and producing the desired outcomes.

The following sections describe some ongoing efforts to develop such criteria in the fields of public health and quality improvement. The intent of the committee is not to endorse these particular models, but rather to illustrate the challenges associated with making these distinctions and establishing standard criteria.

Public Health Practice Versus Public Health Research

The Belmont Report defined *health practice* as "interventions designed solely to enhance the well-being of the person, patient or client, and which have reasonable expectation of success" (CDC, 1999). To apply this definition to "public" health practice, the targeted beneficiary of the intervention must be expanded to include benefit to the community, rather than just a particular person. Neither the Common Rule nor the Privacy Rule provides

---

[32] Another type of oversight board defined by the Privacy Rule. See Chapter 4.

[33] Under the Privacy Rule, consent is referred to as authorization. See Chapter 4.

[34] Personal communication, C. Heide, Office for Civil Rights, HHS, May 29, 2008.

a specific definition for public health research; rather public health research is included in the general definition of research. However, the Privacy Rule regulates public health practice differently from public health research (see Chapter 4).

An early model for distinguishing public health research from public health practice focused on the intent for which the activity was designed, noting that the intent of public health research is to "contribute to or generate generalizable knowledge," while the intent of public health practice is to "conduct programs to prevent disease and injury and improve the health of communities" (Snider and Stroup, 1997). The Centers for Disease Control and Prevention developed a similar method with an expanded assessment of intent. For example, the model posits that in public health research, the intended benefits of the project extend beyond the study participants, and the data collected exceed the requirements for the care of the study participants. But for public health practice, the intended benefits of the project are primarily for the participants in the activity, or for the participants' community, and the only data collected are those needed to assess or improve a public health program or service, or the health of the participants and their community. The model also assumes that public health practice is based on well-established medical interventions and is nonexperimental (CDC, 1999). However, these models both have been criticized as too subjective and too dependent on the opinion of the person conducting the activity (Gostin, 2008; Hodge, 2005).

A new, more comprehensive model incorporating much of the previous two was recently proposed as a more objective checklist to be used by IRBs, Privacy Boards, and interested parties (Hodge, 2005; Hodge and Gostin, 2004). The foundations for this model are specific definitions of public health research: "the collection and analysis of identifiable health data by a public health authority for the purpose of generating knowledge that will benefit those beyond the participating community who bear the risks of participation," and public health practice: "the collection and analysis of identifiable health data by a public health authority for the purpose of protecting the health of a particular community, where the benefits and risks are primarily designed to accrue to the participating community."

The model is based on two primary assumptions. First, the actor performing the activity in question is a governmental public health official, agent, agency, or entity at the federal, tribal, state, or local level. Second, the activity in question involves the acquisition, use, or disclosure of personally identifiable health data. The model is then divided into two stages. Stage 1 is applied to all activities, and can be used to distinguish practice from research in the easiest cases. Stage 2 is only applied to those cases that are hard to distinguish, and where Stage 1 failed to lead to a definitive IRB/Privacy Board decision (Box 3-6).

**BOX 3-6
A Model for Distinguishing Public
Health Practice from Research**

Stage 1

Public health practice:

- "Involves specific legal authorization for conducting the activity as public health practice at the federal, state, or local levels;
- Includes a corresponding governmental duty to perform the activity to protect the public's health;
- Involves direct performance or oversight by a governmental public health authority (or its authorized partner) and accountability to the public for its performance;
- May legitimately involve persons who did not specifically volunteer to participate (i.e., they did not provide informed consent);
- Supported by principles of public health ethics that focus on populations while respecting the dignity and rights of individuals."

Public health research:

- "Involves living individuals;
- Involves, in part, identifiable private health information;
- Involves research subjects who voluntarily participate (or participate with the consent of their guardian) absent a waiver of informed consent;
- Supported by principles of research ethics that focus on the interests of individuals while balancing the communal value of research."

Stage 2

Legal authority: If authorized by a specific legal authority, the activity is health care practice. If authorized by general legal authority, analysis depends on whether the scope and limits of the authorization include research.

Specific intent: The intent of research is to "test a hypothesis and seek to generalize the findings or acquired knowledge beyond the activity's participants." The intent of public health practice is "to assure the conditions in which people can be healthy through public health efforts that are primarily aimed at prevention of known or suspected injuries, diseases, or other conditions, or promoting the health of a particular community." If the intent of an activity meets both definitions, the activity should follow research provisions.

Responsibility: In research, the principal investigator is responsible for the "health, safety, and well-being" of the research participants. In public health practice, a government entity often takes that responsibility.

continued

BOX 3-6 Continued

Participant benefits: In research, participants usually do not receive or expect any direct benefit from the activity. Public health practice is premised on providing some benefit to the participants or the population involved in the activity.
Experimentation: Research is experimental, and usually involves a nonstandard intervention or data analysis. Public health practice uses "standard, accepted, and proven interventions to address known or suspected public health problems."
Subject selection: In research, subjects are often selected randomly to ensure the generalizability of the results and reduce the potential for selection bias. Participants are selected for public health practice because they have or are at risk of having a particular disease or condition, and can likely benefit from the activity.

SOURCES: Hodge (2005); Hodge and Gostin (2004).

Quality Improvement Versus Health Research

Quality improvement has been defined as "systematic, data-guided activities designed to bring about immediate, positive change in the delivery of health care in a particular setting" (Baily, 2008). Quality improvement activities do not require IRB or Privacy Board approval under the Common Rule or the Privacy Rule, which classify quality improvement as a component of health care operations.[35]

However, in many cases, it is difficult for health care providers, IRBs, and Privacy Boards to determine whether a particular activity is purely for quality improvement, or whether it also entails research. One survey[36] exploring opinions in the health care community about the need for IRBs to review various quality-related activities found that physicians conducting quality improvement were less likely than IRB chairs to believe that IRB

---

[35] The Privacy Rule defines the term "health care operations" by listing a number of specific activities that qualify as health care operations. These include "conducting quality assessment and improvement activities, population-based activities relating to improving or reducing health care costs, and case management and care coordination." See 45 C.F.R. § 164.501 (2006).

[36] A total of 444 surveys were mailed to the medical directors of quality improvement and IRB chairs at hospitals with 400 or more beds that belong to the Council of Teaching Hospitals of the Association of American Medical Colleges, and to the editors of all U.S.-based medical journals that publish original research and appear in the Abridged Index Medicus. 236 surveys were returned, for a 53 percent response rate. The survey consisted of six brief scenarios that asked respondents to determine whether the described project needed IRB review and informed consent.

review was required for a given hypothetical activity, or that informed consent was necessary (Lindenauer et al., 2002). Recently, a highly publicized case has again brought the issue to the forefront for all the stakeholders (Box 3-7).

Some members of the health care community have proposed requiring that all prospective quality improvement activities go through external review (Bellin and Dubler, 2001), while others have outlined specific criteria to differentiate quality improvement activities from research.

For example, Casarett and colleagues developed a two-part test to identify quality improvement activities. The first test is whether the majority of

---

BOX 3-7
A Case Study of Quality Improvement and Research

Peter Pronovost of Johns Hopkins University (JHU) led a quality improvement effort at 103 intensive care units (ICUs) in Michigan hospitals to reduce the number of catheter-related bloodstream infections. This effort relied on promoting five medical procedures recommended by the Centers for Disease Control and Prevention (CDC) to reduce infection. The investigators recorded the number of infections that occurred at the ICU level; no data were recorded at the individual level.

Prior to starting the quality improvement effort, the investigators submitted an application to the Johns Hopkins Institutional Review Board (IRB), and classified the project as exempt from the requirements of the Common Rule. The IRB approved the project as exempt, and did not review the proposal further. After a description of the quality improvement effort was published in the *New England Journal of Medicine*, the Office for Human Research Protections (OHRP) received a letter of complaint that this was research without IRB approval and without informed consent. OHRP opened a compliance oversight evaluation, and initially determined that the project was research and needed to go through the IRB review process. OHRP stated that "quality improvement activities can also be research activities" and that "JHU failed to ensure the requirements for obtaining and documenting the legally effective informed consent of the subjects."

On February 15, 2008, OHRP reversed its initial decision, and concluded that this activity was a quality improvement effort and was not required to comply with the regulations governing human subjects research. The Michigan hospitals have been allowed to continue implementing and studying the effectiveness of the CDC-recommended procedures in ICUs, and have not been required to get IRB approval or informed consent. Also at this time, OHRP announced that it was going to review its policies on quality improvement.

SOURCE: OHRP (2008b).

patients are expected to benefit directly from "the knowledge to be gained" from the initiative. This means that the patients must actually benefit from the *knowledge* learned during the evaluation, not just from being a recipient of the protocol itself. If the patients are generally expected to directly benefit from the knowledge gained during the activity, then the activity is quality improvement. If not, the activity is research. The second test is whether the participants would be subjected to additional risks or burdens, including the risk of privacy breach, beyond the usual clinical practice in order to make the results of the initiative generalizable. If yes, then the initiative should be reviewed as research (Casarett et al., 2000).

More recently, the Hastings Center published a report exploring the similarities and differences between research and quality improvement. The report emphasized three fundamental characteristics of quality improvement and three fundamental characteristics of research. The authors argue that individuals have a responsibility to participate in the quality improvement activities because all patients have an interest in receiving high-quality medical care, and the success of a quality improvement activity depends on the cooperation of all patients. In addition, the report notes that quality improvement activities are a low risk to the patient, so there is little justification for not participating. The report also assumes that quality improvement activities are based on existing knowledge about human health and should lead to immediate local improvements in the provision of medical care.

In contrast, the report notes that participation in research should be voluntary, and decisions to participate should be based on researchers' full disclosure of all the potential risks and benefits. In addition, the authors assert that research is designed to create new knowledge about human health, rather than relying solely on existing knowledge, and that most research does not result in any direct benefit to the institution where the research is being conducted.

The authors concluded that IRBs are not the appropriate body for the ethical oversight of quality improvement activities. They argue that IRBs unnecessarily impose high transaction costs on these activities because of the difference in the way they are conducted compared to research. For example, in research, any changes in methodology require further IRB approval. In contrast, quality improvement activities involve frequent adjustments in the intervention, measurement, and goals of the activity based on the experience of the investigators. Requiring the investigator to revisit an IRB every time a small adjustment is needed in such an activity significantly increases the amount of time and effort required to conduct the initiative and to produce meaningful data. Also, the investigators involved in quality improvement activities ordinarily are already involved in the clinical care of participants and bear responsibility for the quality and safety of an intervention. Thus, the authors argue that there is no need for the additional oversight by an IRB to protect participant safety.

Rather, the report recommended integrating the ethical oversight of quality improvement activities into the ongoing management of an institution's health care delivery system, suggesting that oversight of quality improvement could be left with the managers of clinical care organizations, and that consent to receive treatment should include consent to participate in any quality improvement project that is minimal risk. However, the report stated that if a project has the characteristics of both quality improvement and research, the project should be reviewed as both human subjects research and quality improvement (Baily et al., 2006; Lynn et al., 2007).

In response to the ongoing confusion over when quality improvement rises to the level of research and requires IRB review, the IOM jointly hosted a meeting with the American Board of Internal Medicine in May 2008 to discuss this issue. Key members of the quality improvement community attended, and short- and long-term solutions to this problem were proposed. However, no written report from this meeting was produced and no general consensus was reached.

THE IMPORTANCE OF EFFECTIVE
COMMUNICATION WITH THE PUBLIC

As noted previously in this chapter, surveys indicate that the vast majority of Americans believe that health research is important and are interested in the findings of research studies. The majority of patients also appear to be willing to participate in health research, either by volunteering for a study to test a medical intervention or by allowing access to their medical records or stored biospecimens, under certain conditions. Their willingness to participate depends on trust in researchers to safeguard the rights and well-being of patients, including assurance of privacy and confidentiality, and the belief that it is a worthwhile endeavor that warrants their involvement. Yet patients often lack information about how research is conducted, and are rarely informed about research results that may have a direct impact on their health. The committee's recommendations in this section are intended to address both the public's desire for more information about health research and to help fulfill two of the committees overarching goals of the report: (1) improving the privacy and security of health information, and (2) improving the effectiveness of health research.

Disseminating Health Research Results

Ethicists have long suggested greater community involvement in health research studies, including more communication about research results (reviewed by Shalowitz and Miller, 2008a,b). In addition, the IOM committee identified transparency—the responsibility to disclose clearly how and why personally identifiable information is being collected—as an important component of comprehensive privacy protections. A previous IOM report also recommended improved communication with the public and research participants to ensure that the protection process is open and accessible to all interested parties (IOM, 2002). Effective communication would build the public's trust of the research community and is consistent with the principles of fair information practices.

When patients consent to the use of their medical records in a particular study, health researchers should make greater efforts at the conclusion of the study to inform study participants about the results, and the relevance and importance of those results. Learning about clinically relevant findings from a study in which a patient has participated could make patients feel more integrated into the process and could encourage more to participate in future studies. A recent United Kingdom report on the use of personal data in health research concluded that public involvement in research is necessary for the success of information-based research, and that a public informed about the value of research is likely to have greater enthusiasm and confidence in research and the research community (AMS, 2006). Moreover, direct feedback with study participants could lead to improved health care for the individuals if the results indicate that an altered course of care is warranted.

Nonetheless, there are multiple impediments, beyond cost, to providing meaningful feedback to participants. A summary of the results alone, while necessary and reasonable, can be seen as a token, and also raises questions about issues such as how best to write summaries, the stage at which results should be disseminated, and how to present research with uninformative outcomes. For example, one recent study found that sharing results directly with study participants was met with overwhelmingly favorable reactions from patients, but the study also revealed some obstacles (Partridge et al., 2008). In a survey of women who had participated in a randomized trial of breast cancer therapy and had received a summary of the study results by mail, 95 percent reported that they were glad they received the results. Most respondents interpreted the results correctly, although incorrect interpretation of the results was associated with increased anxiety, as was dissatisfaction with treatment.

Although some guidelines for providing and explaining study results to research participants have been proposed, they differ in details because limited data are available on this subject, and thus standards are lacking (Partridge and Winer, 2002; Partridge et al., 2008; Shalowitz and Miller, 2008b; Zarin and Tse, 2008). Because transparency is best achieved by providing graded levels of information and guidance to interested parties

(IOM, 2002), it will be important to develop effective and efficient ways to communicate with various sectors of the population. A commitment to the principles of "plain language"[37] will be important. Broader adoption of electronic medical records may also be helpful in accomplishing this goal.

Research Registries

One way to make information about research studies more broadly available to the public is through registration of trials and other studies in public databases. **HHS should encourage such registration of trials and other studies, particularly when research is conducted with an IRB/Privacy Board approved waiver of consent or authorization** (see Chapter 4). Numerous clinical trial registries already exist, and registration has increased in recent years (reviewed by Zarin and Tse, 2008). In 2000, the National Library of Medicine established a clinical trials registry (ClinicalTrials.gov), which has expanded to include information from several other trial registries and to serve as the FDA-required site for submissions about clinical trials subject to the FDA databank requirement. The FDA Amendments Act of 2007[38] expanded the scope of required registrations at ClinicalTrials.gov and provided the first federally funded trials results database. It mandates registrations of controlled clinical investigations, except for Phase I trials, of drugs, biologics, and devices subject to FDA regulation.

A policy of the International Committee of Medical Journal Editors (ICMJE), adopted in fall 2005, also requires prospective trial registration as a precondition for publication (DeAngelis et al., 2004). This policy led to a 73 percent increase in trial registrations of all intervention types from around the world (Zarin et al., 2005). Nearly 45,000 trials had been registered by fall 2007.

However, although the development of such registries is an important first step toward providing high-quality clinical trial information to the public, no centralized system currently exists to disseminate information about clinical trials of drugs or other interventions, making it difficult for consumers and their health care providers to identify ongoing studies. The current statutory requirements for registration and data reporting in the United States are not as broad as the transnational policies of the ICMJE or the World Health Organization, which call for the registration of all interventional studies in human beings regardless of intervention type (Laine et al., 2007; Sim et al., 2006). Moreover, noninterventional studies, such as observational studies that play an increasingly critical role in biomedical research, are not generally included in these databases. Because

---

[37] See http://plainlanguage.gov/index.cfm.
[38] FDA, Public Law 110–85 § 801 (2007).

many noninterventional studies are conducted with an IRB/Privacy Board approved waiver of consent or authorization, including those studies in a registry could be an important method for increasing public knowledge of such studies.

Informing the Public About the Methods and Value of Research

As noted previously, clinical trials are the most visible of the various types of health research, but a great deal of information-based health research entails analysis of thousands of patient records to better understand human diseases, to determine treatment effectiveness, and to identify adverse side effects of therapies. This form of research is likely to increase in frequency as the availability of electronic records continues to expand. As we move toward the goal of personalized medicine, research results will be even more likely to be directly relevant to patients, but more study subjects will be necessary to derive meaningful results.

However, many patients probably are not aware that their medical records are being used in information-based research. For example, the recent study that used focus groups to examine the views of veterans toward the use of medical records in research found that the majority of participants (75 percent) were not aware that "under some circumstances, [their] medical records could be used in some research studies without [their] permission," despite the fact that a notice of privacy practices, which included a statement that such research could occur, had been mailed to all participants less than a year prior to the study (Damschroder et al., 2007).

Moreover, surveys show that many patients desire not only notice, but also the opportunity to decide whether to consent to such research with medical records. Those surveys further indicate that patients who wish to be asked for consent for each study are most concerned about the potentially detrimental affects of inappropriate disclosure of their personally identifiable health information, including discrimination in obtaining health or life insurance or employment.

As noted in Chapter 2, strengthening security protections of health data should reduce the risk of security breaches and their potential negative consequences, and thus should help to alleviate patient concerns in this regard. But educating patients about how health research is conducted, monitored, and reported on could also help to ease patient concerns about privacy and increase patients' trust in the research community, which as noted above is important for the public's continued participation in health research. For example, datasets are most often provided to researchers without direct identifiers such as name and Social Security number. Furthermore, identifiers are not included in publications about research results. Also, under both the Privacy Rule and the Common Rule, a waiver of consent and authorization is possible only under the supervision of an IRB or Privacy Board, and a waiver is granted only when the research entails minimal risk and when obtaining individual consent and authorization is impracticable (see the previous section and also Chapter 4). Finally, professional ethics dictate that researchers safeguard data and respect privacy.

Conveying the value of medical records research to patients will be important. Surveys show that people are more supportive of research that is relevant to them and their loved ones. At the same time, educational efforts should stress the negative impact of incomplete datasets on research findings. Representative samples are essential to ensure the validity and generalizability of health research (Box 3-8), but datasets will not represent the entire population if some people withhold access to their health information.

In addition, an educated public could also decrease the potential for biased research samples. A universal requirement for consent or authorization in medical records research leads to incomplete datasets, and thus to biased results and inaccurate conclusions. Some large medical institutions with a strong research history and reputation (e.g., Mayo Clinic) can obtain authorization and consent rates as high as 80 percent, but the 20 percent

---

BOX 3-8
Selection Bias in Health Research

When researchers are required to obtain consent or authorization to access each individual's medical record for a research study, it is likely that individuals' willingness to grant access will not be random, and will vary in a way that may bias the study results—a phenomenon known as selection bias. A study sample is biased if certain members are underrepresented or overrepresented relative to others in the population. A biased sample causes problems because any statistic computed from that sample has the potential to be consistently erroneous. The bias can lead to an over- or underrepresentation of the corresponding parameter being studied in the population. Typically this causes measures of statistical significance to appear much stronger than they are, but it is also possible to cause completely illusory artifacts. In either case, conclusions drawn from a biased sample are likely to be invalid. The requirement to obtain consent or authorization may lead to a biased study sample because those who decline to participate may be more or less likely than average to have a particular health problem. This may be especially problematic if the research topic entails sensitive or potentially embarrassing information, such as HIV infection.

SOURCES: Casarett et al. (2005); Jacobsen et al. (1999).

who refuse have distinct demographic and health characteristics. In fact, even a refusal rate of less than 5 percent can create selection bias in the data (Jacobsen et al., 1999; see Chapter 5 for more detail). Conveying to the public the importance of health care improvements derived from medical records research and stressing the negative impact of incomplete datasets on research findings may increase the public's participation in research and their willingness to support information-based research that is conducted with IRB or Privacy Board oversight, under a waiver of patient consent or authorization.

Numerous examples of important research findings from medical records research would not have been possible if direct patient consent and authorization were always required (Box 3-1). For example, analysis of medical records showed that infants exposed to diethylstilbesterol (DES) during the first trimester of pregnancy had an increased risk of breast, vaginal, and cervical cancer as well as reproductive anomalies as adults. Similarly, studies of medical records led to the discovery that folic acid supplementation during pregnancy can prevent neural tube defects.

Thus, HHS and the health research community should work to educate the public about how research is done and the value it provides. All stakeholders, including professional organizations, nonprofit funders, and patient organizations, have different interests and responsibilities to make sure that their constituencies are well informed. For example, the American Society of Clinical Oncology and the American Heart Association already have some online resources to help patients gather information about research that may be relevant to their conditions. But coordination and identification of best practices by HHS would be helpful, and research is needed to identify which segments of the population would be receptive to and benefit from various types of information about how research is done and its value in order to create and implement an effective plan.

Greater use of community-based participatory research, in which community-based organizations or groups bring community members into the research process as partners to help design studies and disseminate the knowledge gained,[39] could help achieve this goal. These groups help researchers to recruit research participants by using the knowledge of the community to understand health problems and to design activities that the community is likely to value. They also inform community members about how the research is done and what comes out of it, with the goal of providing immediate community benefits from the results when possible.

---

[39] See http://www.ahrq.gov/research/cbprrole.htm.

CONCLUSIONS AND RECOMMENDATIONS

Based on its review of the information described in this chapter, the committee agreed on a second overarching principle to guide the formation of recommendations. The committee affirms the importance of maintaining and improving health research effectiveness. Research discoveries are central to achieving the goal of extending the quality of healthy lives. Research into causes of disease, methods for prevention, techniques for diagnosis, and new approaches to treatment has increased life expectancy, reduced infant mortality, limited the toll of infectious diseases, and improved outcomes for patients with heart disease, cancer, diabetes, and other chronic diseases. Patient-oriented clinical research that tests new ideas makes rapid medical progress possible. Today, the rate of discovery is accelerating, and we are at the precipice of a remarkable period of investigative promise made possible by new knowledge about the genetic underpinnings of disease. Genomic research is opening new possibilities for preventing illness and for developing safer, more effective medical care that may eventually be tailored for specific individuals. Further advances in relating genetic information to predispositions to disease and responses to treatments will require the use of large amounts of existing health-related information and stored tissue specimens. The increasing use of electronic medical records will further facilitate the generation of new knowledge through research and accelerate the pace of discovery. These efforts will require broad participation of patients in research and broad data sharing to ensure that the results are valid and applicable to different segments of the population. Collaborative partnerships among communities of patients, their physicians, and teams of researchers to gain new scientific knowledge will bring tangible benefits for people in this country and around the world.

Surveys indicate that the majority of Americans believe that health research is important, are interested in the findings of research studies, and are willing to participate in health research. But patients often lack information about how research is conducted and are rarely informed about research results that may have a direct impact on their health. Effective communication could build the public's trust of the research community, which is important because trust is necessary for the public's continued participation in research. Moreover, direct feedback could lead to improved health care for study participants if the results indicate that an altered course of care is warranted.

Thus, the committee recommends that when patients consent to the use of their medical records in a particular study, health researchers should make greater efforts when the study ends to inform study participants about the results, and the relevance and importance of those results. Broader adoption of electronic health records may be helpful in accomplishing this goal, but standards and guidelines for providing and explaining study results to research participants or various sectors of the public are needed.

HHS should also encourage registration of trials and other studies in public databases, particularly when research is conducted with an IRB/ Privacy Board approved waiver of consent or authorization, as a way to make information about research studies more broadly available to the public. Numerous clinical trial registries already exist, and registration has increased in recent years, but no centralized system currently exists for disseminating information about clinical trials of drugs or other interventions, making it difficult for consumers and their health care providers to identify ongoing studies. Moreover, noninterventional studies, such as observational studies that play an increasingly critical role in biomedical research, are not generally included in these databases. Because many noninterventional studies are conducted with an IRB/Privacy Board approved waiver of consent or authorization, including such studies in a registry could be an important method for increasing public knowledge of those studies.

Interventional clinical trials are the most visible of the various types of health research, but a great deal of information-based health research entails analysis of thousands of patient records to better understand human diseases, to determine treatment effectiveness, and to identify adverse side effects of therapies. This form of research is likely to increase in frequency as the availability of electronic health records continues to expand. As we move toward the goal of personalized medicine, research results will be even more likely to be directly relevant to patients, but more study participants will be necessary to derive meaningful results.

However, many patients are likely not aware that their medical records are being used in information-based research, and surveys show that many patients desire not only notice, but also the opportunity to decide about whether to consent to such research with medical records. As noted in Chapter 2, strengthening security protections of health data should reduce the risk of security breaches and their potential negative consequences, and thus should help to alleviate patient concerns in this regard. But educating patients about how health research is conducted, monitored, and reported could also increase patients' trust in the research community. **Thus, HHS and the health research community should work to educate the public about how research is done.**

It will also be important for HHS and researchers to convey the value of health care improvements derived from medical records research, and to stress the negative impact of incomplete datasets on research findings. Representative samples are essential to ensure the validity and generalizability of health research, but datasets will not be representative of the entire population if some people withhold access to their health information. A universal requirement for consent or authorization in information-based research may lead to incomplete datasets, and thus to biased results and inaccurate conclusions. Numerous examples of important research findings from medical records research would not have been possible if direct patient consent and authorization were always required.

To ensure that beneficial health research and related activities continue to be undertaken with appropriate oversight under federal regulations, it will be important for HHS to also provide more guidance on how to distinguish the various activities. The Privacy Rule makes a distinction between health research and some closely related endeavors, such as public health and quality improvement activities, which also may involve collection and analysis of personally identifiable health information. Under the Privacy Rule (as well as the Common Rule), these activities, which aim to protect the public's health and improve the quality of patient care, are considered health care "practice" rather than health research. Therefore, they can be undertaken without consent or authorization, or an IRB/Privacy Board waiver of consent or authorization. However, it can be a challenge for IRBs and Privacy Boards to distinguish among activities that are or are not subject to the various provisions of the Privacy Rule and the Common Rule, and inappropriate decisions may prevent important activities from being undertaken or could potentially allow improper disclosure of personally identifiable health information.

To address these difficulties, a number of models have been proposed that outline the criteria IRBs and Privacy Boards should use to distinguish practice and research. For example, one recent model provides a detailed checklist for IRBs and Privacy Boards to use in determining whether an activity is public health research and required to comply with the research provisions of the Privacy Rule, or public health practice that does not need IRB/Privacy Board review. The committee believes that standardizing the criteria is essential to support the conduct of these important health care activities.

Thus, HHS should convene the relevant stakeholders to develop standard criteria for IRBs and Privacy Boards to use when making decisions about whether protocols entail research or practice. There should be flexibility in the regulation to allow important activities to go forward with appropriate levels of oversight. Also, it will be important to evaluate whether these criteria are effective in aiding IRB/Privacy Board reviews of proposed protocols, and whether they lead to appropriate IRB/Privacy Board decisions.

These changes suggested above could be accomplished without any changes to HIPAA by making them a condition of funding from HHS and other research sponsors and by providing some additional funds to cover the cost.

REFERENCES

AMS (Academy of Medical Sciences). 2006. *Personal data for public good: Using health information in medical research.* http://www.acmedsci.ac.uk/images/project/Personal.pdf (accessed August 28, 2008).

Baily, M. A. 2008. Harming through protection? *New England Journal of Medicine* 258(8):768–769.

Baily, M. A., M. Bottrell, J. Lynn, and B. Jennings. 2006. The ethics of using QI methods to improve health care quality and safety. *A Hastings Center Special Report* 36(4): S1–S40.

Bates, D. W., L. L. Leape, D. J. Cullen, N. Laird, L. A. Petersen, J. M. Teich, E. Burdick, M. Hickey, S. Kleefield, B. Shea, V. M. Vander, and D. L. Seger. 1998. Effect of computerized physician order entry and a team intervention on prevention of serious medication errors. *JAMA* 280(15):1311–1316.

Bellin, E., and N. N. Dubler. 2001. The quality improvement-research divide and the need for external oversight. *American Journal of Public Health* 91(9):1512–1517.

Big Health. 2008. *Big health consortium.* http://www.bighealthconsortium.org/about/ (accessed October 29, 2008).

Braunstein, J. B., N. S. Sherber, S. P. Schulman, E. L. Ding, and N. R. Powe. 2008. Race, medical researcher distrust, perceived harm, and willingness to participate in cardiovascular prevention trials. *Medicine* 87(1):1–9.

Brown, D. R., M. N. Fouad, K. Basen-Engquist, and G. Tortolero-Luna. 2000. Recruitment and retention of minority women in cancer screening, prevention and treatment trials. *Annals of Epidemiology* 10:S13–S21.

Burris, S., L. Gable, L. Stone, and Z. Lazzarini. 2003. The role of state law in protecting human subjects of public health research and practice. *Journal of Law, Medicine & Ethics* 31:654.

Casarett, D., J. Karlawish, and J. Sugarman. 2000. Determining when quality improvement initiatives should be considered research: Proposed criteria and potential implications. *JAMA* 284(7):2275–2280.

Casarett, D., J. Karlawish, E. Andrews, and A. Caplan. 2005. Bioethical issues in pharmacoepidemiological research. In *Pharmacoepidemiology,* 4th ed., edited by B. L. Strom. West Sussex, England: John Wiley & Sons, Ltd. Pp. 417–432.

CDC (Centers for Disease Control and Prevention). 1999. *Guidelines for defining public health research and public health non-research.* http://www.cdc.gov/od/science/regs/hrpp/researchdefinition.htm (accessed March 4, 2008).

CHSR (Coalition for Health Services Research). 2008. *Framework for health services research policy for 2008.* http://www.chsr.org/Policy_Priorities.pdf (accessed August 21, 2008).

Comis, R. L., C. R. Aldige, E. L. Stovall, L. U. Krebs, P. J. Risher, and H. J. Taylor. 2000. *A quantitative survey of public attitudes towards cancer clinical trials.* Philadelphia, PA: Coalition of National Cancer Cooperative Groups, Cancer Research Foundation of America, Cancer Leadership Council, and Oncology Nursing Society.

Corbie-Smith, G., S. B. Thomas, M. V. Williams, and S. Moody-Ayers. 1999. Attitudes and beliefs of African Americans towards participation in medical research. *Journal of General Internal Medicine* 14:537–546.

Damschroder, L. J., J. L. Pritts, M. A. Neblo, R. J. Kalarickal, J. W. Creswell, and R. A. Hayward. 2007. Patients, privacy and trust: Patients' willingness to allow researchers to access their medical records. *Social Science & Medicine* 64(1):223–235.

DeAngelis, C. D., J. M. Drazen, F. A. Frizelle, C. Haug, J. Hoey, R. Horton, S. Kotzin, C. Laine, A. Marusic, A. J. P. M. Overbeke, T. V. Schroeder, H. C. Sox, and M. B. Van Der Weyden. 2004. Clinical trial registration: A statement from the International Committee of Medical Journal Editors. *JAMA* 292(11):1363–1364.

Farmer, D., S. A. Jackson, F. Camacho, and M. A. Hall. 2007. Attitudes of African American and low socioeconomic status white women toward medical research. *Journal of Health Care for the Poor and Underserved* 18:85–99.

FDA (Food and Drug Administration). 1971. Certain estrogens for oral or parenteral use. Drugs for human use; drug efficacy study implementation. *Federal Register* 36(217):21537–21538.

FDA. 2005. *FDA public health advisory, deaths with antipsychotics in elderly patients with behavioral disturbances.* http://www.fda.gov/cder/drug/advisory/antipsychotics. htm (accessed August 18, 2008).

FDA. 2008. FDA alert [6/16/2008]: *Information for healthcare professionals. Antipsychotics.* http://www.fda.gov/cder/drug/infosheets/hcp/antipsychotics_conventional.htm (accessed August 18, 2008).

Finkelstein, E. A., I. C. Fiebelkorn, and G. Wang. 2003. National medical spending attributable to overweight and obesity: How much, and who's paying? *Health Affairs Web Exclusive.* http://content.healthaffairs.org/cgi/content/abstract/hlthaff.w3.219v1 (accessed August 21, 2008).

Furrow, B. R., T. L. Greaney, S. H. Johnson, T. S. Jost, and R. L. Schwartz. 2004. *Bioethics: Health care law and ethics.* 5th ed. St. Paul, MN: Thomson/West.

GAO (Government Accountability Office). 1996. *Scientific research: Continued vigilance critical to protecting human subjects.* Washington, DC: GAO.

Genetics & Public Policy Center. 2007. *U.S. public opinion on uses of genetic information and genetic discrimination.* http://www.dnapolicy.org/resources/GINAPublic_Opinion_ Genetic_Information_Discrimination.pdf (accessed August 21, 2008).

Gill, S., S. Bronskill, S. Normand, G. Anderson, K. Sykora, K. Lam, C. Bell, P. Lee, H. Fischer, N. Herrmann, J. Gurwitz, and P. Rochon. 2007. Antipsychotic drug use and mortality in older adults with dementia. *Annals of Internal Medicine* 146:775–786.

Giuliano, A. R., N. Mokuau, C. Hughes, G. Tortelero-Luna, B. Risendal, R. C. S. Ho, T. E. Prewitt, and W. J. McCaskill-Stevens. 2000. Participation of minorities in cancer research: The influence of structural, cultural, and linguistic factors. *Annals of Epidemiology* 10:S22–S34.

Goldman, J., and A. Choy. 2001. Privacy and confidentiality in health research. In *Ethical and policy issues in research involving human participants.* Bethesda, MD: National Bioethics Advisory Commission. Pp. C1–C34.

Gostin, L. O. 2008. Surveillance and public health research: Personal privacy and the "right to know." In *Public health law: Power, duty, restraint.* Berkeley, CA: University of California Press.

Grady, C., L. A. Hampson, G. R. Wallen, M. V. Rivera-Goba, K. L. Carrington, and B. B. Mittleman. 2006. Exploring the ethics of clinical research in an urban community. *American Journal of Public Health* 96(11):1996–2001.

Hatfield, M., H. F. Sonnenschein, and L. E. Rosenberg. 2001. *Exceptional returns: The economic value of America's investment in medical research.* http://www.laskerfoundation. org/advocacy/pdf/exceptional.pdf (accessed August 21, 2008).

Herbst, A. L., H. Ulfelder, and D. C. Poskanzer. 1971. Adenocarcinoma of the vagina. Association of maternal stilbestrol therapy with tumor appearance in young women. *New England Journal of Medicine* 284(15):878–881.

HEW (Department of Health, Education and Welfare). 1979. *The Belmont Report: Ethical principles and guidelines for the protection of human subjects of research.* http://ohsr. od.nih.gov/guidelines/belmont.html (accessed August 21, 2008).

HHS (Department of Health and Human Services). 2003. *Institutional review boards and the HIPAA Privacy Rule.* http://privacyruleandresearch.nih.gov/pdf/IRB_Factsheet.pdf (accessed August 21, 2008).

HHS. 2004. *Guidance on research involving coded private information or biological specimens.* http://www.hhs.gov/ohrp/humansubjects/guidance/cdebiol.pdf (accessed August 21, 2008).

Hodge, J. G., Jr. 2005. An enhanced approach to distinguishing public health practice and human subjects research. *Journal of Law, Medicine & Ethics* 33(1):125–141.

Hodge, J. G., and L. O. Gostin. 2004. *Public health practice vs. research: A report for public health practitioners including cases and guidance for making distinctions.* Atlanta, GA: Council of State and Territorial Epidemiologists.

IOM (Institute of Medicine). 1995. *Health services research: Work force and educational issues.* Washington, DC: National Academy Press.

IOM. 2000a. *Protecting data privacy in health services research.* Washington, DC: National Academy Press.

IOM. 2000b. *To err is human: Building a safer health system.* Washington, DC: National Academy Press.

IOM. 2002. *Responsible research: A systems approach to protecting research participants.* Washington, DC: The National Academies Press.

Jacobsen, S., Z. Xia, M. Campion, C. Darby, M. Plevak, K. Seltman, and L. Melton, 3rd. 1999. Potential effect of authorization bias on medical record research. *Mayo Clinic Proceedings* 74:330–338.

Laine, C., R. Horton, C. D. DeAngelis, J. M. Drazen, F. A. Frizelle, F. Godlee, C. Haug, P. C. Hébert, S. Kotzin, A. Marusic, P. Sahni, T. V. Schroeder, H. C. Sox, M. B. Van Der Weyden, and F. W. A. Verheugt. 2007. Clinical trial registration—looking back and moving ahead. *New England Journal of Medicine* 356(26):2734–2736.

Lee, B. 2000. *Comparison of FDA and HHS human subject protection regulations.* http://www.fda.gov/oc/gcp/comparison.html (accessed August 21, 2008).

Lindenauer, P. K., E. M. Benjamin, D. Naglieri-Prescod, J. Fitzgerald, and P. Pekow. 2002. The role of the institutional review board in quality improvement: A survey of quality officers, institutional review board chairs, and journal editors. *The American Journal of Medicine* 113:575–579.

Lowrance, W. W. 2002. *Learning from experience, privacy and the secondary use of data in health research.* London: The Nuffield Trust.

Lowrance, W. W., and F. S. Collins. 2007. Identifiability in genomic research. *Science* 317:600–602.

Lynn, J., M. A. Baily, M. Bottrell, B. Jennings, R. J. Levine, F. Davidoff, D. Casarett, J. Corrigan, E. Fox, M. K. Wynia, G. J. Agich, M. O'Kane, T. Speroff, P. Schyve, P. Batalden, S. Tunis, N. Berlinger, L. Cronenwett, M. Fitzmaurice, N. N. Dubler, and B. James. 2007. The ethics of using quality improvement methods in health care. *Annals of Internal Medicine* 146(6):666–674.

Mandelblatt, J., S. Saha, S. Teutsch, T. Hoerger, A. L. Siu, D. Atkins, J. Klein, and M. Helfand. 2003. The cost-effectiveness of screening mammography beyond age 65: A systematic review for the U.S. Preventive Services Task Force. *Annals of Internal Medicine* 139:835–842.

Mick, S., L. L. Morlock, D. Salkever, G. de Lissovoy, F. Malitz, C. G. Wise, and A. Jones. 1994. Strategic activity and financial performance of U.S. rural hospitals: A national study, 1983 to 1988. *Journal of Rural Health* 10(3):150–167.

Mosconi, P., P. Poli, A. Giolo, and G. Apolone. 2005. How Italian health consumers feel about clinical research: A questionnaire survey. *European Journal of Public Health* 15(4):372–379.

Murphy, K., and R. Topel. 1999. *The economic value of medical research.* Chicago, IL: University of Chicago Press.

NCI (National Cancer Institute). 2008. *Getting connected with caBIG: Data sharing and security framework.* https://cabig.nci.nih.gov/working_groups/DSIC_SLWG/data_sharing_policy/ (accessed October 27, 2008).

NCURA (National Council of University Research Administrators). 2007. *Report on research compliance.* http://www.reportonresearchcompliance.com (accessed March 4, 2008).

NCVHS (National Committee on Vital and Health Statistics). 2007a. Enhanced protections for uses of health data: A stewardship framework for "secondary uses" of electronically collected and transmitted health data. http://ncvhs.hhs.gov/071221lt.pdf (accessed December 19, 2007).

NCVHS, Ad Hoc Work Group on Secondary Uses of Health Data. 2007b. Testimony of the cancer Biomedical Informatics Grid (caBIG) Data Sharing and Intellectual Capital (DSIC) workspace. August 1, 2007.

Needleman, J., P. Buerhaus, S. Mattke, M. Stewart, and K. Zelevinsky. 2002. Nurse-staffing levels and the quality of care in hospitals. *New England Journal of Medicine* 346(22):1715–1722.

NSF (National Science Foundation). 2006. Science and technology: Public attitudes and understanding. In *Science and Engineering Indicators 2006.* Arlington, VA: National Science Foundation. Chapter 7.

OHRP (Office for Human Research Protections). 2008a. *IRB guidebook, part I.A.* http://www.hhs.gov/ohrp/irb/irb_guidebook.htm (accessed August 21, 2008).

OHRP. 2008b. *OHRP concludes case regarding Johns Hopkins University research on hospital infections.* http://www.hhs.gov/ohrp/news/recentnews.html#20080215 (accessed August 21, 2008).

Partridge, A., and E. Winer. 2002. Informing clinical trial participants about study results. *JAMA* 288:363–365.

Partridge, A. H., A. C. Wolff, P. K. Marcom, P. A. Kaufman, L. Zhang, R. Gelman, C. Moore, D. Lake, G. F. Fleming, H. S. Rugo, J. Atkins, E. Sampson, D. Collyar, and E. P. Winer. (2008). The impact of sharing results of a randomized breast cancer clinical trial with study participants. *Breast Cancer Research and Treatment* June 10.

Pitkin, R. 2007. Folate and neural tube defects. *American Journal of Clinical Nutrition* 85(1):285S–288S.

Pritts, J. 2008. *The importance and value of protecting the privacy of health information: Roles of HIPAA Privacy Rule and the Common Rule in health research.* http://www.iom.edu/CMS/3740/43729/53160.aspx (accessed March 15, 2008).

Research!America. 2007. *America speaks: Poll summary.* Vol. 7. Alexandria, VA: United Health Foundation.

Schneeweiss, S., S. Setoguchi, A. Brookhart, C. Dormuth, and P. Wang. 2007. Risk of death associated with the use of conventional versus atypical antipsychotic drugs among elderly patients. *Canadian Medical Association Journal* 176:672–632.

Shalowitz, D. I., and F. G. Miller. 2008a (May 13). Communicating the results of clinical research to participants: Attitudes, practices, and future directions. *PLoS Medicine* 5(5):e91.

Shalowitz, D. I., and F. G. Miller. 2008b (September). The search for clarity in communicating research results to study participants. *Journal of Medical Ethics* 34(9):e17.

Shaul, R. Z., S. Birenbaum, and M. Evans. 2005. Legal liability in research: Early lessons from North America. *BMC Medical Ethics* 6(4):1–4.

Shavers, V. L., C. F. Lynch, and L. F. Burmeister. 2002. Racial differences in factors that influence the willingness to participate in medical research studies. *Annals of Epidemiology* 12:248–256.

Sim, I., A.-W. Chan, A. M. Gülmezoglu, T. Evans, and T. Pang. 2006. Clinical trial registration: Transparency is the watchword. *The Lancet* 367(9523):1631–1633.

Slamon, D., G. Clark, S. Wong, W. Levin, A. Ullrich, and W. McGuire. 1987. Human breast cancer: Correlation of relapse and survival with amplification of the her-2/neu oncogene. *Science* 235(4785):177–182.

Snider, D. E., and D. F. Stroup. 1997. Defining research when it comes to public health. *Public Health Reports* 112:29–32.

Thorpe, K. E., C. S. Florence, D. H. Howard, and P. Joski. 2004. The impact of obesity in rising medical spending. *Health Affairs Web Exclusive.* http://content.healthaffairs.org/cgi/content/abstract/hlthaff.w4.480v1 (accessed August 21, 2008).

Trauth, J. M., D. Musa, L. Siminoff, I. K. Jewell, and E. Ricci. 2000. Public attitudes regarding willingness to participate in medical research studies. *Journal of Health & Social Policy* 12(2):23–43.

Veurink, M., M. Koster, and L. Berg. 2005. The history of DES, lessons to be learned. *Pharmacy World & Science* 27(3):139–143.

Wendler, D., R. Kington, J. Madans, G. Van Wye, H. Christ-Schmidt, L. A. Pratt, O. W. Brawley, C. P. Gross, and E. Emanuel. 2006. Are racial and ethnic minorities less willing to participate in health research? *PLoS Medicine* 3(2):201–210.

Westin, A. 2007. *How the public views privacy and health research.* http://www.iom.edu/Object.File/Master/48/528/%20Westin%20IOM%20Srvy%20Rept%2011-1107.pdf (accessed November 11, 2008).

Williams, E. D. 2005. *Federal protection for human research subjects: An analysis of the Common Rule and its interactions with FDA regulations and the HIPAA Privacy Rule, CRS report for Congress.* Washington, DC: Congressional Research Service.

Williams, I. C., and G. Corbie-Smith. 2006. Investigator beliefs and reported success in recruiting minority participants. *Contemporary Clinical Trials* 27:580–586.

Winston, F. K., D. R. Durbin, M. J. Kallan, and E. K. Moll. 2000. The danger of premature graduation to seat belts for young children. *Pediatrics* 105(6):1179–1183.

WMA (World Medical Association). 1964. *Declaration of Helsinki: Ethical principles for medical research involving human subjects.* http://ohsr.od.nih.gov/guidelines/helsinki.html (accessed August 21, 2008).

Woolley, M., and S. M. Propst. 2005. Public attitudes and perceptions about health-related research. *JAMA* 294(11):1380–1384.

Zarin, D. A., and T. Tse. 2008. Moving toward transparency of clinical trials. *Science* 319:1340–1342.

Zarin, D. A., T. Tse, and N. C. Ide. 2005. Trial registration at ClinicalTrials.gov between May and October 2005. *New England Journal of Medicine* 353(26):2779–2787.

4

HIPAA, the Privacy Rule, and Its Application to Health Research

This chapter provides an overview of the development of the Health Insurance Portability and Accountability Act (HIPAA) Privacy Rule and describes how it applies to health research. A section at the end of the chapter also describes the relationships between HIPAA and other federal and state laws. Because a great deal of health research in the United States is also subject to the Common Rule (described in Chapter 3), disparities between these two federal rules are also noted where relevant throughout the chapter.

OVERVIEW OF HIPAA

HIPAA was passed on August 21, 1996. It was intended to make health care delivery more efficient and to increase the number of Americans with health insurance coverage. These objectives were pursued through three main provisions of the Act: (1) the portability provisions, (2) the tax provisions, and (3) the administrative simplification provisions.

Portability and Tax Provisions

The portability provisions of HIPAA aimed to prevent individuals from losing health care coverage due to a preexisting condition when changing to a new employer's health plan. The portability provisions also aimed to reduce the number of unemployed or self-employed individuals without health insurance by making it easier for individuals to purchase health insurance without their employer.

Similarly, the tax provisions of HIPAA were also intended to make it easier for individuals to maintain health insurance. The tax provisions pursued this goal by modifying existing tax laws to make health insurance more affordable. HIPAA does not regulate the price of health insurance, but rather, it relies on tax breaks and other tax incentives to reduce health care costs (Chaikind et al., 2005).

Administrative Simplification Provisions

The administrative simplification provisions of HIPAA instructed the Secretary of the U.S. Department of Health and Human Services (HHS) to issue several regulations concerning the electronic transmission of health information. These provisions were included in the final version of HIPAA because health plans had requested federal legislation in this area from Congress. The use of electronic health information was expanding in the early 1990s, and the health care industry was unable to standardize the process and use of electronic health information without federal action.[1]

The security standards are one set of regulations mandated by the administrative simplification provisions of HIPAA. The Act instructed the Secretary of HHS to develop nationwide security standards and safeguards for the use of electronic health care information. The resulting HHS regulations spell out specific administrative, technical, and physical security procedures that healthcare plans, providers and clearinghouses must incorporate into their operations to prevent unauthorized access, use, and disclosure of protected health information (CMS, 2005). HHS published the final HIPAA Security Rule in the *Federal Register* on February 20, 2003. Health plans and providers were required to be in compliance with these measures by April 2004 (see Box 2-2).

The administrative simplification provisions of HIPAA also directed the Secretary to develop standards for unique health identifiers for patients, employers, health plans, and providers. Unique health identifiers are national numbers that could be used to identify the individual or organization in standard health transactions. The Centers for Medicare & Medicaid Services (CMS) has issued standards for the unique health identifiers for employers and providers, and unique health identifiers for health plans are under development. However, Congress has prevented CMS from implementing a standard for the unique health identifier for patients by inserting language into the annual appropriations bill every year since HIPAA was enacted (Chaikind et al., 2005).

Finally, the administrative simplification provisions of HIPAA mandated the creation of privacy standards for the protection of personally

---

[1] Personal communication, M. Wilder, Hogan and Hartson, March 17, 2007.

identifiable medical information. Although privacy protections were not a primary objective of the Act, Congress recognized that advances in electronic technology could erode the privacy of health information, and included the privacy provision in HIPAA (IOM, 2006). In accordance with the administrative simplification provisions, HHS developed the Privacy Rule, which constitutes a broad-ranging federal health privacy regulation (see Table 4-1). Incorporating many of the basic fair information practices,[2] the Privacy Rule generally restricts the use or disclosure of protected health information, except as permitted by the individual or as authorized or required by the Privacy Rule. Its provisions also impose on covered entities affirmative requirements to safeguard the information in their possession. The Privacy Rule gives individuals certain rights with respect to their health information (reviewed by Pritts, 2008).

DEVELOPMENT OF THE PRIVACY RULE REGULATIONS

Congress did not include detailed privacy requirements in HIPAA. The terms of HIPAA required the Secretary of HHS to submit detailed recommendations to Congress by August 1997 on ways to protect the privacy of personally identifiable health information. These recommendations were to include suggestions on ways to protect individuals' rights concerning their personally identifiable health information, procedures for exercising such rights, and the uses and disclosures of information that should be authorized or required under HIPAA.[3] If Congress did not enact privacy legislation within 3 years of the passage of HIPAA, the Act required the Secretary of HHS to issue privacy regulations for the protection of personally identifiable health information within 42 months of HIPAA's enactment.[4]

In response to this mandate, HHS submitted recommendations for protecting the privacy of personally identifiable health information to Congress in September 1997. In these recommendations, Secretary Shalala advocated for the passage of federal privacy legislation, rather than relying on HHS to pass a set of privacy regulations. Shalala's report stated, "This report recommends that Congress enact national standards that provide fundamental privacy rights for patients and define responsibilities for those who service them" (Shalala, 1997).

Although numerous bills that attempted to address health information

---

[2] U.S. Secretary of Health and Human Services, *Recommendations on the Confidentiality of Individually-Identifiable Health Information to the Committees on Labor and Human Resources* (September 11, 1997), and Standards for Privacy of Individually Identifiable Health Information: Proposed Rule, 64 Fed. Reg. 59918, 59923 (1999).

[3] Health Insurance Portability and Accountability Act, 45 C.F.R. § 264(a)–(b) (2006).

[4] See 45 C.F.R. § 264(c)(1) (2006).

TABLE 4-1 Timeline of the HIPAA Privacy Rule

Date	Action
August 1996	Health Insurance Portability and Accountability Act (HIPAA) was signed into law by President Clinton
September 1997	Donna Shalala, Secretary of the Department of Health and Human Services (HHS), made recommendations to Congress on the privacy standards mandated in HIPAA
September 1999	Congress failed to enact federal privacy legislation within the 3-year time limit set by HIPAA
November 1999	HHS issued a proposed version of the privacy regulation for public comment
December 2000	HHS published the original Privacy Rule, titled *Standards for Privacy of Individually Identifiable Health Information*
March 2002	HHS published a proposed modification to the Privacy Rule and accepted additional public comments
August 2002	HHS published the Final Privacy Rule
April 2003	Covered entities were required to be in compliance with the Privacy Rule (except small health plans)
	The Association of American Medical Colleges launched a survey examining how research has been affected by the Privacy Rule and proposed recommendations for changes to the Privacy Rule
	In *South Carolina Medical Association v. Tommy Thompson*, plaintiffs lost constitutional challenge to HIPAA
March 2004	The National Committee on Vital and Health Statistics sent a letter to HHS giving detailed recommendations on ways to improve the Privacy Rule's application to research
April 2004	Small health plans were required to be in compliance with the Privacy Rule
September 2004	The Secretary's Advisory Committee on Human Research Protections sent a letter to the Secretary of HHS with recommendations for changes to the Privacy Rule as applied to research
March 2005	In *Citizens for Health v. Michael O. Leavitt*, plaintiffs unsuccessfully challenged the Privacy Rule as being invalid

privacy were introduced, Congress was unable to finalize privacy legislation on the time schedule mandated in HIPAA. During the 1999 congressional session alone, eight such bills were introduced. However, none of these bills was passed. As a result, Congress passed the responsibility of creating health privacy protections to HHS.

Over the course of developing the current Privacy Rule, HHS went through four iterations of the Rule. HHS followed Secretary Shalala's 1997 recommendations to Congress in shaping the regulations (Redhead,

2001). First, HHS issued a proposed version of the Privacy Rule for public comment on November 3, 1999, that drew more than 50,000 comments (Stevens, 2000). Based on these comments, HHS issued the second version of the Privacy Rule, titled *Standards for Privacy of Individually Identifiable Health Information*, in December 2000.[5] Before this version of the Privacy Rule could take effect, the Secretary of HHS was inundated with unsolicited public comments and criticism regarding the Privacy Rule. Health care insurers and providers were concerned that the Privacy Rule would make health care industry operations less efficient. They were particularly concerned about the requirement that they obtain authorization prior to making any routine disclosure of personally identifiable health information for health care operations, treatment, or payment. The comments received also suggested that this version of the Privacy Rule would prevent pharmacists from filling prescriptions and searching for potential drug interactions before patients arrived at pharmacies; interfere with providing emergency medicine in situations where it would be impossible to obtain patient authorization before treatment; and delay the scheduling and preparation of hospital procedures until the doctor could obtain patient authorization.[6]

In March 2002, HHS, under the Bush Administration, published a proposed modification to the Privacy Rule, which reopened the rule-making process and created a new period for submitting public comments. This version of the Privacy Rule drew more than 24,000 comments. Incorporating the suggestions collected through the second notice of proposed rule-making period, HHS issued the final version of the Privacy Rule in August 14, 2002.[7] This is the current, effective, and codified version of the Privacy Rule (45 C.F.R. parts 160 and 164). Most health care providers and health plans were required to be in compliance with this version of the Privacy Rule by April 14, 2003. Small health plans were given until April 14, 2004, to be in compliance.

OVERVIEW OF THE HIPAA PRIVACY RULE[8]

Entities Subject to the Privacy Rule

The Privacy Rule applies to "covered entities,"[9] which are individuals or organizations that electronically transmit health information in the

---

[5] Standards for Privacy of Individually Identifiable Health Information: Final Rule, 65 Fed. Reg. 82461 (2000).

[6] Standards for Privacy of Individually Identifiable Health Information: Final Rule, 67 Fed. Reg. 53181, 53209 (2002).

[7] See 67 Fed. Reg. 53181 (2002).

[8] Some material in this section is adapted from a background paper by Pritts (2008).

[9] See 45 C.F.R. § 160.103 (2006).

course of normal health care practices. Covered entities include health care providers, health plans, and health care clearinghouses. Health plans are entities that provide or pay the cost of medical care, such as private health insurers or managed care organizations, and governmental payors and health programs such as Medicaid, Medicare, or Veterans Affairs. Health care clearinghouses generally refer to billing services, and health care providers include hospitals, doctors, and other health care professionals and facilities that provide treatment (Table 4-2).

If an entity that meets one of the categories of a covered entity also performs functions unrelated to health care, it can become a hybrid entity by designating in writing its "health care components."[10] Only these health care components are then bound by the Privacy Rule. For example, if a university includes an academic medical center with a hospital, the entire university will be classified as a covered entity unless the university elects to be a hybrid entity by designating only the hospital as the health care component. By doing this, only the hospital has to comply with the Privacy Rule. The classification of researchers within a hybrid entity depends on the nature of the work performed (e.g., whether the researchers are within the health care component, providing health care, or conducting electronic transactions) (HHS, 2004c).

Type of Information Protected

The Privacy Rule protects all personally identifiable health information, known as protected health information (PHI), created or received by a covered entity. Personally identifiable health information is defined as information, including demographic information, that "relates to past, present, or future physical or mental health or condition of an individual, the provision of health care to an individual, or the past, present, or future payment for the provision of health care for the individual" that either identifies the individual or with respect to which there is a reasonable basis to believe the information can be used to identify the individual."[11]

The Privacy Rule does not protect personally identifiable health information that is held or maintained by an organization other than a covered entity (HHS, 2004c). It also does not apply to information that has been deidentified in accordance with the Privacy Rule[12] (see later section on Deidentified Information).

---

[10] See 45 C.F.R. § 164.105(a)(2)(iii)(c) (2006).
[11] See 45 C.F.R. § 160.103 (2006).
[12] See 45 C.F.R. § 164.502(d) (2006).

TABLE 4-2 The Uneven Application of the HIPAA Privacy Rule: Examples of HIPAA Covered Entities and Non-Covered Entities

Covered Entities	Non-Covered Entities
• Health maintenance organizations (HMOs) • Group health plans • Medicare and Medicaid programs • Veterans health care program • Civilian Health and Medical Program of the Uniformed Services • Indian Health Service program under the Indian Health Care Improvement Act • Pharmacies • Researchers who are employed by a covered entity • Some universities (or parts of universities, such as health centers) • A public health clinic that is part of a public health agency	• Independent consent management companies • Contract research organizations • Research foundations • Data warehousing/data management companies • Student health services (if they do not bill for services) • Pharmaceutical companies • Researchers who are not employed by a covered entity • Some universities (or parts of universities) • A public health agency that does not perform activities subject to the provisions of the Privacy Rule

Restrictions on Use and Disclosure

Covered entities may not use or disclose PHI except as permitted or required by the Privacy Rule.[13] A covered entity may disclose PHI without the individual's permission for treatment, payment, and health care operations purposes. For other uses and disclosures, the Privacy Rule generally requires the individual's written permission, which is an "authorization" that must meet specific content requirements. The Privacy Rule then establishes a number of exceptions to this general rule, allowing covered entities to use and disclose PHI without the individual's authorization in certain situations. For example, the Privacy Rule permits the disclosure of PHI without the individual's authorization in the following circumstances:

- To business associates[14]
- For public health purposes as required by state and federal law[15]
- To public agencies for health oversight activities, such as audits;

---

[13] See 45 C.F.R. § 164.502(a) (2006). A covered entity is required to make a reasonable effort to use and disclose only the minimum amount of PHI needed for the intended purpose. See 45 C.F.R. § 164.502(b) (2006).

[14] See 45 C.F.R. § 164.506(e) (2006).

[15] See 45 C.F.R. § 164.510(b) (2006).

inspections; civil, criminal, or administrative proceedings; and other activities necessary for the oversight of the health care system[16]

- To law enforcement officials[17]
- For judicial and administrative proceedings, if the request for information is made through a court order[18]
- For research[19]

Most of these permitted uses and disclosures are subject to detailed conditions. For example, the Privacy Rule allows covered entities to disclose PHI without individual authorization to its "business associates," which are defined as persons or entities that perform, on behalf of the covered entity, certain functions or services[20] that require the use or disclosure of PHI, provided adequate safeguards are in place.[21] As a general rule, these safeguards take the form of a business associate agreement whereby the business associate agrees not to use or disclose the PHI it receives except as permitted by the agreement or by law (Box 4-1).

In the case of public health practice, the Privacy Rule notes that there is a legitimate need for public health authorities and others working to ensure the health and safety of the public to have access to PHI. As a result, the Privacy Rule permits, but does not require,[22] covered entities to disclose PHI without authorization for specified public health purposes (Box 4-2). Disclosures for research are discussed in detail in subsequent sections of this chapter.

Individual Rights

The Privacy Rule also confers rights on individuals with respect to their PHI (reviewed by Pritts, 2008). Under the Privacy Rule, individuals have the right to[23]:

- Receive a notice of privacy practices from a health care provider or a health plan that must, among other things, inform patients of

---

[16] See 45 C.F.R. § 164.510(c) (2006).

[17] See 45 C.F.R. § 164.510(f) (2006).

[18] See 45 C.F.R. § 164.510(d) (2006).

[19] See 45 C.F.R. § 164.512 (2006).

[20] Some common functions that business associates perform for covered entities include recruiting subjects, data analysis, processing, or administration; utilization review; quality assurance; and practice management.

[21] See 45 C.F.R. § 164.502(e) (2006).

[22] Only states have the authority to require mandatory public health reporting.

[23] See 45 C.F.R. § 164.520 (2006).

BOX 4-1
Business Associate Agreements

A covered entity must obtain assurances in writing that the business associate will: (1) use the information only for the purposes for which it was engaged by the covered entity; (2) safeguard the information from misuses; and (3) help the covered entity comply with some of the covered entity's duties under the Privacy Rule. Business associate agreements must include:

- A description of the permitted and required uses of the PHI by the business associate.
- A statement that the business associate will not use or disclose the PHI other than as permitted or required by the contract, or as required by law.
- A statement that the business associate will use appropriate safeguards to prevent the use or disclosure of PHI other than as provided for by the contract.

SOURCE: 45 C.F.R. § 160.103 (2006).

BOX 4-2
The HIPAA Privacy Rule and Public Health Practice

The Privacy Rule defines public authorities as any "federal, tribal, or local agency or person or entity acting under a grant of authority or contract with the agency, including state and local health departments, the Food and Drug Administration (FDA), the Centers for Disease Control and Prevention, and the Occupational Safety and Health Administration."

A covered entity can release PHI to a public health authority, without authorization or waiver of authorization, in the following circumstances:

- Monitoring health threats and diseases
- Child abuse or neglect
- Products regulated by the FDA
- Persons at risk of contracting or spreading a disease
- Workplace surveillance

State laws may also permit or require the release of PHI for activities other than those listed above.

SOURCES: 45 C.F.R. § 164.501 (2006); 45 C.F.R. 164.512(b)(i)–(v) (2006); 45 C.F.R. 160.203(c) (2006).

the anticipated uses and disclosures of their health information that may be made without the patients' consent or authorization.[24]

- See and obtain a copy of their own health information.[25]
- Request an amendment of information that is incomplete or inaccurate.[26]
- Obtain an accounting of certain disclosures that the covered entity made of their PHI over the past 6 years.[27]

HIPAA AND RESEARCH

Although health research was not a focus of HIPAA, Congress recognized the important role that health records play in conducting health research and wanted to ensure that privacy protections would not impede researchers' continued access to such data. This is reflected in two House Reports on HIPAA with identical language, stating:

"The conferees recognize that certain uses of individually identifiable information are appropriate, and do not compromise the privacy of an individual. Examples of such use of information include . . . the transfer of information from a health plan to an organization for the sole purpose of conducting health care-related research. As health plans and providers continue to focus on outcomes research and innovation, it is important that the exchange and aggregated use of health care data be allowed" (U.S. Congress, 1996a,b).

In creating the current research provisions of the Privacy Rule, HHS considered several options. One option considered was exempting PHI used in research from the regulations, but HHS rejected this option, noting some reported shortcomings of the protection of the privacy and confidentiality of health information in research (reviewed by Pritts, 2008).[28] A U.S. General Accounting Office report prepared in anticipation of federal health privacy legislation noted that confidentiality protections were not a major thrust of the Common Rule, and oversight boards tended to give confidentiality less attention than other research risks because they had the flexibility to decide when it was appropriate to review confidentiality protection issues (GAO, 1999). The report noted that although "[t]he actual number of instances in which patient privacy is breached is not fully known . . . in

---

[24] See 45 C.F.R. § 164.520 (2006).

[25] See 45 C.F.R. § 164.524 (2006).

[26] See 45 C.F.R. § 164.526 (2006).

[27] See 45 C.F.R. § 164.528 (2006).

[28] U.S. Secretary of Health and Human Services, *Recommendations on the Confidentiality of Individually-Identifiable Health Information to the Committees on Labor and Human Resources* (September 11, 1997) (hereinafter "Secretary Recommendations"); 64 Fed. Reg. 59918, 59968 (1999); 65 Fed. Reg. 82461, 82691 (2000).

an NIH [National Institutes of Health] sponsored study, IRB [Institutional Review Board] chairs reported that complaints about the lack of privacy and confidentiality were among the most common complaints made by research subjects." In addition, the compliance staff of the HHS Office for Protection from Research Risks (now Office of Human Research Protections) related that they had investigated several allegations involving human subjects protection violations resulting from a breach of confidentiality over the past several years and that the complaints related to (1) research subject to IRB review and (2) research outside federal protection (GAO, 1999).

HHS also considered requiring researchers to obtain individual authorization in all situations where a covered entity might want to disclose PHI for research. But this option would have made many research projects nearly impossible to carry out. Instead, HHS created the current system, which attempted to protect individual privacy while still allowing researchers access to data.

In proposing the Privacy Rule, HHS acknowledged that ideally, it would have preferred to directly regulate researchers by extending the protections of the Common Rule to nonfederally funded research and imposing additional criteria for the waiver of authorization in research.[29] However, HHS recognized that it did not have the authority to do so, and therefore, it attempted to protect the health information released to researchers indirectly (but within the scope of its limited authority) by imposing disclosure restrictions on covered entities.

The following sections provide a detailed overview of the Privacy Rule provisions regulating research, along with comparisons to the provisions of the Common Rule (see Chapter 3 for a general overview of the Common Rule).

Research Uses and Disclosures with Individual Authorization

Individuals may voluntarily authorize the use and disclosure of their PHI for essentially any reason, including for research purposes. To be valid under the Privacy Rule, an authorization must be "specific and meaningful"[30]—that is, it must provide a clear description of the information to be used or disclosed. The authorization must also be written in plain language, and contain core elements (e.g., signature of the individual, description of purpose of requested use or disclosure) and statements addressing the individual's right to revoke authorization, as well as

---

[29] See Secretary Recommendations (1997) and 64 Fed. Reg. 59918, 59968 (1999).
[30] See 45 C.F.R. § 164.508(c)(1)(i) (2006).

circumstances under which services or payment may be conditioned on signing the authorization.[31]

Authorization under the Privacy Rule differs from informed consent in research (reviewed by Pritts, 2008). Authorization states how, why, and to whom the PHI will be used and/or disclosed for research, and seeks permission for that use or disclosure. In contrast, informed consent describes the potential risks and benefits of research and seeks permission to involve the subject, although it also provides research participants with a description of how the confidentiality of the research records will be protected. The Privacy Rule permits, but does not require, review of authorization forms by an IRB or a Privacy Board (see Box 4-3). In contrast, under the Common Rule, IRBs are required to review and approve informed consent documents for human subjects research. However, if the authorization is combined in the same document as the informed consent document, then IRB approval must be sought for the combination (HHS, 2004c).

Authorization of Future Research

Under the Common Rule, it is permissible to obtain patient consent for future research with biological samples or information stored in databases, with oversight by an IRB, if such future uses are described in sufficient detail to allow an informed consent. Historically, IRBs typically have tried to craft informed consent language on a case-by-case basis to allow for some measure of consent to future, largely unspecified research uses, but also to require some level of detail with respect to the categories of types of uses of the information or specimens, and to emphasize confidentiality protections for identified data and tissues (Barnes and Heffernan, 2004). For example, a consent form may specify that the tissue will be kept for research to learn about, prevent, or treat the type of cancer that affects the subject.

However, such language is too general to comply with the more stringent HIPAA authorization requirements. Under the Privacy Rule, authorizations for the use or disclosure of PHI must include "[a] description of each purpose of the requested use or disclosure."[32] In the August 2002 Final Rule, HHS commented that research-related purposes described in the authorization must be "study specific" and indicated that authorizations for "unspecified future research" would be considered overly broad and

---

[31] As a general rule, covered entities may not condition the provision of treatment payment or eligibility for benefits on the provision of an authorization (with the exception of research-related treatment). See 45 C.F.R. § 164.508(b)(4) (2006).

[32] See 45 C.F.R. § 164.508(c)(1)(iv) (2006).

BOX 4-3
IRBs and Privacy Boards

Institutional Review Boards (IRBs) and Privacy Boards have different scopes of review. The Common Rule requires IRBs to review research projects involving human subjects for risk of harm to the subjects and to ensure that the appropriate process of informed consent is followed for all research participants. The Privacy Rule added to IRBs' jurisdiction by giving them the responsibility of granting waivers of authorization. In contrast, Privacy Boards did not exist under the Common Rule. Privacy Boards were created by the Privacy Rule and only have authority to review applications for waivers of authorization.

The Privacy Rule did not change the IRB membership requirements from the Common Rule (see also Box 3-3). Privacy Boards have similar membership requirements to IRBs, and must be made up of members with varying backgrounds and have appropriate professional competency to review the research protocol. There must be one member who is not affiliated with any entity conducting or sponsoring the research project and not related to any person who is affiliated with any of these entities. Also, all members with conflicts of interest must be removed.

SOURCE: 45 C.F.R. § 164.512(i)(1)(i)(A) and (B) (2006).

---

invalid.[33] In other words, HHS regards all future uses of PHI as inherently nonspecific, and the Privacy Rule does not permit an individual to grant authorization to nonspecific research.

For example, the creation and maintenance of a biospecimen bank or database is considered a specific research activity under the Privacy Rule, but authorization for any future studies undertaken with the data or materials cannot be sought at the time of collection. However, the process of recontacting individuals whose biospecimens are stored to obtain consent for each and every research project for which the samples could be used is widely viewed as impractical, if not impossible, especially as more and more samples are collected. This situation can be quite problematic for studies using stored biological samples (Barnes and Heffernan, 2004; Bledsoe, 2004; Rosati, 2008; Rothstein, 2005).

HHS received comments suggesting that general descriptions of future research could meet the requirement of "meaningful and specific" authorization, but HHS noted that the Privacy Rule does not require IRB or Privacy Board review of uses and disclosures made with individual authori-

---

[33] See 67 Fed. Reg. 53181, 53226 (2002).

zation, and thus covered entities would be left to decide whether or not the initial authorization was broad enough to cover subsequent research.[34] The HHS response went on to note that authorization for future research would not be required if a waiver of authorization was granted for a subsequent study by an IRB or a Privacy Board (see the section regarding Waiver of Authorization).

However, the committee recommends that this discordance between the Privacy Rule and the Common Rule be eliminated through guidance explicitly stating that future research may go forward if the authorization describes the types or categories of research that may be conducted with the PHI stored in a biospecimen bank or database, and if an IRB or Privacy Board determines that the proposed new research is not incompatible with the initial consent and authorization and poses no greater than minimal risk to the privacy of individuals (Wendler, 2006). Future consent for research is ethically valid if appropriate security measures are in place, donors have the right to withdraw consent, and new studies are reviewed and approved by an IRB or Privacy Board (Hansson et al., 2006). Furthermore, a prohibition on future consent actually limits individual autonomy. If individuals desire to authorize the use of their PHI for future research, they should be able to do so.

Compound Authorization

If a covered entity plans to collect and store PHI in a research repository in conjunction with a clinical trial, HHS has stated that the HIPAA authorization for storage of the PHI in the repository must be separate from the HIPAA authorization for disclosure of PHI associated with participation in the clinical trial. HHS came to this conclusion through a complex series of interpretive steps (reviewed by Rosati, 2008). First, it is generally not permissible to condition treatment on the provision of an authorization, although the Privacy Rule does permit a covered entity to condition treatment in a clinical trial on signing an authorization.[35] Second, although the Privacy Rule generally permits researchers to combine an authorization form with any other type of written permission (including another authorization), the Privacy Rule prohibits combining authorizations where the covered entity conditions the provision of treatment on signing only one of the authorizations, but not the other.[36] Because HHS has concluded that collection of PHI for a clinical trial and for a repository are separate research activities, researchers cannot condition participation in the clini-

---

[34] Id.
[35] See 45 C.F.R. § 164.508(b)(4)(i) (2006).
[36] See 45 C.F.R. § 164.508(b)(3) (2006).

cal trial on signing authorization to include PHI in the repository (HHS, 2004d). Thus, HHS has determined that the two authorizations cannot be combined in one form unless the form has separate signature lines for each authorization, and the text clearly delineates the two activities and states that the participant is not required to sign the portion authorizing the contribution of PHI to the repository.

Ideally, all relevant information pertaining to authorization should be integrated into one simple document, but there is much confusion about these complex provisions of the HIPAA Privacy Rule (Rosati, 2008). Misperceptions about restrictions on individuals' ability to provide compound authorization for the related activities of clinical trial participation and biospecimen donation are widespread. Some institutions require two complete authorization forms with all the attendant language rather than two signature lines on the same form. The excess paperwork that results is burdensome for patients, can reduce the informed nature of authorization by confusing patients, and may reduce patient participation in research. **The committee believes that guidance from HHS to clearly indicate that a single authorization form with two signature lines is permissible in such circumstances would reduce variability and increase the informed nature of authorization.**

Research Uses and Disclosures Without Individual Authorization

Documented IRB or Privacy Board Approval of Such Use or Disclosure

In crafting the Privacy Rule, HHS acknowledged that it is not always possible to obtain authorization for using or disclosing PHI for research, particularly in fields such as health services research and epidemiological research, where thousands of records may be involved (Pritts, 2008). It also recognized the potential for selection bias (see Box 3-8) when authorization is required. In light of these factors, HHS concluded that there were circumstances under which it is appropriate to disclose PHI for research without authorization. HHS noted, however, "[T]he privilege of using individually identifiable health information for research purposes without individual authorization requires that the information be used and disclosed under strict conditions that safeguard individuals' confidentiality."[37]

One situation in which the Privacy Rule permits a covered entity to use and disclose PHI for research purposes without obtaining authorization from each patient is when an IRB or a Privacy Board (Box 4-3) reviews a

---

[37] See 64 Fed. Reg. 59918, 59967 (1999).

research proposal to use PHI and determines whether to grant a "waiver" of authorization to the researcher for that particular research protocol.[38]

The Privacy Rule sets out complex standards for IRBs and Privacy Boards to apply in deciding whether to grant a waiver of authorization for a particular research study. The IRBs and Privacy Boards must determine whether a study meets all of the following criteria[39]:

(A) The use or disclosure of PHI involves no more than a minimal risk to the privacy of individuals, based on, at least, the presence of the following elements:
(1) An adequate plan to protect the identifiers from improper use and disclosure;
(2) An adequate plan to destroy the identifiers at the earliest opportunity consistent with conduct of the research, unless there is a health or research justification for retaining the identifiers or such retention is otherwise required by law; and
(3) Adequate written assurances that the PHI will not be reused or disclosed to any other person or entity, except as required by law, for authorized oversight of the research study, or for other research for which the use or disclosure of PHI would be permitted by this subpart;
(B) The research could not practicably be conducted without the waiver or alteration; and
(C) The research could not practicably be conducted without access to and use of the PHI.

An IRB or a Privacy Board may waive the authorization requirement in whole or in part. A complete waiver of authorization means that no authorization is required for the covered entity to use and disclose PHI. A partial waiver means that the IRB or Privacy Board determined that a covered entity does not need authorization for the uses and disclosure of the PHI for one part of a research project, but does need to obtain authorization from patients for another part of the project. For example, an IRB or a Privacy Board often grants a partial waiver to allow PHI to be disclosed to researchers to access PHI to identify potential subjects for a study. However, if only a partial waiver of authorization is granted, the researchers will need to obtain HIPAA authorization before the PHI for each individual patient is used for the research project. An IRB or Privacy Board may also approve a request for an alteration that removes some, but not all, required elements of an authorization, using the same criteria for a waiver of authorization.

---

[38] See 45 C.F.R. § 164.512(i)(1)(i) (2006).
[39] See 45 C.F.R. § 164.512(i)(2)(ii) (2006).

The final and codified provisions above share only some of the language used in the Common Rule[40] to determine whether it is allowable to alter the elements of informed consent or to waive the requirement of obtaining informed consent. This difference can create a challenge for the IRB decision-making process (Rothstein, 2005).

The concept of "practicability" is used in both the Common Rule and in the HIPAA authorization criteria, but there is no guidance as to what factors (e.g., feasibility or cost) should be considered in determining whether the criteria are met (IOM, 2006; IPPC, 2008; Rothstein, 2005). HHS commentary in the December 2000 Final Rule briefly mentioned cost as one factor that could be considered in determining practicability[41] (HHS, 2000), but guidance documents do not define what is "practicable" or "impracticable." As a result, institutions apply varying standards independently, often too conservatively to allow even low-risk research to proceed (see also Chapter 5). For example, some institutions interpret impracticable as "not at all possible" and require researchers to demonstrate that a study will fail without a waiver of authorization.

Moreover, stakeholders across the board, from researchers to individual patients, have questioned the meaning of the "practicability" standard (Pritts et al., 2008; Tovino, 2004). One focus group study indicated that patients may find it appropriate to consider two factors in determining whether it is practicable to conduct the research without the waiver of authorization: whether having to contact each patient first would (1) make the study less scientifically valid or (2) make the results less useful in improving medical care (i.e., would produce selection bias) (Pritts et al., 2008).

There are also no clear standards regarding what constitutes adequate protection of privacy, or what constitutes a minimal risk to privacy. The concept of minimal risk implies that there is a risk threshold, above which protections should be stricter. However, clearly defining the threshold is problematic. The terms "adequate plan" and "adequate written assurance" are highly subjective, and thus different institutions are likely to set varying thresholds for "minimal risk." **Thus, to facilitate appropriate authorization requirements for responsible research, the committee recommends that HHS simplify the criteria that IRBs and Privacy Boards use in making determinations for when they can waive the requirements to obtain authorization from each patient whose PHI will be used for a research study.**

In the 2000 version of the Privacy Rule, one of the criteria for waiver of authorization was that "the privacy risks to individuals whose PHI is to be used or disclosed are reasonable in relation to the anticipated benefits, if any, to the individual, and the importance of the knowledge that may rea-

---

[40] See 45 C.F.R. § 116(d) (2005).
[41] See 65 Fed. Reg. 82461, 82697 (2000).

sonably be expected to result from the research."[42] In 2002, HHS deleted this criterion from the Final Rule, stating that it was "unnecessarily duplicative of other provisions to protect patients' confidentiality interests."[43] It may have been more appropriate to retain this criterion and omit the criteria for impracticability.

If the current waiver criteria are to be retained, the IOM committee believes that a clear and reasonable definition of practicability, along with specific case examples of what should or should not be considered impracticable or of minimal risk, could perhaps reduce variability and overly conservative interpretation of these provisions.

Simplification or clarification of the waiver criteria would be especially helpful for multi-institutional studies, which fall under the jurisdiction of multiple IRBs or Privacy Boards. Covered entities are permitted to rely on a waiver of authorization approved by a single IRB or Privacy Board with jurisdiction. However, covered entities often decide to require approval from their own IRB or Privacy Board prior to disclosing PHI to the requesting researcher, regardless of whether another IRB or Privacy Board already granted a waiver of authorization. This leads to delays and variability in the protocol at different sites (see also Chapter 5). Simplification would also be very helpful for smaller or community-based institutions that do not have internal counsel or regulatory affairs specialists, and are thus more likely to opt out of research that requires decisions about authorizations.

Activities Preparatory to Research

A second situation where a covered entity is permitted to use and disclose PHI without obtaining authorization is for activities that are preparatory to research.[44] Review by an IRB or a Privacy Board is also not required for activities preparatory to research. A covered entity may permit researchers to look through its medical records in order to develop research protocols and to aid the recruitment of research participants if it obtains from the researcher representations that the information sought is necessary for the research purpose, that information will be reviewed only for the stated purposes preparatory to research, and that no PHI will be removed from the covered entity by the researcher in the course of the review[45] (HHS, 2004a,c).

Many research studies, especially those focused on rare conditions with limited eligible patient populations, rely on large-scale medical chart reviews and searches of patient databases to identify patients who might

---

[42] See 65 Fed. Reg. 82461, 82816 (2000).
[43] See 67 Fed. Reg. 53181, 53229 (2002).
[44] See 45 C.F.R. § 164.512(i)(1)(ii) (2006).
[45] See 45 C.F.R. § 164.512(ii) (2006).

be eligible for and might benefit from a particular study. Sufficient patient enrollment in a timely fashion is essential to ensure the meaningfulness and reliability of the research results. However, confusion regarding what is permitted under this component of the Privacy Rule is widespread (SACHRP, 2004), and surveys and studies indicate that patient recruitment has become more difficult and costly under the varying interpretations of the Privacy Rule (see Chapter 5).

HHS has issued multiple guidance statements on this topic, but these statements, some of which have been contradictory, have failed to eliminate confusion (reviewed by SACHRP, 2004). According to current HHS guidance on the Privacy Rule, researchers (both internal and external to a covered entity) may conduct a review of medical records under the preparatory to research exception. However, only internal researchers (an employee or member of the covered entity's workforce) may contact potential subjects about the possibility of enrolling in a study under this provision of the Privacy Rule. HHS guidance on the Privacy Rule indicates that external researchers are not allowed under the preparatory to research exception to record or remove contact information of patients from a covered entity. External researchers must get an IRB/Privacy Board approved waiver of authorization to perform any recruitment activities. This creates an artificial distinction between internal and external researchers that actually provides less privacy protection than that afforded by the Common Rule, which requires that any activities preparatory to research involving human subjects, or related to initial recruitment of subjects for research studies, be reviewed and approved by an IRB (HHS, 2003). Thus, the Privacy Rule permits conduct that is prohibited by the Common Rule (Rothstein, 2005).

IRBs historically have required all communications about an available research study to come from the individual's caregivers, not from an investigator unknown to the potential subjects (SACHRP, 2004). Moreover, research shows that patients prefer to be approached by their clinician or an associated nurse as opposed to a stranger (Damschroder et al., 2007; Kass et al., 2003; Robling et al., 2004; Westin, 2007; Willison et al., 2007), and HHS has reported that most allegations of violations of the Privacy Rule related to research come from patients upset at receiving recruitment calls from unknown researchers (Heide, 2007).

According to the Secretary's Advisory Committee on Human Research Protections (SACHRP), "The consequence of these confused and complex interpretations of research recruitment requirements has been to layer unnecessary, and extremely burdensome, tasks onto human subjects research. It appears, for example, that in some institutions, boilerplate business associate contracts are being signed, and that template applications for partial waivers of authorization are being routinely granted, as methods of perfunctory compliance with these confusing Privacy Rule requirements. Another effect of the enormous confusion has been that other institutions are hesitant to permit many recruitment activities critical to the continuation of the research enterprise, out of fear that they are in some way misinterpreting the government's current positions on research recruitment. SACHRP is very concerned that the bureaucratic complexities here undermine, rather than enhance, the attention that needs to be paid to the welfare and interests of subjects in the research recruitment process" (SACHRP, 2004).

The IOM committee believes that new guidance documents from HHS that clarify and simplify the rules for activities preparatory to research, and harmonize them with the Common Rule—by requiring IRB/Privacy Board approval for all researchers (internal and external) prior to contacting potential subjects—would help to eliminate this confusion and facilitate ethical research that protects patient privacy.

Research on Protected Health Information of Decedents

The third situation where a covered entity is permitted to disclose PHI without authorization is for research using the PHI of decedents. Covered entities are not required to obtain authorization from the personal representative or next of kin to conduct research on a decedent's PHI, nor are they required to receive a waiver of authorization. These provisions are similar to the Common Rule, which defines a "human subject" as a "living individual."[46]

However, the Privacy Rule does require that researchers make several representations, either in writing or orally, to the covered entity prior to the covered entity granting the researcher access to a decedent's PHI. These representations include:

- The use or disclosure being sought is solely for research on the PHI of decedents
- The PHI is necessary for research
- The death of the individual is documented, if requested by the covered entity[47]

Apparently some covered entities interpret the Privacy Rule more conservatively by requiring researchers to obtain authorization from next of kin, or a waiver of authorization from an IRB or Privacy Board, in order to access the PHI of decedents (Ness, 2007).[48]

---

[46] See 45 C.F.R. § 102(f) (2005).

[47] See 45 C.F.R. § 164.512(i)(1)(iii) (2006).

[48] Personal communication, J. Bailey-Wilson, National Institutes of Health, National Human Genome Research Institute, April 29, 2007. Personal communication, Rachel Nosowsky, Miller, Canfield, Paddock and Stone, PLC, October 23, 2008.

Deidentified Information

Researchers can also access deidentified health information stored by covered entities without obtaining authorization, waiver of authorization, or IRB/Privacy Board approval. Deidentified information does not qualify as PHI, and therefore is not protected under the Privacy Rule—it can be disclosed to researchers at any time (HHS, 2004c). The Privacy Rule offers two methods to deidentify personal health information. Under the statistical method, a statistician or person with appropriate training verifies that enough identifiers have been removed that the risk of identification of the individual is very small. Under the "safe harbor" method, data are considered deidentified if the covered entity removes 18 specified personal identifiers from the data (Box 4-4).[49] In the process of deidentifying information, the covered entity may assign a code to the deidentified information so that it may reidentify it, but the code may not be derived from information related to the individual (e.g., Social Security number). Furthermore, the covered entity may not disclose the key to the code to anyone else.[50] These provisions of the Privacy Rule are based on the federal statistical agencies' policy of using statistical methods to assess and protect the confidentiality of individuals' data they collect and release (Interagency Confidentiality and Data Access Group, 1999; Subcommittee on Disclosure Limitation Methodology, 1994).

These provisions are more stringent than those of the Common Rule, leading to situations in which some coded data might be subject to the Privacy Rule, but not the Common Rule (Rothstein, 2005). The Common Rule does not apply to research if "the identity of the subject is [not] or may [not] be readily ascertained by the investigator or associated with the information accessed by the researcher" (see Chapter 3).[51] In practice, this can mean that a covered entity may no longer routinely disclose for research data that have been anonymized according to the Common Rule (Pritts, 2008). This discrepancy between deidentification standards under the two rules can give rise to situations in which research with anonymized data that are exempt from IRB oversight under the Common Rule may still require a decision by an IRB or a Privacy Board to determine if a waiver of individuals' authorization of disclosure for the use of their information for research purposes is appropriate under the Privacy Rule. But because IRBs have not had to review these protocols in the past, they may find it difficult to make appropriate decisions about waivers.

The Privacy Rule restrictions put greater emphasis on the possibility that health data could be reidentified using publicly available databases.

---

[49] See 45 C.F.R. § 164.514(b) (2006).
[50] See 45 C.F.R. § 164.514(c) (2006).
[51] See 45 C.F.R. § 46.102(f) (2005).

BOX 4-4
HIPAA "Safe Harbor" Deidentification Method

The HIPAA "safe harbor" method of deidentification requires that each of the following identifiers of the individual or of relatives, employers, or household members of the individual must be removed from medical record information in order for the records to be considered deidentified:

1. Names.
2. All geographical subdivisions smaller than a state, including street address, city, county, precinct, ZIP Code, and their equivalent geocodes, except for the initial three digits of a ZIP Code, if according to the current publicly available data from the Bureau of the Census: (1) the geographic unit formed by combining all ZIP Codes with the same three initial digits contains more than 20,000 people; and (2) the initial three digits of a ZIP Code for all such geographic units containing 20,000 or fewer people is changed to 000.
3. All elements of dates (except year) for dates directly related to an individual (including birth date, admission date, discharge date, date of death) and all ages over 89 and all elements of dates (including year) indicative of such age, except that such ages and elements may be aggregated into a single category of age 90 or older.
4. Phone numbers.
5. Fax numbers.
6. Electronic mail addresses.
7. Social Security numbers.
8. Medical record numbers.
9. Health plan beneficiary numbers.
10. Account numbers.
11. Certificate/license numbers.
12. Vehicle identifiers and serial numbers, including license plate numbers.
13. Device identifiers and serial numbers.
14. Web Uniform Resource Locators.
15. Internet Protocol address numbers.
16. Biometric identifiers, including finger and voice prints.
17. Full-face photographic images and any comparable images.
18. Any other unique identifying number, characteristic, or code (note this does not mean the unique code assigned by the investigator to code the data).

SOURCE: 45 C.F.R. § 164.514(b) (2006).

Determining what information can be released without inappropriately compromising the privacy of the individual respondents is inherently a statistical issue (Fienberg, 2005) (see also discussion on privacy-preserving data mining and statistical disclosure limitation in Chapter 2). Record linkage technology has advanced rapidly in the past 10 years, and large public list searches are readily available for integration with "deidentified" data, making it easier to reidentify data than when the Common Rule was implemented (De Wolf et al., 2006; Pritts, 2008). For example, an academic exercise showed that it was possible to identify the names and addresses of 97 percent of the registered voters in Cambridge, Massachusetts, using the birth date and full postal code (Sweeney, 1997). In a nonacademic setting, *New York Times* reporters were also able to identify "anonymous" AOL clients whose search habits had been posted on the web for research projects by linking their search history to other available data (Barbarq and Zeller, 2006).

Studies indicate that even after removal of the 18 identifiers required under the safe harbor method of the Privacy Rule, recipients could reidentify individuals in a study dataset with a moderately high expectation of accuracy by applying only diagnosis and medication combinations (Clause et al., 2004). In short, even the Privacy Rule's deidentification standard may not be stringent enough to protect the anonymity of data in today's technological environment (Pritts, 2008). However, strong security measures (as recommended in Chapter 2) and the implementation of legal sanctions against the unauthorized reidentification of deidentified data (as recommended in subsequent sections of this chapter) may be more effective in protecting privacy than more stringent deidentification standards.

Limited Datasets

Many researchers have argued that removal of all 18 data categories as required by the HIPAA Privacy Rule's deidentification standards can render the dataset unusable for many research projects (Casarett et al., 2005; HHS, 2002; Kulynych and Korn, 2002; SACHRP, 2004) (see also Chapter 5).[52] For example, general areas of origin, residence, and work may be essential to epidemiological and other studies of topics such as disease incidence. Likewise, treatment dates are essential information for determining treatment effects, including adverse side effects. Concerns were also raised that deidentification would impede longitudinal studies, and subsequent research has indicated that information deidentified using the safe harbor method of removing all of the listed identifiers results in lost chronological spacing of episodes of care (Clause et al., 2004).

Because of these concerns, some stakeholders urged HHS "to permit covered entities to disclose PHI for research if the protected information is facially deidentified, that is, stripped of direct identifiers, so long as the research entity provides assurances that it will not use or disclose the information for purposes other than research and will not identify or contact

---

[52] See 67 Fed. Reg. 53181, 53232 (2002).

the individuals who are subjects of the information."[53] Others were more specific and requested that the Privacy Rule be amended to allow the use of keyed-hash message authentication code (HMAC), asserting that this mechanism would be valuable for researchers because it allows the recipient to link clinical information about the individual from multiple entities over time. In direct response to these requests, HHS modified the Privacy Rule and created a category[54] of partially deidentified data called the "limited dataset," which may be used and disclosed for research without obtaining individual authorization or IRB/Privacy Board approval.[55]

To qualify as a limited dataset, 16 of the more direct identifiers— such as names, addresses, Social Security numbers, and medical telephone numbers—must be removed from the data. However, the following elements may be included in a limited dataset: city, state, ZIP Code, elements of date, and other numbers, characteristics, or codes not listed as direct identifiers in the regulation (including HMAC). A limited dataset may be created by a covered entity or the covered entity can enter into a business associate agreement with another party, including the intended recipient, to create the limited dataset on its behalf.[56]

To disclose a limited dataset for research without individual authorization, the covered entity must enter into a data use agreement with the recipient. These contracts specify the recipient of the limited dataset and require the recipient to agree to a number of conditions, including:

- Not to use or disclose the limited dataset other than as permitted by the agreement or as required by law
- To use appropriate safeguards to prevent the use or disclosure of the information other than as provided for in the data use agreement
- To report to the covered entity any use or disclosure of the information not provided for by the data use agreement of which the recipient becomes aware
- To ensure that any agents to whom the recipient provides the limited dataset agree to the same restrictions and conditions as the original recipient
- Not to identify the information or contact the individuals whose records are included in the dataset[57]

---

[53] See 67 Fed. Reg. 53181, 53234 (2002).
[54] See 45 C.F.R. § 164.514(e)(3)(i) (2006).
[55] See 67 Fed. Reg. 53181, 53234 (2002).
[56] See 45 C.F.R. § 164.514(e)(3)(ii) (2006).
[57] See 45 C.F.R. § 164.514(e)(1) (2006).

Although some researchers have indicated that the use of limited data-sets may be "enticing" (Pace et al., 2005), there do not appear to be any studies about the use of limited datasets in the United States (Pritts, 2008). France reportedly uses the equivalent of limited datasets from numerous hospitals to conduct epidemiologic research (Berman, 2002), but the French health care system and legal environment are quite different than in the United States. In testimony at an Institute of Medicine workshop on the HIPAA Privacy Rule and health research, legal experts noted the shortcomings of the limited dataset (IOM, 2006). For example, in some health care settings, it can be challenging to identify an individual who will sign a data use agreement on behalf of the covered entity and thus manage the contract according to the perceived risk and obligation to monitor how that limited dataset is used. At the other extreme, it was noted that some covered entities were signing data use agreements as a matter of course, and thus providing little meaningful privacy protection to the patient (IOM, 2006).

Thus, the committee recommends that HHS encourage greater use of limited datasets and develop clear guidance on how to set up and comply with the associated data use agreements more efficiently and effectively.

Linking Data from Multiple Sources

A single database may not provide a complete picture of a patient's condition or health history, so combining information from multiple sources is often necessary (IOM, 2000). HHS stated that one intent of the limited dataset provisions was to permit data to be used and disclosed in a coded manner such that the recipient of the data could link one person's data longitudinally over multiple settings.[58] However, linking data continues to be problematic for researchers under the HIPAA Privacy Rule (IOM, 2006; IPPC, 2008).

The Privacy Rule addresses data aggregation only with respect to health care operations,[59] not research. However, it is possible in principle under the Privacy Rule for a researcher to aggregate PHI from multiple covered entities with authorization or IRB/Privacy Board waiver of authorization. Obtaining individuals' authorization for research that entails the review of thousands of medical records is unrealistic, though, and even with a waiver of authorization, covered entities with large datasets are often reluctant to allow researchers access to PHI, as noted above (see also Chapters 5 and 6). More commonly, data are provided to researchers with direct identifiers removed. But because datasets from multiple sources cannot be linked to generate a more complete record of

---

[58] See 67 Fed. Reg. 53181, 53235 (2002).
[59] See 45 C.F.R. § 164.501 and 164.504(e)(2)(i) (2006).

a patient's health history without a unique identifier, such datasets often are of minimal value to researchers and are not frequently used. A third party may also collect PHI from covered entities and aggregate the data for research by establishing business associate agreements (BAs) with the various data sources, but in practice, BAs are used infrequently for this purpose (AcademyHealth, 2008). This approach is complicated and impractical to set up for individual research projects. Moreover, BAs can be established by covered entities to gain competitive advantage, rather than to collaborate in research.

The committee believes that a better approach would be to establish secure, trusted, nonconflicted intermediaries that could develop a protocol, or key, for routinely linking data without direct identifiers from different sources and then provide more complete and useful deidentified datasets to researchers. One way this could be accomplished, for example, might be through data warehouses that are certified for the purpose of linking data from different sources (IOM, 2000). The organizations responsible for such linking would be required to use strong security measures and would maintain the details about how this linkage was done, should another research team need to recreate the linked dataset. Using such intermediaries would increase patient privacy protections and allay concerns of covered entities, and thus would facilitate greater use of health data for research and also lead to more meaningful study results.

CMS provides a similar service for Medicare and Medicaid data, via contractors who create standardized data files that are tailored for research (Box 4-5). The agency has begun pilot projects to aggregate Medicare claims data with data from commercial health plans and, in some cases, Medicaid, in order to calculate and report quality measures for physician groups. A broader effort to link data from diverse sources has been initiated by the Agency for Healthcare Research and Quality (AHRQ), called the National Health Data Stewardship Entity.[60] AHRQ is also involved in implementing the Patient Safety and Quality Improvement Act of 2005, which encourages creation of Patient Safety Organizations to receive information from hospitals, doctors, and health care providers on a privileged and confidential basis, for analysis and aggregation.[61] Although the purpose of the latter two initiatives is for monitoring health care quality, they could provide a model for data aggregation applicable to health research as well.

The HIPAA administrative simplification provisions specifically provided for the creation of a unique individual identifier, but work on this project has been halted because there is a great deal of controversy regarding how it could be implemented without comprising individual privacy.

---

[60] National Health Data Stewardship: Request for Information, 72 Fed. Reg. 30803 (2007).

[61] Patient Safety and Quality Improvement: Final Rule, 73 Fed. Reg. 70732 (2008).

BOX 4-5
The Chronic Conditions Warehouse

Section 723 of the Medicare Prescription Drug, Improvement, and Modernization Act of 2003 instructed the Secretary of the U.S. Department of Health and Human Services to make Medicare data more readily available to researchers studying chronic illness in the Medicare population, with the intent to help "identify areas for improving the quality of care provided to chronically ill Medicare beneficiaries, [and] reduce program spending." The Centers for Medicare & Medicaid Services (CMS) contracted with the Iowa Foundation for Medical Care to create the Chronic Conditions Warehouse (CCW) to implement the requirements of the Act.

The Data: The CCW contains fee-for-services claims, enrollment/eligibility, and assessment data. Researchers can efficiently access data on 21 predefined chronic health conditions, such as diabetes, breast cancer, Alzheimer's, and depression. Data files can also be extracted for other cohorts on request. Every data file includes a unique, encrypted CCW beneficiary identifier that allows the researcher to link a beneficiary's data across data sources and types within the CCW system.

The Process: A researcher must submit to CMS a data release request that includes a research design and objectives, which are reviewed by a CMS Privacy Board to ensure that the project will assist CMS "in monitoring, managing, and improving the Medicare and Medicaid programs or the services provided to beneficiaries." The Privacy Board is instructed to "balance the potential risks to the beneficiary confidentiality with the probable benefits gained from the completed research," as well as to consider the researchers' demonstrated expertise and experience in conducting such a study.

Once the request for data release is approved, the researcher must sign a CMS data use agreement that describes how the data can be used and how the data should be destroyed or returned to CMS at the conclusion of the study. If a researcher wishes to publish the study results, the manuscript must be submitted to CMS for review prior to publication to ensure that the privacy of all beneficiaries is maintained.

SOURCES: CMS (2008); IFMC (2008).

Federal agencies are also under pressure from the Office of Management and Budget to reduce the use of Social Security numbers as unique identifiers. But the development of some type of linking key (not based on Social Security numbers) would make linkages more efficient, standardized, and reliable and less costly. Moreover, this type of linkage could greatly facilitate many types of information research, provide more extensive health histories and facilitate public health surveillance, and improve quality of care (HHS, 1998; Hillestad et al., 2008).

Genetic Information and the Privacy Rule

Research involving genetic information presents perhaps some of the most challenging areas for protecting the privacy of health information (Bregman-Eschet, 2006; Farmer and Godard, 2007; Greely, 2007; NBAC, 1999). With recent technological advances in biomedical research, it is now possible to learn a great deal about disease processes and individual variations in treatment effectiveness or susceptibility to disease from genetic analyses because the DNA sequences comprising a person's genome strongly influence a person's health. New knowledge of the human genome, combined with advances in computing capabilities, are expected to help decipher the roles that genetics and the environment play in the origins of complex but common human diseases, such as cancer, heart disease, and diabetes. In this genomic age of health research, patient samples stored in biospecimen banks can provide a wealth of information for addressing long-standing questions about health and disease, and efforts are underway to create large genomic databases for that purpose (Adams, 2008; Greely, 2007; Lowrance, 2002; Lowrance and Collins, 2007). However, it is particularly difficult to assess the potential harms to individuals who are the subjects of research in these rapidly advancing areas (NBAC, 1999; Pritts, 2008), and precedent does not appear to provide sufficient guidance in this relatively uncharted territory (Lowrance, 2002; Lowrance and Collins, 2007). Moreover, HHS has not issued clear guidance on how the Privacy Rule applies to DNA samples or sequences (IOM, 2005).

HHS guidance documents indicate that tissue or blood itself is not protected under the Privacy Rule unless it contains or is associated with HIPAA identifiers (HHS, 2004b). HHS has further stated that the results of an analysis of blood or tissue, if containing or associated with personally identifiable information, would be PHI. However, the research community remains uncertain about whether genetic information accompanying biospecimens is protected under the Privacy Rule because the list of identifiers includes "biometric identifiers" and "unique identifying characteristics"[62] (NCVHS, 2004).

The European Union, which has a more restrictive privacy regime than the United States, does not consider DNA in and of itself to be a direct identifier (DPWP, 2007). Genetic information does not itself identify an individual in the absence of other identifying information. However, in some circumstances, a person's genetic code could be construed as a unique identifier in that it could be used to match a sequence in another biospecimen bank or databank that does include identifiers (Lin et al., 2004; Malin and Sweeney, 2004).

---

[62] See 45 C.F.R. § 164.514 (2006).

As genetic information becomes more prevalent in research and health care, the latter scenario is more likely to occur. For example, in January 2008, the NIH began requiring data from the Genome Wide Association Study[63] to be submitted to a central databank in an anonymous and aggregated form. That database was publicly accessible until August 2008 when officials at NIH removed the database from the public Website, citing concerns about patient confidentiality (Couzin, 2008; Zerhouni and Nabel, 2008). Those concerns stemmed from a study showing that a new type of DNA analysis could confirm the identity of an individual in a pool of similarly masked data if that person's genetic profile was already known (Homer et al., 2008). NIH intends to move the aggregate genotype data to a secure, controlled-access database with policies for review and approval of data access requests (Zerhouni and Nabel, 2008).

Also, as we enter the era of personalized medicine, genetic information is more likely to be included in a person's health records. But at the same time, realization of the promises of personalized medicine will require research on DNA from a great many diverse individuals whose medical histories are well documented. Therefore, the committee believes that the establishment of consistent standards for use and protection of genetic information is important and advocates a focus on strong security measures. **To facilitate appropriate use of DNA in health research, the committee recommends that HHS clarify the circumstances under which DNA samples or sequences are considered PHI. In addition, it recommends the adoption of strict prohibitions on the unauthorized reidentification of individuals by anyone from DNA sequences.**

Regardless of how genetic information is regulated under the HIPAA Privacy Rule, a federal prohibition of genetic discrimination is necessary to allay privacy concerns and diminish potential negative consequences of unintended disclosure of genetic information. Many people are concerned about genetic discrimination—the misuse of genetic information by insurance companies, employers, and others to make decisions based on a person's DNA—so it is important both to protect the privacy of genetic information and to protect people against such discrimination. The Genetic Information Nondiscrimination Act (GINA), recently signed into law, hopefully will begin to address some of these concerns.

Accounting of Research Disclosures

The "accounting of disclosures" provision of the HIPAA Privacy Rule gives individuals the right to receive a list of certain disclosures that a covered entity has made of their PHI in the past 6 years, including disclosures

---

[63] See http://www.genome.gov/20019523/.

made for research purposes.[64] The accounting of disclosures (AOD) must also include certain substantive information related to each disclosure, including the date of the disclosure, the identity of the person who received the information, a description of the information disclosed, and a statement of the purpose of the disclosure.

The AOD requirement was intended "as a means for the individual to find out the nonroutine purposes for which his or her PHI was disclosed by the covered entity, so as to increase the individual's awareness of persons or entities other than the individual's health care provider or health plan in possession of this information."[65] This requirement does not actually protect privacy; it merely requires covered entities to record disclosures that have already happened. In addition, the AOD requirement does not constitute an audit trail, as there are numerous exceptions to the requirement, including disclosures for health care operations, pursuant to an authorization, as part of a limited dataset, for national security or intelligence purposes, and to correctional institutions or law enforcement official. Therefore, AOD cannot provide individuals with some of the information they may want, such as a list of employees who looked at their medical record when they were in the hospital (AHIC, 2007; Pritts, 2008).

Disclosures made for research purposes under a waiver of authorization, or for public health purposes as required by law, must be included in the AOD. In fact, HHS has noted that "making a set of records available for review by a third party constitutes a disclosure of the PHI in the entire set of records, regardless of whether the third party actually reviews any particular record." The Privacy Rule has an exception for research involving groups of 50 or more subjects, which allows the generation of a general list of all protocols for which a person's PHI may have been disclosed, but even in that case, there is a considerable administrative obligation. Furthermore, in many medical facilities, that list is very extensive, and thus is relatively meaningless to a particular patient.

This aspect of the Privacy Rule places a heavy administrative burden on health systems and health services research that achieves little in terms of protecting privacy. Moreover, HHS has not given covered entities any guidance on practical ways to fulfill this requirement in an efficient manner. Annual surveys of health care privacy officers undertaken by the American Health Information Management Association (AHIMA) since 2004 have found that many facilities report difficulties with the AOD requirement (AHIMA, 2006). Furthermore, the surveys have found that the demand for AOD is extremely low. Two-thirds of respondents reported receiving no requests at all. Nearly a third indicated that they would like to see a change

---

[64] See 45 C.F.R. § 164.528 (2006).
[65] See 67 Fed. Reg. 53181, 53245 (2002).

to the AOD provisions—the most frequently cited Privacy Rule provision among all respondents, and by far among those with more than 20,000 admissions/discharges per year. Based on these results, AHIMA concluded that "for many, this provision is not only burdensome but also significantly inefficient."

The National Committee on Vital and Health Statistics (NCVHS), the Association of American Medical Colleges (AAMC), and SACHRP have all recommended changes to the AOD provisions (see Appendix A). Witnesses at the first public hearing held by the NCVHS Subcommittee on Privacy and Confidentiality, held in August 2001, suggested that covered entities were likely to refuse to share PHI because of the burden of the AOD provisions. NCVHS stated that it supported an individual's right to an AOD, but suggested that HHS issue guidance to provide covered entities with ways to fulfill this requirement in a convenient and practical manner. To date, no efforts have been undertaken to identify organizations that have successfully implemented the AOD requirement, or the practices that they have put in place (Pritts, 2008).

Case reports gathered for AAMC's database also indicated that this provision is a tremendous burden to providers and researchers and has resulted in many covered entities refusing to make PHI available to researchers. AAMC recommended that the AOD requirement be eliminated for research, if IRB/Privacy Board approval is given, asserting that most AOD do not provide any meaningful information to the individual and that it would be better to investigate any questionable disclosures as they occur.

SACHRP made a similar recommendation, stating that the Privacy Rule imposes sufficient privacy protections without applying this portion of the Privacy Rule to research. Indeed, SACHRP concluded that the cost and burden of compliance with AOD requirements was so high that institutions were likely to accept the risk of noncompliance rather than incur the cost of compliance. Noting that researchers must establish a certain standard of privacy protections before an IRB or a Privacy Board will grant a waiver of authorization, or before a covered entity will permit a researcher to access PHI preparatory to research, SACHRP recommended that covered entities should inform patients in the HIPAA "Notice of Privacy Practices" that their PHI may be used and disclosed for research purposes without their authorization if sufficient privacy safeguards are in place. The IOM committee concurs, and **recommends that HHS reform the requirements for the accounting of disclosures of protected health information for research.** In the interest of transparency, institutions should maintain a list, accessible to the public, of all studies approved by an IRB or Privacy Board, in place of the AOD requirement. However, as the health care system moves toward broader implementation of electronic health records, automatic tracking of audit trails will be an important component to incorporate.

ENFORCEMENT OF THE PRIVACY RULE

The Privacy Rule sets out both civil and criminal penalties for covered entities that breach the Rule.[66] The civil penalty provision allows a $100 fine per violation for disclosure made in error, with a maximum fine of up to $25,000 per year. The criminal penalties for persons who knowingly obtain or disclose personally identifiable information include fines of up to $50,000 and imprisonment for up to 1 year. If the crime is committed under false pretenses, the individual or organization faces fines up to $100,000 and 5 years of imprisonment. Penalties for the sale or use of PHI for commercial advantage, personal gain, or malicious harm are fines of up to $250,000 and 10 years of imprisonment.

The Privacy Rule does not provide for a private right of action by patients or research participants.[67] Thus, an individual whose privacy is violated under the Privacy Rule cannot sue the covered entity or individual who breached his or her privacy. Rather, an individual can file a claim with HHS's Office for Civil Rights (OCR). OCR is in charge of enforcement and decides whether and when to pursue a regulatory investigation and penalties against a covered entity (Stevens, 2003). In addition, it is important to note that this does not prevent an individual from pursuing a private right of action under state law (Pritts, 2008).

The Compliance and Enforcement regulations stress cooperative compliance over the imposition of penalties (reviewed by Pritts, 2008). The regulations specifically provide that the Secretary will, to the extent practicable, seek the cooperation of the covered entity in obtaining compliance.[68] If an investigation indicates a failure to comply, the regulations provide that the Secretary will first attempt to resolve the matter by informal means.[69] Such informal resolutions include demonstrating compliance, a completed corrective action plan, or a resolution agreement (HHS, 2007).[70] Only if a covered entity does not take action to resolve the noncompliance will HHS contemplate imposing civil monetary penalties on the covered entity.[71]

---

[66] See 45 C.F.R. part 160, subparts C and E (2006).

[67] See, for example, *Doe v. Bd. of Trustees of Univ. of Illinois*, 429 F. Supp. 2d 930, 944 (N.D. Ill. 2006); *Poli v. Mt. Valley's Health Ctrs., Inc.*, 2006 U.S. Dist. LEXIS 2559, No. 05-2015, 2006 WL 83378, at 13-14 (E.D. Cal. January 11, 2006); *Haranzo v. Dep't of Rehabilitative Servs.*, 2005 U.S. Dist. LEXIS 27302, No. 7:04-CV-00326, 2005 WL 3019240, at 4 (W.D. Va. November 10, 2005); *Dominic J. v. Wyo. Valley West High Sch.*, 362 F. Supp. 2d 560, 573 (M.D. Pa. 2005); *Univ. of Colo. Hosp. Auth. v. Denver Publ. Co.*, 340 F. Supp. 2d 1142 (D. Colo. 2004); *O'Donnell v. Blue Cross Blue Shield of Wyo.*, 173 F. Supp. 2d 1176, 1179-80 (D. Wyo. 2001).

[68] See 45 C.F.R. §160.304 (2006).

[69] See 45 C.F.R. §160.312(a)(1) (2006).

[70] *Id.*

[71] *Id.*

Also, a covered entity that is itself in compliance with the Privacy Rule will not be held liable for the actions of a business associate that breaches the terms of its business associate agreement. A covered entity that knows of a pattern of activity or practice of a business associate that constitutes a material breach of its contract must take reasonable steps to cure the breach or end the violation.[72] If such efforts are unsuccessful, the covered entity must terminate the contract if feasible.[73] If termination is not feasible, the covered entity must report the problem to the Secretary.[74] So long as a covered entity complies with these procedures, it is not liable for the actions of its business associates and will not be assessed civil monetary penalties (HHS, 2006).[75]

Between April 2003 and March 2008, OCR received more than 33,000 complaints alleging violations of the Privacy Rule (Barr, 2008). Most of the complaints have been filed against health care providers, including physician practices, general hospitals, pharmacies, and outpatient clinics, and largely deal with health information uses, disclosures, and safeguards. The number of complaints OCR has received that relate to research is unclear (NCVHS, 2005). In the majority of cases, OCR determined that the complaint did not present an eligible case for enforcement, either because OCR lacked jurisdiction, the complaint was untimely, or the activity did not violate the Privacy Rule.

To date, there have been no civil penalties imposed against any covered entity for breaching the Privacy Rule. Similarly, there have only been three criminal prosecutions under the Privacy Rule of individuals involved in medical identity theft (Rahman, 2006).[76] In spite of this enforcement record, many covered entities remain hesitant to share health information due to concerns about liability (Pritts, 2008).

In surveys, many providers and payors self-report that they are not in compliance with the Privacy Rule. In a recent survey by Phoenix Health Systems, 20 percent of providers and 13 percent of payors reported that they have had insufficient incentives to incur the cost of implementing all the requirements of the Privacy Rule. In the survey, none of the participating providers was able to show that it had complied with every provision of the Privacy Rule. Payors only reported doing marginally better (Phoenix Health Systems, 2006). In surveys by AHIMA, about 40 percent of hospitals and health systems reported full compliance with HIPAA regulations, while about 15 percent believed they were less than 85 percent compliant (AHIMA, 2006). More than half the respondents indicated that resources

---

[72] See 45 C.F.R. § 164.504(e)(1)(ii) (2006).

[73] *Id.*

[74] *Id.*

[75] See 45 C.F.R. § 160.402(b) (2006).

[76] See *U.S. v. Gibson*, 2004 WL 2188280 (W.D. Wash. 2004) and *U.S. v. Ramirez*, Warrant, Criminal No. M-05-708, McAllen Division.

were the most significant barrier to full privacy compliance, noting a particular need to support education and training of new staff.

RELATIONSHIP BETWEEN HIPAA AND OTHER LAWS

Federal Research Statutes

Several other federal statutes regulate research and affect the types of research projects that can be carried out in the United States. The federal regulations most relevant to health research are the Common Rule[77] and the Food and Drug Administration (FDA) Protection of Human Subjects Regulations, which have similar origins and intent[78] (see Chapter 3). Both the Common Rule and the FDA regulations are concerned primarily with the physical risks to humans associated with participation in a research study. Neither set of regulations provides detailed and prescriptive regulations for the protection of privacy (HHS, 2002). Nonetheless, there are numerous instances in which the Privacy Rule and the Common Rule diverge, as described above.

General Federal Laws

The Privacy Rule also often interacts with other federal laws. In the preamble to the Privacy Rule, HHS stated that there should be few instances where the Privacy Rule conflicts with existing statutes or regulations. Where potential conflicts do exist, HHS stated that an attempt should be made to resolve the conflict so that both laws apply. For example, if a statute or regulation permits the dissemination of PHI, but the Privacy Rule prohibits the use or disclosure of PHI without authorization, the covered entity is able to comply with both sets of laws. The entity could obtain HIPAA authorization prior to disseminating the information as permitted by the other law (HHS, 2000).

The fact that a covered entity is permitted to use or disclose PHI "as required by law" under the Privacy Rule reduces a number of potential conflicts between the Privacy Rule and other federal rules.[79] HHS provided an example to explain this point. If a previous statute or regulation requires a specific use or disclosure of PHI that the Privacy Rule appears to prohibit, the section of the Privacy Rule that permits uses or disclosures "as required by law" would allow this disclosure to be made. Also, HHS specifically stated that if a statute or regulation prohibits a use or disclo-

---

[77] See 45 C.F.R. part 46(a) (2005).
[78] See 21 C.F.R. parts 50 and 56 (2008).
[79] See 45 C.F.R. § 164.512(a) (2006).

sure of PHI that the Privacy Rule permits, the earlier, more specific statute applies (HHS, 2000).

As a result, covered entities are often subject to both the Privacy Rule and other federal statutes and regulations simultaneously. In many situations, researchers must comply with the Privacy Rule and the Common Rule or the FDA Protection of Human Subjects Regulations. Medicare providers must comply with the requirements of the Privacy Rule and the Privacy Act of 1974. Health care providers in schools, colleges, and universities must comply with the Privacy Rule and the Family Educational Rights and Privacy Act. Substance abuse treatment facilities must comply with the Privacy Rule and the Substance Abuse Confidentiality provisions of the Public Health Service Act, Section 543 and its regulations. There are innumerable examples where the Privacy Rule and another federal statute both must be followed (HHS, 2000).

State Laws

Similar to the Privacy Rule's relationship to other federal statutes, the relationship between the Privacy Rule and state privacy laws is also complicated. In general, the Privacy Rule preempts contrary state laws relating to the privacy of health information. Generally, this means that if it is impossible for a covered entity to comply with both the Privacy Rule and the state law in question, the Privacy Rule will be applied in the situation and the state law will be considered void.[80]

This general rule has three exceptions. First, any state law that is not contrary to the Privacy Rule is not preempted. If it is possible for a covered entity to comply with both the Privacy Rule and the state law simultaneously, there is no preemption of the state law, and the covered entity must comply with both sets of privacy rules.

Second, state laws that are contrary to the Privacy Rule, but provide more protection to the privacy of health information, are not preempted by the Privacy Rule. The Privacy Rule sets a national floor for the protection of PHI, not a national ceiling. More stringent means that the state law: (1) prohibits or restricts a use or disclosure in circumstances that would be permitted under HIPAA; (2) permits greater rights of access or amendment for the individual who is the subject of the PHI; (3) provides an individual with a greater amount of information regarding disclosure, rights, and remedies; (4) narrows the scope or duration of any legal permission to use PHI, or increases the privacy protections afforded to PHI; (5) provides for the retention or reporting of more detailed information for longer durations;

---

[80] See 45 C.F.R. part 160, subpart B (2006).

or (6) provides greater privacy protection for the individual with respect to any other matter.

The third exception to the general preemption rule is in the public health arena. State laws that are contrary to the Privacy Rule—but provide for the reporting of disease or injury, child abuse, birth, or death, or for conducting public health surveillance, investigation, and intervention—are not preempted by the Privacy Rule. States are permitted to set their own rules regarding what type of information can be collected by public health agents and how that information is used (HHS, 2004c).

Applying this preemption rule and determining what privacy laws must be followed in any given state can be a difficult task for covered entities. All states provide some protection for the privacy of health information. However, they differ greatly in what type of protection they provide, and thus, interact differently with the federal Privacy Rule. To successfully conduct a preemption analysis, a covered entity must become familiar with both the state laws and the Privacy Rule, interpret how the state and federal regulations interact with each other, and correctly determine the situations in which the Privacy Rule preempts state law. Many of the provisions in the Privacy Rule do not have directly corresponding provisions in state laws. This makes comparing the two sets of rules a technical and tedious task. One of the main impediments to a covered entity complying with the Privacy Rule is likely the lack of understanding of what the Privacy Rule actually requires in each state (Pritts, 2002).

CONCLUSIONS AND RECOMMENDATIONS

The HIPAA Privacy Rule was written to provide consistent standards in the United States for the use and disclosure of PHI by covered entities, including the use and disclosure of such information for research purposes. In its current state, however, the HIPAA Privacy Rule is difficult to reconcile with other federal regulations, including HHS regulations for the protection of human subjects (the Common Rule), FDA regulations pertaining to human subjects,[81] and other applicable federal or state laws.

Inconsistencies, for example, in federal regulations and their interpretations governing the deidentification of personal health information, obtaining individuals' consent for future research, and the recruitment of research volunteers make it challenging for health researchers seeking to comply with all these regulations to undertake important research activities. In addition, there is substantial variation in the way in which institutions interpret and apply the Privacy Rule (see also Chapter 5).

Additional guidance from HHS, along with some changes in interpreta-

---

[81] See 21 C.F.R. parts 50 and 56 (2008).

tion by HHS, would reduce misunderstandings of the Privacy Rule provisions by covered entities, IRBs, and Privacy Boards and help to harmonize federal regulations governing health research, which would in turn reduce complexity for researchers and covered entities, and thereby help to ensure consistent and appropriate privacy protections for patients. **Thus, HHS should develop revised and expanded guidance materials for the Privacy Rule.**

For example, HHS should develop guidance to clearly state that future research with repositories can go forward under the Privacy Rule with IRB/Privacy Board oversight. Many institutions create and maintain databases with patient health information as well as repositories with biological materials collected from patients, and use them for many types of health research, including studies to understand diseases or to compare patient outcomes following different treatments. Once created, these collections offer a cost-effective resource for rapidly addressing new research questions as technologies and knowledge advance. Collecting the samples and data necessary to address each new research question as it arises could take years, or even decades, at great expense. Thus, the pace and efficiency of medical progress is significantly enhanced by using established resources whenever feasible. Under the Common Rule, it is permissible to obtain patient consent for future research, with IRB oversight, as long as such future uses are described in sufficient detail to allow an informed consent.

However, the provisions of the Privacy Rule, as interpreted by HHS, have made it more difficult to effectively use these valuable resources for research. As a result, patients must be recontacted to obtain individual authorization for any additional studies undertaken with the data and samples collected unless the researchers obtain a waiver or alteration of authorization from an IRB or a Privacy Board. Recontacting patients for additional authorization is not only impractical, but even in those instances when it is possible, it can be intrusive and burdensome for patients and their families. The committee believes that authorization for future use of these databases and biospecimen banks should be appropriate for protecting privacy as long as there is an IRB or a Privacy Board overseeing the research. **Thus, HHS should eliminate the discordance between the Privacy Rule and the Common Rule through guidance explicitly stating that future research may go forward if the authorization describes the types or categories of research that may be conducted with the PHI stored in the biospecimen bank and if an IRB or a Privacy Board determines that the proposed new research is not incompatible with the initial consent and authorization, and poses no greater than minimal risk.**

Because science is evolving very quickly, one cannot adequately anticipate what knowledge will be gained in the future, and significant opportunities for beneficial research could be lost without some alterations to the way in which this portion of the Privacy Rule is interpreted. Databanks and biospecimen banks created and maintained with federal funds in particular should be used for multiple studies as often as feasible, given the high cost of such activities and the high value of investigating and comparing multiple scientific questions from the same pool of data.

Additional guidance from HHS is also needed to clarify the circumstances under which DNA samples or sequences are considered PHI. The research community remains uncertain about whether genetic information accompanying biospecimens is protected under HIPAA because the list of HIPAA identifiers includes "biometric identifiers" and "unique identifying characteristics."[82] Although genetic information does not itself identify an individual, a person's genetic code could be construed as a unique identifier in that it could be used to match sequence in another biospecimen bank or databank that does include identifiers. As genetic information becomes more prevalent in research and health care, concerns regarding genetic privacy and discrimination are likely to intensify. Thus, the establishment of consistent standards for use and protection of genetic information is important. The committee advocates a focus on strong security measures, with the goal of realizing the full potential of personalized medicine. **In addition, unauthorized reidentification of individuals from DNA sequences, by anyone, should be strictly prohibited.**

The committee also recommends that HHS issue guidance to clearly indicate that when researchers seek to store data and materials collected in conjunction with a clinical trial, a single authorization form with two signature lines is permissible if the text clearly delineates the two activities and states that the participant is not required to sign the portion authorizing the contribution of PHI to the repository. Informed consent and authorization are essential for the protection of individuals who volunteer to participate in clinical trials. Thus, it is imperative that the informed consent and authorization documents are easily understood and meaningful to the individuals involved. Ideally, all relevant information should be integrated into one simple document, but the HIPAA Privacy Rule's complex provisions have generated misperceptions about restrictions on individuals' ability to provide compound authorization for the related activities of clinical trial participation and biospecimen donation, and some institutions require two complete authorization forms with all the attendant language rather than two signature lines on the same form. Such misperceptions can diminish the informed nature of consent and authorization because they can lead to patient confusion and misunderstanding.

HHS should also simplify the procedures for the identification and recruitment of potential research participants and harmonize them with the

---

[82]See 45 C.F.R. § 164.514 (2006).

Common Rule. The provisions regarding these activities that are preparatory to research are complex, confusing, and actually provide less privacy
protection than the Common Rule. The committee believes that IRBs and
Privacy Boards can protect research participants, including their privacy
and confidentiality interests, and thus recommends that IRB/Privacy Board
approval (as required under the Common Rule) should be required for all
researchers (internal and external to the covered entity) prior to contacting potential subjects. When making a decision about whether to approve
research projects, the IRB or Privacy Board should review and consider
the investigator's plans for contacting patients, and also ensure that the
information will be used only for research projects approved by the IRB or
Privacy Board and not be disclosed to anyone else.

**HHS should also take steps to facilitate greater use of data with direct
identifiers removed.** Because the Privacy Rule and the Common Rule define
personally identifiable information and deidentification differently, there is
a discrepancy between what research is exempt from the Common Rule and
what research is exempt from the Privacy Rule. This discrepancy can give
rise to situations in which research with anonymized data that are exempt
from IRB oversight under the Common Rule may still require a decision by
an IRB or a Privacy Board to determine if a waiver of individuals' authorization for the use of their information for research purposes is appropriate
under the Privacy Rule.

Also, there appears to be a great deal of confusion about how to meet
conditions of data use agreements for limited datasets, which have been
stripped of the 16 most direct identifiers and can be used and disclosed for
research without obtaining individuals' authorization or an IRB/Privacy
Board waiver of authorization. **HHS could help to ameliorate this situation by issuing clear guidance on how to set up and comply with data use
agreements more efficiently and effectively.**

New tools are also needed to facilitate important health research by
allowing new hypotheses to be tested with existing data. One major challenge of using data from which direct identifiers have been removed is that
a patient's health information is rarely stored in one single location, and
data from multiple sources cannot be linked to generate a more complete
record of a patient's health history without a unique identifier. As a result,
these datasets often are of minimal value to researchers and are not frequently used. A trusted intermediary that could link data from different
sources and then provide more complete and useful deidentified datasets to
researchers would facilitate the greater use of health data for research and
lead to more meaningful study results while also increasing patient privacy
protections and allaying concerns of covered entities. **Thus, HHS should
develop a mechanism for linking data from multiple sources so that more
useful datasets can be made available for research in a manner that protects**

privacy, confidentiality, and security. Similar efforts have been initiated by AHRQ for the purpose of monitoring health care quality.

The committee also concluded that for some provisions of the Privacy Rule the burdens are heavy and the privacy protections are small. Reconsideration of such provisions may be necessary if society is to derive maximal benefits from health research. In particular, the required accounting of disclosures entails a heavy administrative burden on health systems and health services research that achieves little in terms of protecting privacy. **The committee recommends that the Privacy Rule permit medical facilities to inform patients in advance that PHI might be used for health research (with IRB/Privacy Board oversight) or for public health purposes, and the Privacy Rule should be altered to exempt these activities from AOD requirements.**

Robust safeguards are already in place to protect the privacy of PHI disclosures in health research via IRBs and Privacy Boards. As the health care system moves toward broader implementation of electronic health records, however, automatic tracking of audit trails will be important to incorporate. Technology advances will likely make automatic AOD tracking feasible, affordable, and widely available in the future. **Until then, the committee recommends that disclosures of PHI made for health research and public health purposes be exempted from the HIPAA Privacy Rule's AOD requirement. However, in the interest of transparency, institutions should maintain a list, accessible to the public, of all studies approved by its IRB or Privacy Board.**

HHS should also simplify the criteria that IRBs and Privacy Boards use in making determinations for when they can waive the requirements to obtain authorization from each patient whose PHI will be used for a research study. If the current criteria for waiver of authorization are to be retained, a clear and reasonable definition of impracticability from HHS, along with specific case examples of what should or should not be considered impracticable or of minimal risk, could reduce variability and overly conservative interpretations among IRBs and Privacy Boards.

Case examples should help delineate what IRBs and Privacy Boards should do to facilitate research, rather than just defining what is permissible. For example, it is appropriate to allow use of registries, clinical databases, and biospecimen banks for justifiable scientific inquiries. HHS should clearly state that IRBs and Privacy Boards should not impede research that is permissible under the Privacy Rule without a compelling concern (for example, if participant solicitation plans are inappropriate or if the principal investigator is unqualified).

Simplification or clarification of the waiver criteria would be especially helpful for multi-institutional studies, which fall under the jurisdiction of multiple IRBs or Privacy Boards, and for smaller or community-based institutions that do not have internal counsel or regulatory affairs specialists, and are thus more likely to opt out of research that requires decisions about authorizations. With better guidance, all covered entities would have more confidence in their decisions, and might be more willing to rely on a lead IRB/Privacy Board decision in the case of multi-institutional studies.

REFERENCES

AcademyHealth. 2008. PowerPoint presentation to the Institute of Medicine Committee on Health Research and the Privacy of Health Information: The HIPAA Privacy Rule, on AcademyHealth survey results.

Adams, R. 2008. Progress vs. privacy. *CQ Weekly* May 26, 1404.

AHIC (American Health Information Community). 2007. *Confidentiality, privacy, and security workgroup, summary of the 14th web conference.* http://137.187.25.8/healthit/ahic/materials/summary/cpssum_100407.html (accessed August 27, 2008).

AHIMA (American Health Information Management Association). 2006. *The state of HIPAA privacy and security compliance.* http://www.ahima.org/emerging_issues/2006StateofHIPAACompliance.pdf (accessed April 20, 2008).

Barbarq, M., and T. Zeller, Jr. 2006. Confidentiality issues for data miners. *Artificial Intelligence in Medicine* 26:25–36.

Barnes, M., and K. G. Heffernan. 2004. The "future uses" dilemma: Secondary uses of data and materials by researchers and commercial research sponsors. *Medical Research Law and Policy Report* 3:440–452.

Barr, S. 2008. HIPAA enforcement of Privacy Rule stresses voluntary compliance, HHS official says. *BNA Privacy and Security Law Report* 7(13):479.

Berman, J. J. 2002. Confidentiality issues for data miners. *Artificial Intelligence in Medicine* 26(1):25–36.

Bledsoe, M. 2004. HIPAA models for repositories. *ISBER Newsletter: International Society for Biological and Environmental Repositories* 4(1):1–4.

Bregman-Eschet, Y. 2006. Genetic databases and biobanks: Who controls our genetic privacy? *Santa Clara Computer & High Technology Law Journal* 23:1.

Casarett, D., J. Karlawish, E. Andrews, and A. Caplan. 2005. Bioethical issues in pharmaco-epidemiological research. In *Pharmacoepidemiology*, 4th ed., edited by B. L. Strom. West Sussex, England: John Wiley & Sons, Ltd. Pp. 417–432.

Chaikind, H., J. Hearne, B. Lyke, and C. S. Redhead. 2005. *CRS report for congress: The Health Insurance Portability and Accountability Act (HIPAA) of 1996: Overview and guidance on frequently asked questions.* http://www.law.umaryland.edu/marshall/crsreports/crsdocuments/RL3163401242005.pdf (accessed August 27, 2005).

Clause, S. L., D. M. Triller, C. P. H. Bornhorst, R. A. Hamilton, and L. E. Cosler. 2004. Conforming to HIPAA regulations and compilation of research data. *American Journal of Health-System Pharmacy* 61(10):1025–1031.

CMS (Centers for Medicare & Medicaid Services). 2005. *Overview: Security standards.* http://www.cms.hhs.gov/SecurityStandard/ (accessed March 27, 2007).

CMS. 2008. *Criteria for review of requests for CMS research identifiable data.* http://www.cms.hhs.gov/PrivProtectedData/02_Criteria.asp#TopOfPage (accessed April 23, 2008).

Couzin, J. 2008. Whole-genome data not anonymous, challenging assumptions. *Science* 321:1278.

Damschroder, L. J., J. L. Pritts, M. A. Neblo, R. J. Kalarickal, J. W. Creswell, and R. A. Hayward. 2007. Patients, privacy and trust: Patients' willingness to allow researchers to access their medical records. *Social Science & Medicine* 64(1):223–235.

De Wolf, V. A., J. E. Sieber, P. M. Steel, and A. O. Zarate. 2006. Part II: HIPAA and disclosure risk issues. *IRB: Ethics and Human Research* 28(1):6–11.

DPWP (Data Protection Working Party). 2007. *Opinion 4/2007 on the concept of personal data.* http://ec.europa.eu/justice_home/fsj/privacy/docs/wpdocs/2007/wp136_en.pdf (accessed August 28, 2008).

Farmer, Y., and B. Godard. 2007. Public health genomics (PHG): From scientific considerations to ethical integration. *Genomics, Society and Policy* 3:14–27.

Fienberg, S. E. 2005. Confidentiality and disclosure limitation. *Encyclopedia of Social Measurement* 1:463–469.

GAO (Government Accounting Office). 1999. *Medical records privacy: Access needed for health research but oversight of privacy protections is limited.* Washington, DC: GAO.

Greely, H. 2007. The uneasy ethical and legal underpinnings of large-scale genomic biobanks. *Annual Review of Genomics and Human Genetics* 8:346.

Hansson, M., J. Dillner, C. Bartram, J. Carlson, and G. Helgesson. 2006. Should donors be allowed to give broad consent to future biobank research? *Lancet Oncology* 7(3):266–269.

Heide, C. 2007. PowerPoint presentation to the Institute of Medicine Committee on Health Research and the Privacy of Health Information: The HIPAA Privacy Rule, on the HIPAA Privacy Rule & research: Update from HHS Office for Civil Rights.

HHS (Department of Health and Human Services). 1998. White paper on unique identifiers.

HHS. 2000. Standards for privacy of individually identifiable health information; Final Rule. *65 Fed. Reg. 82462.*

HHS. 2002. *OCR guidance explaining significant aspects of the Privacy Rule.* http://www.hhs.gov/ocr/hipaa/privacy.html (accessed August 27, 2008).

HHS. 2003. *Institutional review boards and the HIPAA Privacy Rule.* http://privacyruleandresearch.nih.gov/pdf/IRB_Factsheet.pdf (accessed August 21, 2008).

HHS. 2004a. *Clinical research and the HIPAA Privacy Rule.* http://privacyruleandresearch.nih/gov/pdf/clin_research.asp (accessed August 27, 2008).

HHS. 2004b. *Guidance on research involving coded private information or biological specimens.* http://www.hhs.gov/ohrp/humansubjects/guidance/cdebiol.pdf (accessed August 21, 2008).

HHS. 2004c. *Protecting personal health information in research: Understanding the HIPAA Privacy Rule.* http://privacyruleandresearch.nih.gov/pr_02.asp (accessed April 17, 2007).

HHS. 2004d. *Research repositories, databases, and the HIPAA Privacy Rule.* http://privacyruleandresearch.nih.gov/research_repositories.asp (accessed August 27, 2008).

HHS. 2006. *Frequently asked questions: Is a covered entity liable for, or required to monitor, the actions of its business associates?* http://www.hhs.gov/hipaafaq/providers/business/236.html (accessed August 27, 2008).

HHS. 2007. *How OCR enforces the HIPAA Privacy Rule.* http://www.hhs.gov/ocr/privacy/enforcement/hipaarule.html (accessed August 27, 2008).

Hillestad, R., J. H. Bigelow, B. Chaudhry, P. Dreyer, M. D. Greenberg, R. C. Meili, M. S. Ridgely, J. Rothenberg, and R. Taylor. 2008. *Identity crisis: An examination of the costs and benefits of a unique patient identifier for the U.S. health care system.* RAND Corporation.

Homer, N., S. Szelinger, M. Redman, D. Duggan, W. Tembe, J. Muehling, J. V. Pearson, D. A. Stephan, S. F. Nelson, and D. W. Craig. 2008. Resolving individuals contributing trace amounts of DNA to highly complex mixtures using high-density SNP genotyping microarrays. *PLoS Genetics* 4(8):e1000167. doi:10.1371/journal.pgen.1000167.

IFMC (Iowa Foundation for Medical Care). 2008. *Chronic condition data warehouse: User manual.* Version 1.3. http://www.ccwdata.org/downloads/CCW%20User%20Manual. pdf (accessed August 27, 2008).

Interagency Confidentiality and Data Access Group. 1999. *Checklist on disclosure potential of proposed data releases.* http://www.fcsm.gov/committees/cdac/checklist_799.doc (accessed January 13, 2009).

IOM (Institute of Medicine). 2000. *Protecting data privacy in health services research.* Washington, DC: National Academy Press.

IOM. 2005. *Implications of genomics for public health: Workshop summary.* Washington, DC: The National Academies Press.

IOM. 2006. *Effect of the HIPAA Privacy Rule on health research: Proceedings of a workshop presented to the National Cancer Policy Forum.* Washington, DC: The National Academies Press.

IPPC (International Pharmaceutical Privacy Consortium). 2008. Comments to the Institute of Medicine Committee on Health Research and the Privacy of Health Information: The HIPAA Privacy Rule, on the impact of the HIPAA Privacy Rule on pharmaceutical research.

Kass, N. E., M. R. Natowicz, S. C. Hull, R. R. Faden, L. Plantinga, L. O. Gostin, and J. Slutsman. 2003. The use of medical records in research: What do patients want? *Journal of Law, Medicine & Ethics* 31:429–433.

Kulynych, J., and D. Korn. 2002. The effect of the new federal medical-Privacy Rule on research. *New England Journal of Medicine* 346(3):201–204.

Lin, Z., A. B. Owen, and R. B. Altman. 2004. Genomic research and human subject privacy. *Science* 305(5681):183.

Lowrance, W. W. 2002. *Learning from experience, privacy and the secondary use of data in health research.* London: The Nuffield Trust.

Lowrance, W. W., and F. S. Collins. 2007. Identifiability in genomic research. *Science* 317:600–602.

Malin, B., and L. Sweeney. 2004. How (not) to protect genomic data privacy in a distributed network: Using trail re-identification to evaluate and design anonymity protection systems. *Journal of Biomedical Informatics* 37:179–192.

NBAC (National Bioethics Advisory Commission). 1999. *Research involving human biological materials: Ethical issues and policy guidance, report and recommendations.* Vol. 1. Rockville, MD: NBAC.

NCVHS (National Committee on Vital and Health Statistics). 2004. *Letter to Secretary Thompson—recommendation on the effect of the Privacy Rule.* http://ncvhs.hhs.gov/040305l2.htm (accessed August 27, 2008).

NCVHS. 2005. *Seventh annual report to congress on the implementation of the administrative simplification provisions of the Health Insurance Portability and Accountability Act (HIPAA).* http://ncvhs.hhs.gov/050908rpt.htm (accessed August 27, 2008).

Ness, R. 2007. Influence on the HIPAA Privacy Rule on health research. *JAMA* 298(18): 2164–2170.

Pace, W. D., E. W. Staton, and S. Holcomb. 2005. Practice-based research network studies in the age of HIPAA. *Annals of Family Medicine* 3(Supp. 1):S38–S45.

Phoenix Health Systems. 2006. *US healthcare industry HIPAA compliance survey results: Summer 2006.* http://www.hipaadvisory.com/action/surveynew/ (accessed April 5, 2007).

Pritts, J. 2002. *Testimony before the National Committee on Vital and Health Statistics, Subcommittee on Privacy and Confidentiality: Implementation of the federal standards for privacy of individually identifiable health information.* http://www.ncvhs.hhs.gov/021030p6.htm (accessed August 27, 2008).

Pritts, J. 2008. *The importance and value of protecting the privacy of health information: Roles of HIPAA Privacy Rule and the Common Rule in health research.* http://www.iom.edu/CMS/3740/43729/53160.aspx (accessed March 15, 2008).

Pritts, J., M. Neblo, L. Damschroder, and R. Hayward. 2008. Veterans' views on balancing privacy and research in medicine: A deliberative democratic study. *Michigan State University Journal of Medicine and Law* 12:17–31.

Rahman, N. 2006. Medical: Reflections on privacy: Recent developments in HIPAA Privacy Rule. *I/S: A Journal of Law and Policy for the Information Society* 2(3):685.

Redhead, C. S. 2001. *CRS report for congress: Health information standards, privacy and security: HIPAA's administrative simplification regulations.* Washington, DC: Congressional Research Service.

Robling, M. R., K. Hood, H. Houston, R. Pill, J. Fay, and H. M. Evans. 2004. Public attitudes towards the use of primary care patient record data in medical research without consent: A qualitative study. *Journal of Medical Ethics* 30:104–109.

Rosati, K. 2008. PowerPoint presentation to the Institute of Medicine Committee on Health Research and the Privacy of Health Information: The HIPAA Privacy Rule, on the challenges with biorepositories, databases, and future research.

Rothstein, M. A. 2005. Research privacy under HIPAA and the Common Rule. *Journal of Law, Medicine & Ethics* 33(1):154–159.

SACHRP (Secretary's Advisory Committee on Human Research Protections). 2004. *Letter to Secretary Thompson.* http://www.hhs.gov/ohrp/sachrp/hipaalettertosecy090104.html (accessed August 27, 2008).

Shalala, D. E. 1997. *Confidentiality of individually-identifiable health information: Recommendations of the Secretary of Health and Human Services, pursuant to section 264 of the Health Insurance Portability and Accountability Act of 1996.* http://aspe.hhs.gov/admnsimp/pvcrec0.htm (accessed August 27, 2008).

Stevens, G. M. 2000. *CRS report for Congress: Summary of the proposed rule for the privacy of individually identifiable health information.* Washington, DC: Congressional Research Service.

Stevens, G. M. 2003. *CRS report for Congress: Compliance with the HIPAA medical Privacy Rule.* Washington, DC: Congressional Research Service.

Subcommittee on Disclosure Limitation Methodology, Federal Committee on Statistical Methodology. 1994. *Statistical policy working paper 22: Report on statistical disclosure limitation methodology.* http://www.ciser.cornell.edu/NYCRDC/helpful_links/WP-22-OMB-totalreport.pdf (accessed January 13, 2009).

Sweeney, L. 1997. Weaving technology and policy together to maintain confidentiality. *Journal of Law, Medicine & Ethics* 25:98–110.

Tovino, S. A. 2004. The use and disclosure of protected health information for research under the HIPAA Privacy Rule: Unrealized patient autonomy and burdensome government regulation. *South Dakota Law Review* 49(3):447–502.

U.S. Congress, House of Representatives, Committee of Conference. *Health Insurance Portability and Accountability Act of 1996.* 104th Cong., 2d Sess. July 31, 1996.

U.S. Congress, House of Representatives, Committee on Ways and Means. *Health Coverage Availability and Affordability Act of 1996.* 104th Cong., 2d Sess. March 25, 1996.

Wendler, D. 2006. One-time general consent for research on biological samples: Is it compatible with the Health Insurance Portability and Accountability Act? *Archives of Internal Medicine* 166(14):1449–1452.

Westin, A. 2007. *How the public views privacy and health research.* http://www.iom.edu/Object.File/Master/48/528/%20Westin%20IOM%20Srvy%20Rept%2011-1107.pdf (accessed November 11, 2007).

Willison, D. J., L. Schwartz, J. Abelson, C. Charles, M. Swinton, D. Northrup, and L. Thabane. 2007 (September 25–28). *Alternatives to project-specific consent for access to personal information for health research. What do Canadians think?* Paper presented at 29th International Conference of Data Protection and Privacy Commissioners, Montreal, Canada.

Zerhouni, E. A., and E. G. Nabel. 2008. Protecting aggregate genomic data. *Science* 322:44.

5

Effect of the HIPAA Privacy Rule
on Health Research

Since the Health Insurance Portability and Accountability Act (HIPAA) Privacy Rule was implemented by the U.S. Department of Health and Human Services (HHS) in April 2003, health researchers have asserted that the Privacy Rule has had a negative effect on researchers' abilities to conduct meaningful research. The purpose of this chapter is to review the currently available evidence on the effect of the Privacy Rule on research, including surveys as well as other types of studies to measure impact. The chapter begins with an overview of several surveys that examined health researchers' personal experiences with and opinions about the Privacy Rule. Many issues identified by survey respondents were also the focus of other types of studies, so the remainder of the chapter consists of a topical review of the available evidence regarding the effect of the Privacy Rule, and its interpretation, on health research. The following issues are reviewed in detail: (1) selection bias, (2) research efficiency, (3) abandoned research, (4) deidentified information, (5) the authorization process, and (6) concerns about potential legal consequences.

OVERVIEW OF SURVEY RESULTS

As noted in previous chapters (Chapter 1 in particular), the information gained by opinion surveys has limitations. The potential for bias exists because of the way the questions are worded and framed, and respondents may have self-motivated reasons for responding in a particular fashion. For example, individuals responding to surveys conducted by professional societies may be more likely to have encountered difficulties with the Privacy

Rule than those who did not respond. Thus, information gathered from surveys is anecdotal and based on individual's personal opinions; it does not constitute systematic data on the experience of all researchers.

Before discussing the relevant surveys in detail in this chapter, it is also important to recognize the strengths and weaknesses of these survey data. One strength is that multiple surveys addressed similar topics, and many respondents were affiliated with different institutions and different fields of health research. The fact that the respondents to the different surveys reported similar problems with conducting research under the Privacy Rule makes it more likely that results can be generalized and are not specific to a particular institution. Weaknesses include the size and low response rates of some surveys and, in some cases, the lack of a denominator, making it impossible to determine a response rate, which is an important measure to assess the representativeness of the results. Also, three of the surveys discussed below were conducted immediately or shortly after the Privacy Rule was implemented, before covered entities and other stakeholders had adequate time to adapt to the new regulation. However, more recent surveys of researchers' experiences with the Privacy Rule, two of which were commissioned by the Institute of Medicine (IOM) committee, found that researchers were still reporting negative effects of the Privacy Rule on health research (Box 5-1).

Surveys to gauge the impact of the HIPAA Privacy Rule on health research have been undertaken by numerous agencies and organizations with various constituencies, including the Association of American Medical Colleges (NCVHS, 2003), the National Cancer Advisory Board (Ramirez and Niederhuber, 2003), the Agency for Healthcare Research and Quality (Walker, 2005), Epidemiological Societies (Ness, 2007), the HMO Research Network (Greene et al., 2008), AcademyHealth (Helms, 2008), the American Heart Association (Ring, 2007), and the North American Association of Central Cancer Registries (Deapen, 2006). In addition, structured interviews were undertaken by the American Society for Clinical Oncology (ASCO, 2008), and focus groups were organized by the Association of Academic Health Centers (AAHC, 2008). An overview of these projects is provided below (also see Table 5-1).

Association of American Medical Colleges Survey

In 2003, on the day that covered entities were required to be in compliance with the Privacy Rule, the Association of American Medical Colleges (AAMC) launched a survey to examine the Privacy Rule experiences of investigators, Institutional Review Board (IRB) personnel, privacy officials, research administrators, and deans. AAMC then created a database of case reports and research functions affected by the Privacy Rule based on 331 individuals' responses. After analyzing the database, AAMC concluded that

---

BOX 5-1
Health Researchers' Experience with the Privacy Rule:
Survey Results in 2003–2004 and 2007–2008

- The Privacy Rule has increased the cost and time it takes to conduct a research project from start to finish (AAMC, NCAB, AHRQ, Ness, Academy-Health, HMORN, AHA/ACC, AAHC)
- Institutional differences in interpretation of the Privacy Rule have made conducting health research more difficult than in the pre-Privacy Rule era (AAMC, NCAB, AHRQ, Ness, AcademyHealth, HMORN, AAHC)
- The Privacy Rule has made recruitment of research participants more difficult and has increased the likelihood of selection bias (AAMC, AHRQ, Ness, AcademyHealth, AHA/ACC, AAHC)
- The Privacy Rule has increased research participants' confusion regarding their rights and protections (NCAB, Ness, HMORN)
- The Privacy Rule's standards for deidentification have not created an effective way for researchers to collect data (AAMC, AHRQ, Ness, AcademyHealth, HMORN, AHA/ACC)
- The Privacy Rule has led researchers to abandon studies (AAMC, AHRQ, AcademyHealth, HMORN, ASCO)
- The Privacy Rule has created new barriers to the use of patient specimens collected during clinical trials (NCAB, AAHC, ASCO)

Survey Institutions: Association of American Medical Colleges (AAMC), National Cancer Advisory Board (NCAB), Agency for Healthcare Research and Quality (AHRQ), HMO Research Network (HMORN), American Heart Association/ American College of Cardiology (AHA/ACC), Association of Academic Health Centers (AAHC), American Society of Clinical Oncology (ASCO).

SOURCES: AAHC (2008); ASCO (2008); Greene et al. (2006); Helms (2008); NCVHS (2003); Ness (2007); Ramirez and Niederhuber (2003); Ring (2007); Walker (2005).

---

the Privacy Rule affects many types of health research, including clinical, health services, epidemiological, behavioral, biomedical, health economics, and outcomes research. The most common effects of the Privacy Rule on research reported were that the Privacy Rule: (1) reduced patient recruitment, (2) increased the likelihood of selection bias, (3) increased the costs of conducting research by requiring more paperwork and complicating the IRB approval process, (4) increased the number of errors in research when deidentified information was used, (5) made multisite trials more difficult because of variations in IRB interpretation of the Rule, and (6) caused researchers to abandon projects because of the increased number of rules for operating a research study (NCVHS, 2003).

TABLE 5-1 Summary of Relevant Surveys

Survey	Year	Survey Participants	Response Rate[a]
Association of American Medical Colleges	2003	Targeted investigators, institutional review board (IRB) personnel, privacy officials, research administrators, and deans	331 respondents[b]
National Cancer Advisory Board	2003	Individuals suggested from cancer center directors, clinical cooperative group chairs, and principal investigators of Special Programs of Research Excellence	39% (89/226)
Agency for Healthcare Research and Quality	2004	16 health services researchers, and 17 privacy officers, research compliance officers, and IRB directors	77% (33/43)
National Survey of Epidemiologists	2007	Professional members of 13 epidemiological societies	1,527 respondents[c]
HMO Research Network (HMORN): survey of investigators	2008	Scientists working in the 15 HMORN research centers	43% (89/235)
HMORN: survey of IRB administrators	2008	IRB administrators at the 15 HMORN research centers	73% (11/15)
AcademyHealth	2007	Professional members of AcademyHealth	396 respondents[d]
American Heart Association/American College of Cardiology	2007	Professional members of the American Heart Association and the American College of Cardiology	656 respondents[e]
North American Association of Central Cancer Registries	2006	Membership of the North American Association of Central Cancer Registries	66% (47/77)
American Society for Clinical Oncology	2008	27 compliance officials and investigators from 13 institutions	27 respondents (structured interviews)
Association of Academic Health Centers	2007	Researchers and compliance personnel from 5 institutions	5 focus groups
Total Number of Responses from All Entities			3,211 respondents

[a]Where the data are available, the response rate includes the number of survey respondents divided by the total number of individuals invited to participate in the survey.

[b]The total number of individuals invited to complete this survey is unknown.

[c]The epidemiological societies e-mailed the survey to 10,347 e-mail addresses. However, a substantial number of epidemiologists belong to more than one organization, and as a result it is impossible to calculate a response rate. Also, only those members who had submitted an application to an IRB since the Privacy Rule was implemented met the criteria for inclusion in the analysis.

notes continue

TABLE 5-1 Notes continued

*d*All 3,461 AcademyHealth members were invited to participate in the survey, but only members who were principal investigators met the criteria for inclusion in the survey analysis. Calculating a response rate was impossible because the total number of eligible survey participants was unknown.

*e*All 18,261 professional members of the American Heart Association and the American College of Cardiology were invited to complete this survey. Many of these members are practicing physicians, not researchers, and thus were not the intended audience for the survey. As a result, it was impossible to calculate the total number of eligible individuals invited to participate in the survey, or the response rate.

National Cancer Advisory Board Survey

The National Cancer Advisory Board (NCAB)[1] conducted a survey of health researchers' experiences with the Privacy Rule in 2003. NCAB requested the names of Privacy Rule experts from cancer center directors, clinical cooperative group chairs, and principal investigators of Special Programs of Research Excellence. A total of 226 experts were identified. These experts were invited to visit a website and submit public comments on the effect of the Privacy Rule on cancer research. NCAB received 89 responses to the survey, for a 39 percent response rate. The survey showed that the majority of respondents believed that: (1) the Privacy Rule increased patient confusion, (2) the Privacy Rule's complex documentation requirements delayed research, (3) differing interpretations of the Privacy Rule made conducting health research more challenging, and (4) the Privacy Rule created new barriers to the use of patient specimens collected during clinical trials (Ramirez and Niederhuber, 2003).

AHRQ Survey

In 2004, the Agency for Healthcare Research and Quality (AHRQ) interviewed 33 senior health care researchers, privacy officers, research compliance officers, and IRB directors representing a variety of health settings in 18 states that covered all regions of the United States. With a 77 percent response rate, 92 percent of respondents reported an impact of the Privacy Rule on health research. Those reporting substantial impact were often involved in multisite studies where follow-up information from many patients was needed from many sources. Many respondents reported

---

[1]NCAB was appointed by the President of the United States to advise the HHS Secretary and the National Cancer Institute Director regarding the activities of the Institute and policies regarding these activities.

conflicting IRB decisions, difficulties with authorization as well as access to deidentified data, increased cost and time, and lack of participation from small hospitals and provider groups due to lack of resources. More than half of respondents thought that misinterpretations and overly conservative interpretations of the Privacy Rule were the cause of the difficulties (Walker, 2005).

National Survey of Epidemiologists

The IOM committee commissioned a survey by Roberta Ness at the University of Pittsburgh. In 2007, Dr. Ness conducted a web-based survey of 1,527 epidemiologists who had submitted a new application to an IRB for a research project involving human subjects research since the Privacy Rule was implemented (see Appendix B for methodological details). The survey asked respondents to answer a number of questions on a 5-point Likert scale (1 = none, 5 = a great deal). More than 84 percent of respondents ranked the statement "the Privacy Rule made research easier" as a 1 or 2. In contrast, 68 percent of respondents ranked the statement "the degree to which the Rule made research more difficult" as a 4 or 5. Only 11 percent of respondents stated that the Privacy Rule strengthened public trust in research, and 26 percent responded that the Privacy Rule did a great deal to enhance participant confidentiality and privacy (Figure 5-1).

This survey also provided respondents with the opportunity to write in comments regarding their experiences conducting research under the Privacy Rule. A total of 427 comments were received; 90 percent were negative, 5 percent were neutral, and 5 percent were positive. The common themes in the comments were: (1) the Privacy Rule added patient burden without enhancing privacy protections, (2) institutions vary greatly in their interpretations of the Privacy Rule, and (3) many government agencies are confused about the demarcation between public health surveillance, which is exempt from the Privacy Rule, and health research. Finally, the survey found that many respondents believed the Privacy Rule added to research costs, caused delays to research projects, and made recruitment of research participants much more difficult (Ness, 2007).

HMO Research Network Survey

The IOM committee also commissioned data-gathering efforts from the HMO Research Network (HMORN) of investigator and IRB members' experiences operating under the Privacy Rule (see Appendix B for methodological details). The HMORN is a consortium of more than 250 scientists who work in 15 research centers based in health care delivery systems. The data collection efforts consisted of a web-based survey of investigators in

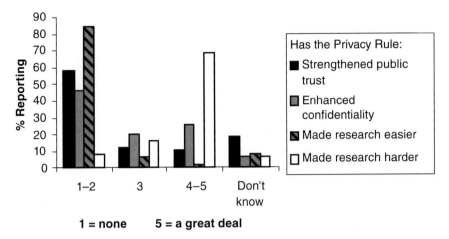

FIGURE 5-1 National Survey of Epidemiologists: Scaled perceptions of the impact of the Health Insurance Portability and Accountability Act Privacy Rule.
SOURCE: Ness (2007).

the Cancer Research Network (conducted in fall 2007), a follow-up telephone survey of those investigators who reported having a study affected by the Privacy Rule, and a mailed survey to IRB administrators at the 15 HMORN sites (conducted in early 2008). The response rate for the investigator survey was 43 percent (235 investigators were invited to participate in the survey, and 89 responses were received). Respondents were mostly doctoral-level scientists, and 72 percent of them had been in research for 10 or more years. Twelve respondents completed telephone interviews. The response rate for the IRB administrator survey was 73 percent (11 of the 15 sites submitted responses).

The results of these surveys are consistent with those of previous surveys. Respondents reported numerous difficulties with conducting health research since the implementation of the Privacy Rule, including increased time required to conduct research, problems with gaining IRB approval for studies, impediments to multicenter research, confusion over the authorization process, and problems with the use of deidentified data. Of the investigators who responded, 74 percent reported having a study affected by the Privacy Rule. Of these respondents, 61 percent reported having a study affected more than once. In addition, 60 percent of the investigators reported difficulty conducting research under the requirements of the Privacy Rule. On the other hand, 59 percent of the investigators reported that the Privacy Rule has strengthened patient privacy.

The IRB administrators were more positive than the investigators regarding the Privacy Rule. Ninety percent of IRB administrators reported that the Privacy Rule strengthened patient privacy. In addition, 46 percent of IRB administrators said it was easy to work within the privacy regulations, as opposed to 36 percent of IRB administrators who said it was not easy to work within the regulations. Nonetheless, 63 percent of IRB administrators reported that the Privacy Rule has made conducting research more difficult. More than 72 percent of IRB administrators reported that the federal government needs to give more guidance to IRBs about interpreting and implementing the Privacy Rule (Greene et al., 2008).

AcademyHealth Survey

To provide input to the IOM study, AcademyHealth conducted a survey in 2007 of researchers' experiences operating under the Privacy Rule. AcademyHealth is a professional society for health services researchers and health policy analysts. Its mission is to strengthen the research infrastructure, promote the use of the best available research, and assist health policy and practice leaders in addressing major health care challenges. The organization conducted a web-based survey of principal investigators. All 3,461 AcademyHealth members were invited to participate in the survey by e-mail. A total 696 members responded. Out of this group, 396 members were principal investigators and met the criteria for inclusion in the survey analysis. In general, 75 percent of the survey respondents reported that their experiences with the Privacy Rule were negative. Only 6 percent of respondents reported that their experiences were positive. Nearly half—48 percent—reported that their institution provided support to assist researchers with HIPAA compliance and IRB issues, and 77 percent of the researchers at these institutions indicated that they used these resources. Respondents were also asked whether they believe the Privacy Rule strikes the correct balance between protecting individual privacy and allowing research to be conducted. A majority—63 percent—of the respondents reported that the Privacy Rule provides protection to individuals at the expense of access to research data; 28 percent reported that the Privacy Rule strikes the right balance between these two goods; and only 1 percent reported that the Privacy Rule provides access to research data at the expense of privacy protection for individuals (Figure 5-2) (Helms, 2008).

American Heart Association/American College of Cardiology Survey

The American Heart Association (AHA) and the American College of Cardiology (ACC) also conducted a survey in 2007. The 18,261 professional members of AHA and ACC were invited to complete a questionnaire by e-mail, and 656 individuals completed the survey. However, it

Does the Privacy Rule:

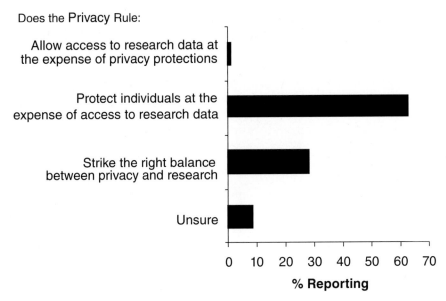

FIGURE 5-2 AcademyHealth Survey: Perspective on the balance of individual protections and research access.
SOURCE: Helms (2008).

is important to note that many professional members of AHA and ACC are practicing physicians, not researchers, and thus were not the intended audience for the survey. Of the individuals completing the survey, 61 percent reported that they had submitted an IRB application since the Privacy Rule was implemented. In general, the respondents indicated that the Privacy Rule had a negative impact on research and did not improve patient privacy. Only 22 percent of respondents reported that the Privacy Rule increased public trust in research, 44 percent reported that it increased confidentiality, 9 percent reported that it decreased privacy breaches, and 14 percent reported that patients' privacy was better protected than before the Privacy Rule. Respondents also indicated that the Privacy Rule had a negative impact on research recruitment, the IRB approval process, the cost and time to conduct research, multicenter research, and the use of deidentified information (Ring, 2007).

North American Association of Central Cancer Registries

In 2006, the North American Association of Central Cancer Registries (NAACCR) conducted a survey of its memberships' experience operating under the Privacy Rule. NAACCR members represent population-based state, regional, and provincial cancer registries in Canada, the United States and its territories. These registries provide cancer incidence data for public health surveillance and research purposes. All 71 members of NAACCR were invited to participate in the survey and 55 responses were received, however, many of the members are not HIPAA covered entities. In general, the respondents indicated that the Privacy Rule has interfered with both basic cancer surveillance and registry-based research (Deapen, 2006).

American Society of Clinical Oncology Interviews

The American Society of Clinical Oncology (ASCO) gathered qualitative information through structured interviews in early 2008 with 27 compliance officials and investigators from 13 institutions about their attitudes toward the Privacy Rule. Participants were presented with three research scenarios prior to their interviews: (1) communication with cancer survivors' family members to request their participation in genetic studies intended to investigate familial cancer syndromes, (2) establishment and use of tissue and data banks that would contain protected health information (PHI), and (3) identification and consent of cancer survivors to participate in long-term survivorship studies. These scenarios were then discussed during the interviews to explore how the Privacy Rule standards are applied at the different institutions, and to gauge the opinions of the researchers and compliance officers toward the regulation.

Unlike some of the surveys, many of the ASCO interview participants indicated that the Privacy Rule had a positive effect on privacy by triggering a reconsideration of how confidential health information is handled in research. However, they also noted that different institutions' IRBs have very different approaches to complying with the Privacy Rule, and this can impede important research. They identified the authorization process as the most significant challenge to complying with the Privacy Rule, especially for future research projects relying on stored tissue and databases. Compliance officers and researchers disagreed on the possibility of obtaining authorization for "future research." Other problems identified included abandoned studies, a lack of training and useful guidance documents on the requirements of the Privacy Rule, and concerns about the security of research databases (ASCO, 2008).

Association of Academic Health Centers Focus Groups

The Association of Academic Health Centers (AAHC) organized focus groups in fall 2007 at five institutions to examine researchers' experiences operating under the HIPAA Privacy Rule. Each focus group included both researchers and compliance personnel from the institution, and all groups were asked the same set of questions. The focus groups reported problems with the Privacy Rule's regulation of research similar to those found in the surveys. Major issues identified included overly conservative interpretation of the Privacy Rule by institutions, diminished ability to recruit research participants, obstacles in accessing stored tissue and genetic datasets, increased cost and time to conduct research, and increased complexity in the IRB review procedures. Participants also indicated that some hospitals and community physicians were opting out of research, rather than attempting to comply with the Privacy Rule (AAHC, 2008)

SELECTION BIAS

Selection bias is created when data are more likely to be collected from one subset of the population than from a representative sample of the entire population (see Box 3-8). This can cause a systematic difference between the characteristics of the individuals included in a study and the individuals not included. Selection bias is problematic for research because it can lead to inaccurate results and it reduces the generalizability of research results to the general population, as indicated by the examples described below.

The Privacy Rule has the potential to contribute to selection bias because it requires researchers to seek patient authorization to access their health records in most situations (see Chapter 4). Selection bias occurs if the individuals who give permission for researchers to access their medical data differ from the group of individuals who are unwilling to give permission for their health information to be used in research. This section provides a detailed overview of the evidence regarding the Privacy Rule's impact on selection bias. It starts with a description of relevant survey data from the researcher surveys described above, then provides a summary of several systematic studies that examined the effect of consent and authorization on selection bias. It concludes with a section summarizing several studies that specifically examined the Privacy Rule's effect on research samples.

Two surveys provide evidence that researchers are concerned about the Privacy Rule introducing selection bias into research. In the AHRQ survey, 74 percent of respondents reported that they had experienced problems with sample representation and bias. One of the most commonly cited reasons for selection bias was that fewer patients have agreed to participate in research since the Privacy Rule was implemented. Respondents indicated that the complicated and lengthy authorization forms required by the Privacy Rule create an impediment to subject recruitment. Also, 42 percent of respondents reported that many small health care entities and other entities serving disadvantaged populations are not participating in research because of an inability to meet all of the Privacy Rule requirements. This results in the underrepresentation of minority populations in many research studies (Walker, 2005).

A survey of NAACCR found similar results, with 36 percent of respondents reporting that the Privacy Rule had introduced selection bias into a research project. The response rate for this survey was 66 percent (Deapen, 2006). A new privacy policy of Veterans Affairs has deepened concern about bias in cancer registries (Kolata, 2007; see also Chapter 6). This policy goes beyond the requirements of the Privacy Rule by requiring each state to sign a national directive setting privacy standards for the use of patients' health information. Some states have refused to sign the directive, asserting that it is not feasible to meet the requirements. As a result, cancer registries will not be representative of the entire U.S. population, and researchers and public health officials will have difficulty interpreting annual cancer statistics published by the National Cancer Institute.

General Studies of Consent and Selection Bias

Numerous studies have directly examined the effect of consent and authorization requirements on selection bias in a systematic manner (Al-Shahi et al., 2005; Harris and Levy, 2008; McCarthy et al., 1999; Trevena et al., 2006; Tu et al., 2004; Ward et al., 2007; Woolf et al., 2000). Woolf and colleagues (2000) at Virginia Commonwealth University studied the effect of requiring patients to give consent on the demographics of research participants at an urban family practice center. Patients were recruited to complete the Health Assessment Survey (HAS). At the end of the HAS, patients were asked to give the researchers permission to contact them by phone or mail, and to review their medical records. Of patients who completed the HAS survey, 67 percent granted researchers consent to complete the follow-up activities, 25 percent actively denied consent, and 8 percent did not answer the question. Patients who gave consent were older, and included fewer women and African Americans than patients who did not give consent. Patients who actively denied consent were younger, included more women, and were more educated than patients giving consent. Also, patients who gave consent differed in health status from patients who denied consent. The researchers concluded that patients willing to release personal health information for health services research differed on important characteristics from patients denying consent (Woolf et al., 2000).

A study conducted by Jack Tu and colleagues (2004) examined the effect of requiring consent on the representativeness of the Registry of the Canadian Stroke Network of the entire population of individuals with stroke. The researchers found that requiring consent before enrollment created a database that was not representative. Patients who agreed to participate in the stroke database were younger, more likely to be alert at admission to the hospital, more likely to be alive at discharge, and were more likely to speak English or French than those patients who did not agree to participate in the database.

In addition, the in-hospital discharge rates differed significantly between enrolled patients (7 percent) and unenrolled patients (22 percent). This difference was likely due to the difficulty in approaching critically ill patients and their family members for recruitment during the ordeal of a stroke. Also, many stroke patients were unable to give or decline to give consent because they were cognitively impaired. The selection bias occurred at hospitals with both high and low participation rates. Based on this study's results, the Registry of the Canadian Stroke Network switched from a consent-based system to a system that uses deidentified patient data and does not require patient consent, to ensure the universality of the registry (Tu et al., 2004). This change, however, eliminated the possibility of follow-up interviews with patients.

In Scotland, a study conducted by Rustam Al-Shahi and colleagues (2005) evaluated the effect of requiring consent on prospective, observational research. The researchers attempted to obtain informed consent to review the medical records and conduct annual follow-up questionnaires of all patients residing in Scotland who presented with intracranial vascular malformation between 1999 and 2002. An ethics board gave the researchers permission to collect baseline and follow-up data on those patients who did not give consent. The researchers found that adults who consented to participate in the study differed on important prognostic variables from patients who did not consent. For example, patients who gave consent were significantly less likely to have intracranial hemorrhage, or to be dependent at presentation. During the yearly follow-ups, patients who gave consent were significantly more likely to have received interventional treatment, less likely to have died, and more likely to have had an epileptic seizure than nonconsenters. The researchers concluded that requiring consent for observational research produced significant selection bias (Al-Shahi et al., 2005).

McCarthy and colleagues (1999) studied a Minnesota law that required patient-informed consent before medical records were permitted to be used by researchers. In this pharmacoepidemiologic study, 73 of 140 potential research participants responded to a request for informed consent, with 26 of the potential research participants authorizing the use of their medical records for the study, and 47 declining. Although it is unclear whether there were important differences between the group of individuals granting informed consent and the group of individuals declining to give informed consent, the authors concluded that the low response rate compromised the generalizability of the study results. In contrast, the researchers achieved a 93 percent recruitment rate for this study in states without a privacy law requiring informed consent, where health care providers could grant access to patient medical records based on a general enrollment authorization. The low participation rate in Minnesota was directly attributed to the state privacy law (McCarthy et al., 1999).

Similar results were found in the study that examined the effect of the recent Australian privacy legislation on selection bias in health research. Trevena and colleagues (2006) conducted a randomized trial comparing recruitment under an opt-out and an opt-in methodology. In the opt-out condition, potential research participants were informed that their physician was participating in a research study, and if they did not wish to be contacted by the researchers they should inform their physician and their contact information would be withheld. Under the opt-in condition, potential research participants could only be contacted by researchers if they affirmatively gave permission in writing, over the phone, or via e-mail to the researchers. This study found that a smaller percentage of potential research participants participated under the opt-in methodology (47 percent) compared to the opt-out methodology (67 percent). Although there was no difference in the age, sex, health status, or socioeconomic status between the opt-in and opt-out populations, individuals in the opt-in group were more likely (75 percent) to prefer an active role in making health care decisions than individuals in the opt-out group (45 percent). The researchers concluded that the opt-in method produced a sample of research participants who differed in important behavioral characteristics from the opt-out method participants (Trevena et al., 2006).

In a study of the United Kingdom Data Protection Act of 1998, epidemiological researchers assessed their ability to recruit potential research participants under this Act. The researchers wrote to a number of physicians and recruited them to participate in the study. If the physicians agreed to participate, the researchers requested the physicians to randomly select 20 of their patients and ask them to consent to being contacted by the researchers. Those individuals granting consent to be contacted were then invited by the researchers to participate in the study. Following this methodology, the researchers were only able to obtain consent from 16 percent of the patients approached. They concluded that such a low participation rate led to selection bias, as well as inadequate statistical power and statistical significance. They documented that health care workers were overrepresented in the resulting study population (Ward et al., 2007).

HIPAA Authorization and Selection Bias

Several studies have explicitly examined whether the provisions of the Privacy Rule contribute to biased research samples. Armstrong and colleagues (2005) at the University of Michigan conducted a 6-month follow-up questionnaire for the Acute Coronary Syndrome Registry. They then compared the percentage of patients who gave consent pre-HIPAA and post-HIPAA for participation in the follow-up survey. In the pre-HIPAA time period, informed consent for the follow-up questionnaire was given over the phone by the patient. In the post-HIPAA era, written informed consent and authorization were required. The percentage of patients consenting to complete the questionnaire decreased from 96 percent in the pre-HIPAA era to 34 percent in the post-HIPAA era. Patients who gave consent post-HIPAA were more likely to be older, married, and white than those who refused to provide consent or did not respond. Patients who gave consent also had lower mortality rates at 6 months than patients who refused consent. The results suggest that implementation of the Privacy Rule led to selection bias in the Registry (Armstrong et al., 2005).

Beebe and colleagues (2007) at the Mayo Clinic College of Medicine in Rochester, MN, followed up on the Armstrong study and conducted a randomized clinical trial that examined the effect of the Privacy Rule on response rate and selection bias. In this study, 6,939 research participants were randomly assigned to one of two research conditions: (1) one condition required patients to complete and return a HIPAA authorization form in order to participate in the study, and (2) in the second condition, patients were not required to complete a HIPAA authorization form to participate. The response rates were significantly different between the condition requiring an authorization form (38 percent) and the condition not requiring an authorization form (55 percent). However, unlike the studies described above, the researchers did not find that the lower response rate translated into a detectable selection bias (Beebe et al., 2007).

The lack of detectable selection bias in this study could be the result of the authorization form used. Beebe and colleagues used a simple one-page authorization form. In the other studies discussed in this section, the authorization forms were much longer than one page and were often written in complex language. Simplifying the authorization form likely minimized the effect of requiring patient authorization on potential research participants' willingness to participate in a study. However, as will be discussed below in the chapter section on the authorization process, a majority of covered entities require lengthy and highly legalistic authorization forms.

Another study that examined the effect of the Privacy Rule on selection bias was conducted by Dunlop and colleagues (2007) at Emory University in Atlanta. In this study the researchers investigated the impact of including an authorization form on the willingness of African Americans to participate in a clinical study of an antihypertensive medication. Research participants were randomly assigned to one of two study conditions in which they received either (1) an informed consent form (informed consent condition), or (2) an informed consent form and an authorization form (authorization condition). The researchers recorded the reasons that potential research participants gave for declining to participate in the study.

The study found that a smaller percentage of research participants in the authorization condition indicated a willingness to participate in the study than in the informed consent condition (27 percent versus 39 percent). This was especially true for individuals over 40 years of age with a high school education or less, and in men. In addition, individuals required to complete an authorization form were more likely to report the following reasons for declining to participate in the study: (1) concerns related to mistrust or fear of research, researchers, or research institutions, and (2) poor comprehension of forms. The researchers concluded that the Privacy Rule's authorization requirement acted as a deterrent for African American participation in research (Dunlop et al., 2007).

EFFICIENCY OF RESEARCH

Substantial evidence indicates that many institution's implementation and interpretation of the Privacy Rule have had a detrimental effect on health researchers' ability to efficiently conduct information-based research. This section reviews the available evidence on the effect of the Privacy Rule, and its interpretation, on the efficiency of research in terms of (1) cost and time, (2) research participant recruitment, (3) IRB oversight of research projects, (4) international collaboration between researchers, and (5) the use of business associate agreements.

Cost and Time

In the 2000 version of the Privacy Rule, HHS estimated that the Privacy Rule would cost the health care industry more than $17.6 billion to implement.[2] The expected costs for research were projected to be more than $40 million the first year, and $585 million over 10 years. The 2002 version of the Privacy Rule reduced the projected costs for implementing the research provisions by $10 million the first year, and $146 million over 10 years.[3] HHS stated that it was difficult to conduct a true cost–benefit analysis of the Privacy Rule because the value of protecting health privacy is difficult to quantify.[4] However, in implementing the Privacy Rule, the agency clearly decided that the benefits of protecting privacy outweighed the economic costs of the Privacy Rule. The aggregate cost to research has

---

[2] Standards for Privacy of Individually Identifiable Health Information: Final Rule, 67 Fed. Reg. 53,255 (August 24, 2002) (codified at 45 C.F.R. parts 160 and 164).

[3] Id. at 53,258.

[4] Id. at 53,255.

not been measured or estimated since April 2003, and as outlined below, researchers' estimates of the increase in cost and time attributable to the Privacy Rule vary widely.

In a recent article published in the *Annual Review of Medicine*, Nosowsky and Giordano (2006) reviewed the existing evidence on the effect of the Privacy Rule on research, and concluded that the costs projected by HHS have more than been realized by covered entities, researchers, and IRBs, although no figures were cited. They attributed the increased research costs to the large amounts of paperwork required by the Privacy Rule, increased staff time, and difficulties in recruiting research participants. They concluded that these additional burdens on research have pushed researchers to reformulate and abandon many studies. Furthermore, the authors speculated that these changes have increased the need for researchers to obtain additional funding, discouraged investigator-initiated research, and caused many smaller research projects to end (Nosowsky and Giordano, 2006).

Many researchers report that the implementation of the Privacy Rule increased the cost of conducting health research and increased the time necessary to conduct a research project from start to finish. The national survey of epidemiologists found that most respondents believe the Privacy Rule increased the cost and time of conducting health research. In this survey, 90 percent of the respondents reported an increase in resource expenditure, with 40 percent indicating that the Privacy Rule increased research costs a great deal (i.e., 4–5 on the Likert scale). Half of the respondents indicated that the additional time required to comply with the Privacy Rule was great (4–5 on the Likert scale) (Figure 5-3a) (Ness, 2007). In the AHA/ACC survey, 78 percent of respondents reported that the Privacy Rule increased the cost of research, and 79 percent reported that it increased the time to conduct research (Ring, 2007).

The AcademyHealth survey results were similar, with 86 percent of respondents reporting that the Privacy Rule increased the time necessary for research, and 8 percent of those reporting that the increase was so great that it led some researchers to forego projects. In terms of cost, 73 percent of respondents reported that the Privacy Rule increased the cost of research (4 percent much more, 24 percent significantly more, and 45 percent somewhat more) (Helms, 2008) (Figure 5-3b).

In the HMORN survey of investigators, 55 percent of respondents reported that study time lines were negatively affected by the Privacy Rule (Figure 5-4). A third of the investigators indicated that the Privacy Rule delayed their research by 1 to more than 3 months. Also, investigators reported that the Privacy Rule led to a median of 20 additional staff hours required to comply with the requirements of the regulation. Twelve percent of respondents reported that 100 or more staff hours were required. In one extreme case in the structured interview portion of this survey, an inves-

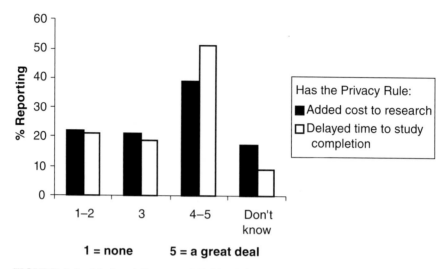

FIGURE 5-3a National Survey of Epidemiologists: Impact on cost and time to complete research.
SOURCE: Ness (2007).

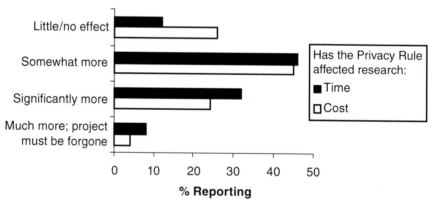

FIGURE 5-3b AcademyHealth Survey: Impact on cost and time to complete research.
SOURCE: Helms (2008).

tigator said that compliance with the HIPAA procedures required about 1,000–2,000 additional hours of staff time, and added $100,000–$200,000 in unanticipated costs (Greene et al., 2008). In the NAACCR survey of cancer registries, 68 percent of respondents reported that the Privacy Rule delayed a research project or caused it to take longer than it would have

Has the Privacy Rule added to:

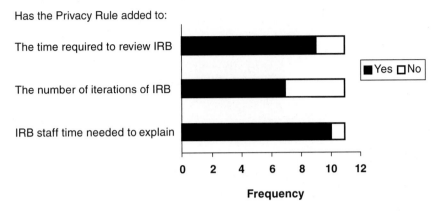

FIGURE 5-4 HMO Research Network Survey of Institutional Review Board Administrators. Responses to the question: Taken as a whole, do you think the Health Insurance Portability and Accountability Act Privacy Rule has added to. . . . SOURCE: Greene et al. (2008).

taken pre-HIPAA. In addition, 66 percent of respondents indicated that the Privacy Rule had been cited as the reason for actions that interfered with nonresearch operations of the cancer registry, such as basic surveillance (Deapen, 2006).

A number of researchers have attempted to quantitatively document the increased time and cost of research attributable to the implementation of the Privacy Rule at their institutions. It is important to note that these studies are site specific and depend on how institutions interpret and implement the Privacy Rule. A recent letter to the editor of *Anesthesiology* reported on the amount of research staff hours spent per month on recruitment and follow-up activities in a randomized clinical trial at the University of Pittsburgh, before and after the Privacy Rule went into effect. Implementation of the Privacy Rule led to a 75-hour increase per month in staff time spent updating work logs, and a 77-hour increase in time spent on HIPAA implementation tasks. According to the authors' calculations, this was a 70 percent increase in staff hours above the monthly base workload. The authors did not try to determine which aspects of the Privacy Rule were responsible for the recorded increases (Williams et al., 2007).

Similarly, the Armstrong study on the Acute Coronary Syndrome Registry documented that the incremental cost for this registry at the University of Michigan of complying with the Privacy Rule was $8,704.50 for the first year, and an additional $4,558.50 for each year thereafter. The authors did not report the total expenditure of the study but suggested that this was a substantial increase in the study's budget (Armstrong et al., 2005).

Johns Hopkins University estimates that the cost of complying with the Privacy Rule is about $2 million annually (Friedman, 2006). Since the Privacy Rule was implemented, the institution calculated that it has required nearly 26,000 of its faculty and staff to pass a written test on their understanding of the Privacy Rule.

Recruitment

A number of researchers have also demonstrated that many interpretations of the Privacy Rule have made research recruitment more difficult (Table 5-2). During a clinical trial evaluating the efficacy of an educational strategy to inform veterans about the National Cancer Institute/Department of Veterans Affairs Selenium and Vitamin E Cancer Prevention Trial (SELECT), Wolf and Bennett (2006) monitored the recruitment of research participants before and after implementation of the Privacy Rule. Several recruitment methods were used throughout this clinical trial, depending on the phase of HIPAA implementation. Before the Privacy Rule was implemented, potential research participants were directly approached by research assistants for informed consent. After the Privacy Rule was implemented, research assistants could no longer approach potential research participants; recruitment was done by hospital staff. The post-HIPAA recruitment protocol was modified once to increase participation rates. Under the modified protocol, potential research participants were introduced to the study by desk staff at the medical clinic where the study was conducted, all clinic staff members were reminded of the study, and a research assistant was stationed prominently in the medical clinic.

The researchers were able to recruit seven patients a week in the pre-HIPAA phase. The average time to recruit a patient was 4.1 hours, for an average cost of $49 per patient. The study was on target to complete recruitment in 60 weeks. Immediately after the Privacy Rule was implemented, recruitment decreased by 73 percent to 1.9 patients per week. The average time to recruit each new patient was 14.1 hours, for a cost of $169 per patient. Meeting the recruitment goals of the study at this rate would require 158 weeks. The modified recruitment protocol increased recruitment to 7.1 patients a week, required 3.9 hours, and cost $52 per patient. The modified recruitment strategy was measured again at a later date in the study to assess whether the modified protocol could be maintained. During this time period, 5.2 patients were recruited per week. Research assistants needed an average of 5.4 hours to recruit each patient, for a cost of $65 per patient.

The authors concluded that the Privacy Rule dramatically hindered researchers' ability to recruit research participants. Implementation of the

TABLE 5-2 Research Participant Recruitment Before and After Implementation of the Privacy Rule

Wolf and Bennett: Selenium and Vitamin E Cancer Prevention Trial in Veterans (2006)	
Pre-HIPAA	7 patients recruited per week
Post-HIPAA	1.9 patients recruited per week
Modified protocol (time period 1)	7.1 patients recruited per week
Modified protocol (time period 2)	5.2 patients recruited per week
Roberta Ness: Pregnancy Exposures and Preeclampsia Prevention (2005)	
Pre-HIPAA (1997–2001)	12.4 patients recruited per week
HIPAA implementation (2002)	0.0 patients recruited per week
No waivers 1 (4/03–9/03)	2.5 patients recruited per week
Waivers of authorization (10/03–6/04)	5.7 patients recruited per week
No waivers 2 (6/04)	3.3 patients recruited per week
Beebe and Colleagues: HIPAA Authorization and Willingness to Participate (2007)	
No authorization	55.0% of potential research subjects participated
Authorization	39.8% of potential research subjects participated
Dunlop and Colleagues: HIPAA Authorization and Willingness to Participate (2007)	
No authorization	39% of potential research subjects participated
Authorization	27% of potential research subjects participated

SOURCES: Beebe et al. (2007); Dunlop et al. (2007); Ness (2005); Wolf and Bennett (2006).

Privacy Rule increased the cost and time required for recruitment and made it more difficult to achieve an appropriate-sized research sample. Although the modified protocol increased recruitment, the fact that the initial recruitment level could not be maintained over time suggests that the new protocol required a great deal of effort and did not completely solve recruitment difficulties. In addition, an intensive evaluation of a study's recruitment process to devise a new strategy, as was required to develop the modified protocol, costs money, takes time, and may not always be possible (Wolf and Bennett, 2006).

A reduced rate of recruitment following implementation of the Privacy Rule was also documented by Roberta Ness in the course of a study on pregnancy exposures and preeclampsia prevention at the University of Pittsburgh. Again, the recruitment methods were divided into several different time periods: (1) pre-HIPAA (1997–2001), (2) 2002, (3) April 2003–September 2003, (4) October 2003–May 2004, and (5) June 2004. In the pre-HIPAA time period, researchers recruited an average of 12.4 women a week. In 2002 recruitment was shut down completely for 4 months while the covered entity where the study was being conducted decided how to implement the requirements of the Privacy Rule.

From April 2003 to September 2003, recruitment was allowed to continue, but the covered entity was unwilling to grant any waivers of authorization. Researchers recruited only 2.5 women a week. In October 2003, the covered entity allowed waivers of authorization to be issued, and the researchers were able to review potential research participants' medical records without obtaining authorization. However, the waivers of authorization required that the researchers obtain the consent of the potential research participants' health care providers before the researchers could approach individuals for participation in the study. Approximately 5.7 women a week were recruited following this protocol. The need for the health care providers' permission prevented recruitment from reaching pre-HIPAA levels. The covered entity merged with another covered entity in June 2004, and the waiver of authorization was retracted. Recruitment immediately fell to 3.3 women a week (Ness, 2005). These recruitment numbers clearly demonstrate that the implementation and interpretation of the Privacy Rule, and the availability of waivers of authorization, can have an enormous influence on recruitment success. They also show that conducting research under changing policies, organization, or interpretations of the Privacy Rule can be problematic.

Several studies that were discussed previously provide further evidence that many interpretations of the Privacy Rule have made research recruitment more difficult. The Beebe study found that the percentage of potential research participants willing to participate declined when HIPAA authorization was required at the Mayo Clinic College of Medicine. More than half—55 percent—of potential research participants participated in the study when authorization was not required, but only 39.8 percent of potential research participants took part if they were required to complete an authorization form (Beebe et al., 2007). In the Dunlop study, 39 percent of potential research participants indicated a willingness to participate in a clinical trial of a hypertensive medication when authorization was not required. Only 27 percent indicated a willingness to participate when authorization was required (Dunlop et al., 2007).

Also, the national survey of epidemiologists found Privacy Rule modifications were needed in 84.8 percent of proposed research protocols. Of these cases, 68 percent of respondents reported that these modifications increased recruitment difficulties a great deal (4–5 on the Likert scale) (Ness, 2007). In the AcademyHealth survey, 47 percent of respondents reported that the Privacy Rule decreased recruitment (Helms, 2008). Similarly, the 49 percent of respondents to the AHA/ACC survey reported that the Privacy Rule decreased recruitment by more than 10 percent (Ring, 2007).

IRB and Privacy Board Oversight

A previous IOM report noted that the workload of IRBs, and the complexity of their work, has been steadily increasing as a result of new and evolving requirements for research regulation and documentation (IOM, 2002), including the HIPAA Privacy Rule. This heavy burden has increased the difficulty of both recruiting knowledgeable IRB members and allowing them sufficient time for the necessary ethical reflection to make appropriate decisions about human research projects. In addition, the report noted that the extreme variability in the approval decisions and regulatory interpretations among IRBs is one of the weaknesses in the current protection system (IOM, 2002). Recent findings from surveys and other studies indicate that these issues are a continuing concern for both IRBs and Privacy Boards. This section provides a detailed review of the evidence that the Privacy Rule, and its interpretation, has had a detrimental effect on the oversight process for reviewing research proposals, including information on: (1) IRB approval, (2) exemption from full IRB review, (3) waiver of authorization, (4) differentiating types of research, and (5) inconsistent interpretation of the Privacy Rule by IRBs and Privacy Boards in multicenter research projects.

IRB Approval

Recent surveys provide evidence that the Privacy Rule, or its interpretation, has reduced the efficiency of health research by affecting researchers' ability to move a study through the IRB approval process. In the AHRQ survey, 94 percent of respondents stated that the Privacy Rule impacted the design and conduct of health services research. The respondents who reported that the Privacy Rule had no impact on study design were all researchers who used only deidentified data and were not required to go through the IRB/Privacy Board review process under the Privacy Rule (Walker, 2005). Similarly, in the national survey of epidemiologists, 87 percent of respondents reported an increase in the time required for preparing a research proposal for review by an IRB (Ness, 2007).

The AcademyHealth survey found that 69 percent of respondents reported difficulty gaining approval from IRBs to collect PHI. Respondents also reported difficulty gaining approval to collect PHI from health plans (32 percent), institution lawyers (29 percent), and physicians (25 percent). In the HMORN survey of investigators, respondents reported that they were required to submit a research project for a median of two additional IRB iterations after the Privacy Rule was implemented. Twenty percent of investigators reported that four or more IRB iterations were required. Also, investigators reported that in one-third of study protocols, modifications were due to an IRB requirement. In that survey, 29 percent of investigators reported that an IRB required them to modify their planned method of identifying potential research participants, 29 percent reported that an IRB put restrictions on the kind of identifiers that could be collected, and 59 percent reported that an IRB required a study to be modified to include additional consent and/or authorization language (Greene et al., 2008). The AHA/ACC survey also found that 67 percent of respondents reported that the IRB submission process was made more complex by the Privacy Rule (Ring, 2007).

Exemption from Full IRB Review

Certain types of research that pose minimal risk to human subjects are exempt from IRB review under the Common Rule (45 C.F.R. § 46.101). For these studies, an IRB chair or member can review an application for exemption and determine if the study meets the criteria for exemption. If the study qualifies for exemption, then no further IRB review is necessary. Expedited IRB review is a process allowed by the Common Rule (45 C.F.R. § 46.110) in which an IRB chair or member reviews the entire study protocol. A study conducted by O'Herrin and colleagues (2004) examined the effect of the Privacy Rule on applications for IRB exemption for proposed research projects at the University of Wisconsin. This study was broken down into three time periods: (1) September 1999–December 2000, during which there was no specific process for handling requests for IRB exemption for medical records studies; (2) January 2001–December 2002, during which the institution followed a standardized procedure for Applications for Exemption; and (3) January 2003–March 2003, during which the IRB became fully compliant with the Privacy Rule.

During Period 1, all the medical records research projects submitted to the IRB were approved under "expedited" IRB review procedures. In Period 2, 89 percent of the applications received an IRB exemption without revision. Of the applications that required revision, 36 percent were revised and successfully approved for exemption within 75 ± 64 days of the original submission. The remaining applications required review by the full IRB committee, but were all ultimately given approval. In Period 3, when the covered entity was in full compliance with the Privacy Rule, 59 percent of proposals received exemption from full IRB review without revision in 12 ± 23 days. Of the projects requiring revision, 50 percent were revised and approved within 29 ± 35 days of the initial submission.

The percentage of projects that required full IRB committee review increased from 0 percent in Period 1, to 7 percent in Period 2, to 16 percent in Period 3. The authors of this study concluded that the Privacy Rule complicated the IRB review process because a larger percentage of studies became ineligible for IRB exemption or expedited IRB review. Also, the complexity of the IRB approval process discouraged many researchers from completing their proposed research study. Of the applications that required full IRB committee review, 77 percent were abandoned by the researchers in Period 3. Most of the abandoned studies were chart reviews, and there was no evidence that the full IRB committee review was justified or a necessary change that safeguarded research participants' privacy (O'Herrin et al., 2004).

Waiver of Authorization

The Privacy Rule allows a covered entity to use and disclose PHI for research purposes without patient authorization if an IRB or Privacy Board determines that a research project meets three criteria, including minimal risk to patient privacy, and whether the study could practicably be conducted without the waiver of authorization and without access to and use of PHI (see Chapter 4). However, surveys indicate that many researchers have experienced difficulty in obtaining a waiver of authorization. In the national survey of epidemiologists, 40 percent of respondents reported that they had attempted to obtain a waiver of authorization under the Privacy Rule. Of these researchers, 31 percent reported a high level of difficulty in obtaining a waiver (4–5 on the Likert scale) (Ness, 2007).

The AcademyHealth survey also examined this issue, with 62 percent of respondents reporting that they had been involved in one or more studies requiring waivers or alterations of authorization requirements by IRBs (65 percent had been involved in 2–5 studies, and 3 percent had been involved in more than 20 studies). Among respondents who had requested waivers or alteration of waivers from IRBs or Privacy Boards, 59 percent reported that the availability of existing datasets has been impacted by the Privacy Rule. Only 40 percent of the respondents who had requested waivers or alterations of authorization reported that they were successful in accessing data from an existing dataset in its original form under an approved waiver of authorization (Helms, 2008). In the AHA/ACC survey, 59 percent of respondents reported attempting to obtain a waiver of authorization. Of those respondents, 69 percent reported the waiver was hard to attain (Ring, 2007).

Differentiating Various Types of Research

Scientific and ethical difficulties may arise when rules that were developed to guide clinical research are applied to other kinds of research (Casarett et al., 2005). Under the Privacy Rule, IRBs are charged with reviewing different types of health research that were previously not in their purview, including many types of health services research that use data that have been anonymized and are thus exempt under the Common Rule, so making judgments about approval and determining which research studies require a waiver of authorization is a challenge. Some evidence indicates that IRBs do not recognize important differences among various types of health research. In the AcademyHealth survey, 44 percent of the respondents reported that IRBs did not correctly differentiate between clinical research and health services research (and 25 percent were unsure). Clinical research often involves the study of a new drug or experimental treatment on human subjects. In contrast, respondents to the AcademyHealth survey reported that most of health services research involves survey or questionnaire data (82 percent), medical record review (70 percent), and administrative data (66 percent). Only a small portion of respondents reported doing health research studies that involved direct human contact; 9 percent reported conducting research that required the collection of specimens, and 5 percent reported conducting research on existing specimens. Also, survey respondents indicated that IRBs often did not differentiate between the cost and time required to conduct health services research compared to clinical research (Helms, 2008).

Inconsistent Interpretation of the Privacy Rule: Multicenter Research

Research studies that entail the collection of data from multiple sites involve the jurisdiction of multiple IRBs or Privacy Boards. The Privacy Rule does not require a researcher to obtain a waiver of authorization from the IRB or Privacy Board of every entity that is contributing PHI. Covered entities are permitted to rely on a waiver of authorization approved by as few as one IRB or Privacy Board with jurisdiction. However, a covered entity may decide to require approval from its own IRB or Privacy Board prior to disclosing PHI to the requesting researcher, regardless of whether another IRB or Privacy Board had already granted a waiver of authorization. The Privacy Rule does not address potential disagreements between IRBs or Privacy Boards, but HHS "strongly encourages" researchers to notify IRBs and Privacy Boards of any prior reviews of a research protocol to reduce the chance of IRBs and Privacy Boards disagreeing.

Surveys indicate that the Privacy Rule has had a detrimental effect on the efficiency of multicenter health research because the participating covered entities, IRBs, and Privacy Boards interpret the Privacy Rule differently (AAHC, 2008; Ring, 2007). Researchers conducting a single study at different locations are routinely required to go through multiple IRB/Privacy Board review processes, and to use different authorization forms and methodology across the various sites, even though the Privacy Rule permits reliance on the review or decision of one IRB or Privacy Board for all sites.

In the AHRQ survey, 65 percent of respondents reported problems satisfying the requirements of multiple IRBs for multisite studies. One area with which researchers reported significant frustration was the lack of consistent consent and authorization forms (Walker, 2005). The Academy-Health survey found that 28 percent of researchers who required a waiver of authorization to conduct a study were required to get the waiver from all research sites involved. Only 9 percent of the respondents reported that the same waiver was used at all sites, and 6 percent reported the waivers were required from more than one, but not all, sites. Three percent of the respondents reported that they were unable to proceed with a multisite study because they were unable to resolve disagreement among sites (Helms, 2008).

In the HMORN survey of investigators, 78 percent of respondents reported participating in multicenter research. Of these respondents 54 percent indicated that different IRBs raised different concerns about the same study protocol, and 45 percent of respondents reported that these different concerns led to protocol variability across the different sites (Figure 5-5). The HMORN survey of IRB administrators found that 4 of the 11 IRBs reported requiring proof of Privacy Rule–related training for all participating investigators in a study, even if they were from another site. This requirement is not a provision of the Privacy Rule (Greene et al., 2008).

The national survey of epidemiologists also confirms that many researchers are frustrated with the process of conducting research at multiple covered entities. In the survey, 76.8 percent of respondents reported difficulties with the Privacy Rule when conducting multicenter research. The problems related to site-specific variability in the research design and method in 40 percent of studies. The survey further explored this issue by presenting survey participants with five case studies that should have been approved without patient authorization either unconditionally or with a waiver of authorization under the Privacy Rule. However, on each of the case studies, 4.7 to 33.8 percent of respondents reported that their IRB would disapprove the study. Only 4.9 to 33.8 percent believed that their IRB would unconditionally approve the studies, and 13.3 to 26.7 percent reported that they did not know what their IRB would require. To further complicate multicenter research, a minority of respondents (17.3 percent) knew of covered entities unwilling to do any clinical research, regardless of the IRB's interpretation of the Privacy Rule (Ness, 2007).

In addition to the survey results, several studies have directly examined the effect of the Privacy Rule, or its interpretation, on multicenter research. Lydon-Rochelle and Holt (2004) at the University of Washington documented their experience in attempting to access medical records from 19 area hospitals during the Privacy Rule implementation period, for a study designed to assess the accuracy of maternally linked birth records. They explained to the participating hospitals that their study protocol met

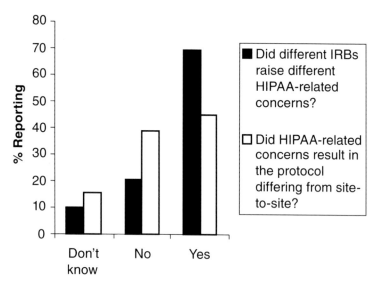

FIGURE 5-5 HMO Research Network Survey of Researchers: Multisite research.
NOTE: HIPAA = Health Insurance Portability and Accountability Act; IRB = Institutional Review Board.
SOURCE: Greene et al. (2008).

the Privacy Rule waiver of authorization requirement and encouraged the hospitals' IRBs to rely on their IRB's approval of the study. However, the 19 IRBs displayed great variability in their willingness to approve the study.

None of the 19 hospitals agreed to rely on the researchers' own institution's IRB approval of the study. Ten hospitals used an expedited in-house IRB review process for the study, and 9 required a full IRB review of the study. The 9 IRBs requiring full review of the study cited concerns over the Privacy Rule's civil and criminal penalties as the main reason for denying expedited review or for not honoring another IRB's decisions. All 19 of the reviewing IRBs required different application forms, content, and procedures for complying with the Privacy Rule. The authors concluded that the Privacy Rule has increased the difficulty of conducting multicenter health research because of the challenges of navigating through many IRBs' review processes (Lydon-Rochelle and Holt, 2004).

A second study that examined the institutional variability in IRB approval processes was conducted by Newgard and colleagues (2005). The researchers sent 27 hospitals an identical research protocol for a study examining a decision rule to identify children seriously injured in motor vehicle crashes in Los Angeles County. This was a minimal risk observational study and clearly met the requirements for a waiver of authorization. However, 6 of the 27 hospitals refused to participate in the study at all. Of the remaining 21 hospitals, the median time for the study to be approved by the covered entities' IRBs was 118 days. Significant differences in approval times were seen across the different covered entities.

The researchers recognized they could not conclusively attribute the hospitals' refusals to participate in the study and the long IRB review processes to the Privacy Rule itself. However, they believed the Privacy Rule was largely responsible for the results. They compared their experience to a previous study conducted in Los Angeles County before the implementation of the Privacy Rule. The same 27 hospitals were approached for participation in a randomized, controlled, interventional trial for emergent airway management in children with a waiver of consent. All 27 hospitals approved the airway protocol without change, while only 21 of the same 27 hospitals approved Newgard and colleagues' minimal risk, noninterventional study. The authors believed this difference was directly attributable to the complex requirements of the Privacy Rule and the perceived institutional risks associated with research (Newgard et al., 2005).

A third study that examined the impact of allowing multiple IRBs to review the same research proposal was conducted by Greene and colleagues (2006). Participants were recruited through a mailed invitation for a survey of psychosocial outcomes after prophylactic mastectomy. A second mailing and a follow-up phone call were made to nonresponders. The study's protocol was reviewed by six IRBs. All of the IRBs requested that the protocol, letters, and phone call script be modified. Resolving all of the IRBs' concerns took two to eight iterations at each site, and achieving a uniform study methodology across the sites was impossible. Also, the response rates at the six institutions varied greatly, ranging from 40.9 to 70.8 percent among living individuals, to 60.7 to 84.6 percent among living individuals with physician consent and correct address.

The authors concluded that having multiple IRBs review the same study protocol lengthened the study time line, adversely affected the budget, and created protocol variability that may have affected response rate (Greene et al., 2006). This study did not specifically focus on the Privacy Rule. However, as demonstrated by the other studies discussed in this section, since the Privacy Rule was implemented, IRBs are often unwilling to honor the decisions of other IRBs. The Privacy Rule likely contributed to the six IRBs in this study all insisting on reviewing the same research protocol and for the resulting variability in study design.

Business Associate Agreements

The AcademyHealth survey indicated that most health services researchers do not use business associate agreements to gain access to health data, but when they do, difficulties often arise. Twenty-two percent of the respondents reported using a business associate agreement to conduct research, and of these respondents, most reported that the business associate agreement negatively impacted research activities because it complicated the research process, made research more time consuming, and added more paperwork. Of the respondents who reported that they have used an existing dataset to conduct research, 28 percent indicated that they had to develop a business associate relationship with the covered entity to gain access to the dataset. Another 14 percent reported use of an intermediary organization that had a business associate relationship with the covered entity to gain access to an existing dataset (Helms, 2008).

International Collaboration

A report by Dutch researchers suggests that the Privacy Rule, or its interpretation, has made it more difficult for international researchers to collaborate with U.S. research centers (Kompanje and Maas, 2006). The authors recorded their experiences operating under the Privacy Rule in an international, multicenter, Phase III trial on the safety and efficacy of a neuroprotective agent in traumatic brain injury. The researchers compared the completion of screening logs between research centers in the United States and Europe. Because of the Privacy Rule, many of the U.S. screening logs had a large amount of missing data. All the European sites reported the actual age of the research participants on their screening logs, but only 5 of the 15 U.S. sites reported the age. The remaining 10 U.S. sites only reported whether the patient met the inclusion criteria for the study. Also, all the European sites reported the date and time of the injury, while only 10 U.S. sites provided this information. Information on secondary insults and the Glasgow Coma Scale were often omitted from the screening logs of U.S. sites.

Overly conservative or variable interpretations of the Privacy Rule prevented many U.S. sites from providing the requisite data to the researchers and made it difficult for the researchers to monitor their study for selection bias and quality (Kompanje and Maas, 2006). In many situations, having international data is important to study a health problem. How often the Privacy Rule, or its interpretation, hinders U.S. collaboration in international research is unclear. But it is very conceivable that other international researchers have experienced frustrations similar to the Dutch researchers over collecting data from U.S. sites, or have even abandoned attempts to work with U.S. research centers due to the restrictions of the Privacy Rule.

ABANDONED STUDIES

Some evidence, mostly in the form of case studies and survey results, shows that researchers have abandoned research studies that they would have pursued prior to the Privacy Rule. The paucity of systematic analysis is likely because abandoned research studies are more difficult to measure and to conclusively document than the other aspects of research that have been affected by the Privacy Rule. Documenting something that did not happen (i.e., an abandoned study) is more challenging than measuring something that did happen (e.g., selection bias, increased inefficiency). One study that examined abandoned studies in a systematic manner was the study by O'Herrin et al. (2004), discussed previously. The researchers determined that 77 percent of research proposals at the University of Wisconsin that were required to be reviewed by the full IRB, rather than being exempted from IRB review or receiving expedited review, were abandoned by investigators. The study did not try to tease out the reasons for abandonment or the appropriateness of abandonment (O'Herrin et al., 2004).

A well-publicized instance of the Privacy Rule leading to studies being abandoned was outlined in the *San Francisco Chronicle*. Reporting of cancer cases to the State of California Cancer Registry is required by law and should not have been affected by the implementation Privacy Rule. However, after the Privacy Rule became effective, 17 hospitals in the Bay area restricted the registry's access to patient data, endangering many studies that relied on the California Cancer Registry for data. For example, a study examining why African Americans in the Bay Area have a higher risk of lung cancer than other racial and ethnic groups was nearly abandoned after the Privacy Rule came into effect because of the difficulty of collecting data (Russell, 2004b). This problem was created by the hospitals' overly conservative interpretation of the Privacy Rule, not the actual requirements of the Privacy Rule. A settlement was eventually reached after 2 years of disagreement, and the California Cancer Registry now has full access to the files and records of cancer patients, as is required in all states (Russell, 2004a).

A second instance of an institution's interpretation of the Privacy Rule leading to an abandoned study was reported in the Minneapolis *Star Tribune*. For more than 25 years, researchers at the University of Minnesota–Twin Cities were allowed to access more than 40,000 Minnesotans' medical records as part of a longitudinal study into heart attacks and cholesterol-lowering drugs. This study depended on researchers viewing the medical records of patients without the individuals' consent. After the Privacy Rule was implemented, data collection for this study was put on hold because the researchers were unable to obtain a waiver of authorization. The researchers decided not to seek additional grant money for the study because it was unclear whether they could continue without a seriously modified protocol under the Privacy Rule (Kaiser, 2006; Shaffer, 2006).

In addition, a significant number of researchers surveyed attribute abandoned studies to the Privacy Rule. In the NAACCR survey, 19 percent of respondents cited the Privacy Rule as a reason for stopping or preventing a research project (Howe et al., 2006). In the AHRQ survey, 45 percent of respondents described a study that had been stopped or altered because the respondents found it was not possible to redesign a study protocol to comply with the Privacy Rule. Examples of studies that were ended included: (1) follow-up studies where patients were tracked through a number of health facilities for services; (2) studies involving community health centers, community-based mental health and substance abuse programs, and rural sites; (3) longitudinal studies, where the Privacy Rule requires researchers to obtain multiple authorizations; and (4) research evaluating government programs and clinical interventions in order to improve patient population health (Walker, 2005).

In the HMORN survey of investigators, 65 percent of respondents agreed that they were hesitant to pursue new study ideas due to the Privacy Rule (Figure 5-6) (Greene et al., 2008). In the AcademyHealth survey, 13 percent of respondents reported that an IRB or Privacy Board has prevented a study in which they were involved from moving forward due to the IRB or Privacy Board's concern about violating the Privacy Rule. Ten percent of respondents said they considered or developed a study, but did not submit it to the IRB or Privacy Board because they thought it would not be approved due to their IRB or Privacy Board's conservative interpretation of the Privacy Rule (Helms, 2008). In addition, in the ASCO survey, six investigators said they had abandoned genetic studies on family members of individuals diagnosed with cancer because of difficulty in moving the projects through the IRB approval process. IRBs were most concerned about the privacy of the cancer patients (ASCO, 2008).

DEIDENTIFIED INFORMATION

In drafting the Privacy Rule, HHS specifically excluded deidentified information from the definition of PHI (see Chapter 4). In principle, researchers can access and use deidentified information without patient authorization. However, many researchers have reported that the deidentification provisions of the Privacy Rule do not provide an effective way to obtain health data for research. The two major problems reported are that researchers have difficulty obtaining deidentified information from covered entities and that data that have been deidentified according to the Privacy Rule provisions (which are more stringent than the Common Rule provisions) are of poor quality and difficult to use in research.

The Privacy Rule makes researchers
hesitant to pursue new studies:

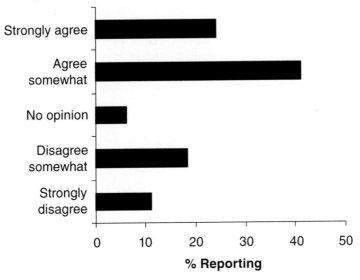

FIGURE 5-6 HMO Research Network Survey of Researchers. Responses to the question: There are study ideas that I have considered pursuing, but am hesitant to do so because of the Health Insurance Portability and Accountability Act regulations.
SOURCE: Greene et al. (2008).

Access to Deidentified Data

Survey data indicate that researchers often have difficulty obtaining deidentified information from covered entities. In the national survey of epidemiologists, half of the respondents reported accessing deidentified information since the Privacy Rule was implemented. Of this half, 40 percent reported a high level of difficulty in gaining access to this deidentified information (i.e., 4–5 on the Likert scale) (Ness, 2007). In addition, the AHRQ survey found that 39 percent of respondents reported problems obtaining deidentified data from covered entities or had problems creating deidentified datasets. Most respondents to the survey also reported concerns about the use of the statistical method to certify deidentified data. Many were looking for an alternative option to the "safe harbor" process of deidentification because they believed the resultant datasets were too restrictive for health services research (Walker, 2005).

The HMORN survey of investigators also found similar results. Of the respondents, 42 percent reported that accessing deidentified data had occasionally been difficult, and 13 percent reported that it was "routinely difficult." However, in the HMORN survey of IRB administrators, 4 of the 11 sites reported having individuals on staff who could assist with the deidentification of data using the statistical method (Greene et al., 2008). In the AHA/ACC survey, only 32 percent of respondents reported attempting to use deidentified data for research. Of these respondents, 76 percent reported that the process was difficult (Ring, 2007).

Quality of Deidentified Data

Clause and colleagues (2004) at the Albany College of Pharmacy designed a study to measure the amount of data that is lost when PHI is deidentified under the safe harbor provision of the Privacy Rule (see Chapter 4). For this study, the researchers first created a limited dataset from the pharmacy, administrative, and financial files of patients discharged from hospitals within the Northeast Health System. A limited dataset is a collection of health information compiled for research in which 16 direct identifiers are removed from the PHI (see Chapter 4). A limited dataset allows researchers to access more information than deidentified information because the Privacy Rule requires that researchers using a limited dataset enter into a data use agreement specifying the permitted uses and disclosures of the limited dataset. The researchers then converted the limited dataset into deidentified information under the safe harbor provision of the Privacy Rule, which requires removal of 18 personal identifiers. They measured data lost as a function of unique data elements (UDEs) for both the limited dataset and the deidentified information.

This study found that a large percentage of data was lost when information was deidentified. The limited dataset represented 4,738 patient discharges and contained 810,456 UDEs in 322,657 records. The deidentified dataset represented 4,733 patient discharges but only contained 562,171 UDEs. This means that the deidentified dataset contained 31 percent fewer UDEs than the limited dataset. The researchers reported that much of the information lost when the information was deidentified was of the type that is of the most interest to researchers, such as time between episodes of care. The researchers concluded that deidentified data removes too much information to produce data useful for conducting good research (Clause et al., 2004).

Results from the AcademyHealth survey also indicate concern about the usefulness of deidentified data for research. In this survey, 62 percent of the respondents reported that the use of deidentified data had a negative impact on research, 38 percent reported that the removal of the required identifiers interfered somewhat with research, and 21 percent reported that the removal of identifiers interfered significantly with research. Only 3 percent of the respondents reported that the removal of identifiers did not interfere with research (Helms, 2008).

AUTHORIZATION PROCESS

The authorization provisions of the Privacy Rule are relevant to health researchers because although there are some situations in which researchers can obtain PHI without authorization (i.e., by obtaining an IRB/Privacy Board waiver of authorization, or using limited datasets or deidentified information), for many research projects, researchers must obtain a signed authorization form from each research participant (see Chapter 4). Many researchers have expressed dissatisfaction with how the authorization process has been interpreted and implemented by covered entities. Researchers report that many IRBs and Privacy Boards require lengthy and complex wording to describe the authorization within consent forms. They claim that the extra language added to consent forms is confusing to research participants, burdens the informed consent process, and undermines research recruitment (AAHC, 2008; Shalowitz and Wendler, 2006).

In the HMORN survey of investigators, 76 percent of respondents reported that they had incorporated the Privacy Rule's requirements for authorization directly into their informed consent forms. However, in the structured interviews of investigators, all four respondents who conducted primary data collection reported that they were obliged by their IRB to augment the consent and authorization procedures for their studies after the Privacy Rule was implemented. All four investigators also stated that the Privacy Rule authorization language had an adverse effect on research recruitment because it increased patient confusion and frustration. Likewise, in the HMORN survey of IRB administrators, 54.6 percent of respondents stated that study participants are unduly burdened by the complexity of authorization forms (Greene et al., 2008).

Studies analyzing the readability of Privacy Rule–compliant authorization forms document the effect of complex authorization forms on individuals' willingness to participate in research. In a letter to the editor of the *Annals of Internal Medicine*, Breese and colleagues (2004) outlined an evaluation of the readability and length of authorization forms. The researchers analyzed the authorization templates from the 125 academic medical centers receiving the most funding from the National Institutes of Health and from 31 independent IRBs. First, the authors determined that the authorization form added an average of two pages of additional material to the informed consent form, or about 744 extra words.

Next, the researchers looked at the authorization forms' readability using three formulas: the Simple Measure of Gobbledegook (SMOG), the Flesch-Kincaid reading level, and the Flesch Reading Ease Score. Using the SMOG formula to evaluate the authorization forms, the researchers found that the median reading level for the authorization templates was 13th grade (i.e., freshman year in college). All of the forms scored above the eighth-grade reading level. Under the Flesch-Kincaid reading-level formula, the researchers found that 97 percent of the forms were written above the eighth-grade reading level. Similarly, using the Flesch Reading Ease Score, the researchers found that 86.5 percent of the forms were "difficult" or "very difficult" to read. Only 3 of 111 authorization forms scored at the "standard English" reading level. The authors concluded that these results are problematic for researchers because half of the U.S. adult population reads at or below the eighth-grade level. A large percentage of potential research participants are likely unable to comprehend much of the information contained in authorization forms. The authors believe that many institutions view authorization forms as liability protection, rather than as a mechanism to inform research participants about a study (Breese et al., 2004).

A similar study was conducted by Nosowsky and Giordano (2006) at the University of Michigan. They analyzed the National Institutes of Health's model authorization form using Microsoft's Flesch-Kincaid scale and found that it was written at a 12th-grade reading level. The authors concluded that many research participants cannot understand the forms they are required to sign. Thus, it is not surprising that researchers are reporting that the authorization process is causing confusion for research participants (Nosowsky and Giordano, 2006).

Another study that examined whether the Privacy Rule authorization requirement has created a barrier to research was conducted by Shen et al. at Governors State University, University Park, IL. The researchers followed the authorization process in a school-based educational program for childhood obesity prevention as a case study. The authorization form used in this case study was as simple as possible. Most of the sentences on the form were taken directly out of the Privacy Rule regulation, and any additional sentences were required by the local IRB. However, despite an attempt to simplify the authorization form, only 21 percent of parents granted authorization for their children to participate in the school-based obesity program. The researchers concluded that the authorization form was overly complex, making many parents reluctant or unwilling to sign it. The authors noted, however, that the low recruitment rate recorded perhaps could have been more easily solved through better communication about the program with the students' parents than through modification of the authorization forms (Shen et al., 2006).

CONCERNS ABOUT POTENTIAL LEGAL CONSEQUENCES

Because many institutions are risk averse, the AcademyHealth survey examined the impact of concerns about the penalty provisions of the Privacy Rule on research. Nineteen percent of the respondents reported that the penalties had no effect on efforts to obtain data from a covered entity, and 24 percent reported that penalties were considered by covered entities but ultimately did not prevent researchers from obtaining data. However, 26 percent of respondents reported that concerns about penalties have impeded access to data—16 percent reported that fear of penalties has prevented covered entities from providing data to researchers, and 10 percent reported that covered entities' concerns about data privacy caused them to forego research activities. Nearly 30 percent of respondents were unsure what impact, if any, penalties have had on efforts to obtain data from covered entities (Helms, 2008). Similar concerns were reported for a study using data from 19 hospitals near the University of Washington, as noted previously. The nine IRBs requiring full review of a study already approved by the IRB of the University cited concerns over the Privacy Rule's civil and criminal penalties as the main reason for denying expedited review or for not honoring another IRB's decisions (Lydon-Rochelle and Holt, 2004).

Fear of civil suits could also lead IRB and Privacy Board members to be overly conservative in their decisions about research proposals brought before them, and could be a significant deterrent in recruiting qualified volunteers to serve on IRBs and Privacy Boards. Effective oversight of health research depends on the recruitment of qualified and knowledgeable volunteers to serve on IRBs and Privacy Boards, but the growth over the past decade of lawsuits naming individual IRB members as defendants[5] has created a chill that threatens the willingness of volunteers to serve on IRBs (Hoffman and Berg, 2005; Icenogle, 2003; IPPC, 2008; Rose and Lodato, 2004; Shaul et al., 2005). Members of IRBs and Privacy Boards are generally indemnified by their institutions, but they are not immune from being named in a suit. Therefore they could still have to devote time and resources to defending themselves for decisions made by an IRB or a Privacy Board on which they served.

POTENTIAL WAYS TO REDUCE INTERPRETIVE VARIABILITY AMONG IRBS, PRIVACY BOARDS, AND COVERED ENTITIES

HHS intended to allow covered entities, IRBs, and Privacy Boards to have some local control in implementing and interpreting the Privacy Rule as it applies to the use and disclosure of PHI for research. Sensitivity to local

---

[5] For examples of specific cases naming IRB members as individual defendants, see *Robertson v. McGee* (2001), *Guckin v. Nagle* (2002), and *Scheer v. Burke* (2003), available at http://www.sskrplaw.com/gene/index.html.

issues can be a desirable feature, particularly when institutions serve special populations or under unusual circumstances. However, variations in IRB and Privacy Board oversight may relate less to true local differences in the research environment than to the administrative differences and variability in the skills and resources of IRBs and Privacy Boards (Casarett et al., 2005). There is no required certification process to ensure that IRB/Privacy Board members have sufficient knowledge and understanding of research ethics and regulation, and funding is often through indirect sources, such as grants.

Based on the evidence presented in this chapter, it is clear that over-interpretation of the Privacy Rule is common and that the substantial variability in interpretation among covered entities and oversight boards is detrimental to health research. More consistent application of the Privacy Rule would facilitate responsible research and also provide more meaningful protection of patient privacy. One potential way to begin to address this issue would be for HHS to regularly identify and disseminate "best practices" for responsible research (IOM, 2000). Guidance materials and models or templates for things such as the authorization form (written at an appropriate reading level), waiver of authorization form, data use agreements, and business associate agreements would make it easier for investigators to appropriately design research projects and put institutions at ease about decisions their IRBs and Privacy Boards make with regard to privacy concerns. This endeavor could perhaps be accomplished as an activity of the National Institutes of Health (NIH) Roadmap,[6] under the direction of the Office for Civil Rights. An informative precedent for this activity is the *National Practitioner Data Bank Guidebook*[7] of the Health Resources and Services Administration, established through Title IV of the Healthcare Quality Improvement Act of 1986, Public Law 99–660. That guidebook, which is frequently updated, provides many case examples of what should be done in various situations.

Stakeholders—including researchers; research institutions, IRBs, and Privacy Boards; sponsors of research; public health practitioners and agencies; patient and consumer organizations; and privacy experts—could have considerable influence on the adoption of best practices once they have been identified and thus could help to make privacy protections and IRB/Privacy Board decisions more uniform. For example, Requests for Proposals and other funding mechanisms could be more instructive on this point. Many

---

[6]The NIH Roadmap was initiated in 2004 as "an integrated vision to deepen our understanding of biology, stimulate interdisciplinary research teams, and reshape clinical research to accelerate medical discovery and improve people's health." See http://nihroadmap.nih.gov/overview.asp (accessed January 13, 2009).

[7]See http://www.npdb-hipdb.hrsa.gov/npdbguidebook.html (accessed January 13, 2009).

academic researchers depend on their ability to procure funding from a source external to their institutions, and research sponsors also have obligations to protect research participants. As a result, major nonfederal funders could be a powerful force for adherence to ethical guidelines, even in the absence of strong federal regulations and enforcement.

Organizations whose primary missions are focused on promoting responsible and ethical research, such as Public Responsibility in Medicine and Research (PRIM&R) and the Association for the Accreditation of Human Research Protection Programs (AAHRPP), featured in Boxes 5-2 and 5-3, could contribute much to the dynamic and ongoing process of developing best practices. These organizations educate IRB professionals, offer voluntary certification programs, and have hosted conferences to address ethical and legal challenges in research, including those related to HIPAA. Increased participation in PRIM&R and AAHRPP could extend understanding of regulatory requirements and foster national discourse about issues of interpretation and application of the Privacy Rule.

An important point to remember is that HHS's policy is to seek compliance first, rather than penalties, when a concern is brought to the agency's attention (see Chapter 5). Institutions might be less inclined to be overly conservative in interpreting the Privacy Rule if this were stated more clearly

---

BOX 5-2
Public Responsibility in Medicine and Research (PRIM&R)

The mission of PRIM&R is to promote ethical research in humans and animals. It tracks and provides input to policy initiatives and regulatory changes relating to ethical standards in research and offers educational opportunities in the fields of biomedical and social/behavioral/educational research. PRIM&R also offers two certification programs, one for administrators for animal care and use committees, and one for IRB professionals.

The latter is designed specifically for individuals participating in and/or overseeing the daily operations of IRBs, including IRB administrators, staff, chairs, and institutional officials. Professionals from institutional IRBs, independent IRBs, and industry, as well as other institutions focused on either biomedical or social/behavioral/educational research, are eligible. Candidates' IRB experience must be "substantial and ongoing" and must reflect the applicant's commitment to applied research ethics in human subjects protections. The exam for certification is administered by the Professional Testing Corporation and is offered at least twice yearly at testing sites across the United States and Canada. Certification is valid for 3 years and can be renewed via reexamination or once in a 6-year period with continuing education credits.

SOURCE: See http://www.primr.org.

BOX 5-3
Association for the Accreditation of Human
Research Protection Programs (AAHRPP)

AAHRPP is an independent, nonprofit entity that accredits organizations' human research protection programs. Its mission is to accredit "high-quality human research protection programs in order to promote excellent, ethically sound research. Through partnership with research organizations, researchers, sponsors, and the public, AAHRPP encourages effective, efficient, and innovative systems of protection for human research participants." To earn and maintain accreditation, an organization must provide evidence that its practices, policies, and procedures promote ethically sound and scientific research every 3 years. AAHRPP provides print, online, and training resources to guide organizations through the accreditation process and to help organizations interpret the required accreditation standards.

SOURCE: See http://www.aahrpp.org/www.aspx.

---

in guidance materials. Simple clarification and clear communication of the way HHS will enforce the Privacy Rule and seek penalties would be helpful.

In addition, some limited protection against civil suits brought pursuant to federal or state law for members of IRBs and Privacy Boards for decisions made within the scope of their responsibilities under the Privacy Rule and the Common Rule could be beneficial. This limited protection should not include protection for willful and wanton misconduct in reviewing the research. Members of IRBs or Privacy Boards who receive limited protection against lawsuits may be less likely to interpret the Privacy Rule too conservatively. A similar provision was incorporated into the Ontario Personal Health Information Protection Act of 2004, under which members of Research Ethics Boards are immune for acts done and omissions made in good faith that are reasonable under the circumstances (see also Chapter 6). This type of immunity for IRB and Privacy Board members would be similar to the precedent of protection for peer review members under state laws and under the Health Care Quality Improvement Act of 1986.

Such protections might also facilitate multi-institutional research by reducing the variability among local IRBs and Privacy Boards because they might be more comfortable accepting the decision of a lead IRB/Privacy Board. But even in the absence of this sort of regulatory or statutory change, a clear statement from HHS regarding the acceptability, and thus the limits, of legal consequences of accepting the decision of another IRB or Privacy Board would help to facilitate multi-institutional research.

CONCLUSIONS AND RECOMMENDATIONS

The evidence presented in this chapter demonstrates that implementation and interpretation of the Privacy Rule has had a significant effect on how health research is conducted in the United States. Although the Privacy Rule may have extended regulatory protections of privacy in health research that were desirable, the numerous studies reviewed here indicate that it has also had an unintended negative effect on health research, often due to variations in how covered entities, IRBs, and Privacy Boards interpret the complex regulations. Nonetheless, even if the effect on research has been negative, carefully considering the effect on privacy of any changes to the Privacy Rule as well as the effect on research is important. Many problems identified in this chapter could potentially be improved by HHS without changing the Privacy Rule itself.

More consistent application of the Privacy Rule would facilitate responsible research and provide more meaningful protection of patient privacy. **Thus, the committee recommends that HHS regularly convene consensus development conferences in collaboration with health research stakeholders to collect and evaluate current practices in privacy protection in order to identify and disseminate best practices for responsible research.** Stakeholders can then enable and encourage researchers to use these best practices in designing and conducting research involving the use of PHI.

Current guidance from HHS addresses only what is permissible under the HIPAA Privacy Rule; the guidance does not identify best practices. A dynamic, ongoing process for the identification and dissemination of best practices in privacy protection for various types of health research by HHS would facilitate reviews by IRBs and Privacy Boards and would lead to more consistent and appropriate decisions. Guidance materials with best practices and models or templates for things such as the authorization form, waiver of authorization form, data use agreements, and business associate agreements would make it easier for investigators to appropriately design research projects and put institutions at ease about decisions their IRBs and Privacy Boards make with regard to privacy concerns. Such guidance materials should be written as clearly and simply as possible, using an inclusive, dynamic, and transparent development process, and should override all prior guidance documents.

Stakeholders—including researchers; research institutions, IRBs, and Privacy Boards; sponsors of research; public health practitioners and agencies; patient and consumer organizations; and privacy experts—could have considerable influence on the adoption of best practices once they have been identified and thus could help to make privacy protections and IRB/Privacy Board decisions more uniform. Organizations whose primary missions are focused on promoting responsible and ethical research, such as PRIM&R and AAHRPP, can contribute much to the process.

Another potential way to reduce inconsistency and overly conservative interpretation would be to provide some limited legal protection for IRB and Privacy Board members, who may be fearful of lawsuits pertaining to IRB/Privacy Board decisions. **The committee recommends that HHS—or, as necessary, Congress—provide reasonable protection against civil suits brought pursuant to federal or state law for members of IRBs and Privacy Boards for decisions made within the scope of their responsibilities under the HIPAA Privacy Rule and the Common Rule. The limitation on liability should not include protection for willful and wanton misconduct in reviewing the research, but should instead be for good-faith decisions, backed by minutes or other evidence, in responsibly applying the legal requirements under the HIPAA Privacy Rule or the Common Rule.**

Recommendations put forth in previous chapters should also help to reduce variability and overinpretation of the regulations. These include facilitating greater use of data with direct identifiers removed and facilitating appropriate IRB and Privacy Board oversight of identification and recruitment of potential research participants (see Chapter 4). Clarifying the distinction between "research" and "practice" to ensure appropriate ethical oversight of the use of protected health information would also help IRBs and Privacy Boards make decisions that adequately protect patient privacy and facilitate responsible research (see Chapter 3).

However, as indicated in Chapter 6, the committee believes that ideally, a bolder approach should be taken, with HHS developing a new approach to protecting privacy in health research that emphasizes privacy, security, accountability, and transparency and that is applicable to all health research in the United States.

REFERENCES

AAHC (Association of Academic Health Centers). 2008. *HIPAA creating barriers to research and discovery: HIPAA problems widespread and unresolved since 2003.* http://www.aahcdc.org/policy/reddot/AAHC_HIPAA_Creating_Barriers.pdf (accessed September 2, 2008).

Al-Shahi, R., C. Vousden, and C. Warlow. 2005. Bias from requiring explicit consent from all participants in observational research: Prospective, population based study. *British Medical Journal* 331:942–945.

Armstrong, D., E. Kline-Rogers, S. M. Jani, E. B. Goldman, J. Fang, D. Mukherjee, B. K. Nallamothu, and K. A. Eagle. 2005. Potential impact of the HIPAA Privacy Rule on data collection in a registry of patients with acute coronary syndrome. *Archives of Internal Medicine* 165(10):1125–1129.

ASCO (American Society of Clinical Oncology). 2008. *The impact of the Privacy Rule on cancer research: Variations in attitudes and application of regulatory standards.* Alexandria, VA: ASCO.

Beebe, T., N. Talley, M. Camilleri, S. M. Jenkins, K. J. Anderson, and G. R. Locke. 2007. The HIPAA authorization form and effects on survey response rate, nonresponse bias, and data quality. *Medical Care* 45(10):959–965.

Breese, P., W. Burman, C. Rietmeijer, and D. Lezotte. 2004. The Health Insurance Portability and Accountability Act and the informed consent process. *Annals of Internal Medicine* 141:897–898.

Casarett, D., J. Karlawish, E. Andrews, and A. Caplan. 2005. Bioethical issues in pharmaco-epidemiological research. In *Pharmacoepidemiology*, 4th ed, edited by B. L. Strom. West Sussex, England: John Wiley & Sons, Ltd. Pp. 417–432.

Clause, S. L., D. M. Triller, C. P. H. Bornhorst, R. A. Hamilton, and L. E. Cosler. 2004. Conforming to HIPAA regulations and compilation of research data. *American Journal of Health-System Pharmacy* 61(10):1025–1031.

Deapen, D. 2006. *Negative impact of HIPAA on population-based cancer registry research: A brief survey.* Springfield, IL: North American Association of Central Cancer Registries.

Dunlop, A., T. Graham, Z. Leroy, K. Glanz, and B. Dunlop. 2007. The impact of HIPAA authorization on willingness to participate in clinical research. *Annals of Epidemiology* 17(11):899–905.

Friedman, D. S. 2006. HIPAA and research: How have the first two years gone? *American Journal of Ophthalmology* 141(3):543–546.

Greene, S. M., A. M. Geiger, E. L. Harris, A. Altschuler, L. Nekhlyudov, M. B. Barton, S. J. Rolnick, J. G. Elmore, and S. Fletcher. 2006. Impact of IRB requirements on a multicenter survey of prophylactic mastectomy outcomes. *Annals of Epidemiology* 16:275–278.

Greene, S. M., S. Bennett, B. Kirlin, K. R. Oliver, R. Pardee, and E. Wagner. 2008. *Impact of the HIPAA Privacy Rule in the HMO Research Network.* Seattle, WA: Group Health Cooperative Center for Health Studies.

Harris, M. A., and A. R. Levy. 2008. Personal privacy and public health: Potential impacts of privacy legislation on health research in Canada. *Canadian Journal of Public Health* 99(4):293–296.

Helms, D. 2008 (February 14). PowerPoint presentation to the Institute of Medicine Committee on Health Research and the Privacy of Health Information: The HIPAA Privacy Rule, on the AcademyHealth survey results.

Hoffman, S., and J. W. Berg. 2005. The suitability of IRB liability. *Case Legal Studies Research Paper No. 05-4.* February. http://papers.ssrn.com/sol3/papers.cfm?abstract_id=671004 (accessed September 2, 2008).

Howe, H. L., A. J. Lake, and T. Shen. 2006. Method to assess identifiability in electronic data files. *American Journal of Epidemiology* 165(5):597–601.

Icenogle, D. L. 2003. IRBs, conflict and liability: Will we see IRBs in court? Or is it when? *Clinical Medicine & Research* 1(1):63–68.

IOM (Institute of Medicine). 2000. *Protecting data privacy in health services research.* Washington, DC: National Academy Press.

IOM. 2002. *Responsible research: A systems approach to protecting research participants.* Washington, DC: The National Academies Press.

IPPC (International Pharmaceutical Privacy Consortium). 2008 (March 30). Comments to the Institute of Medicine Committee on Health Research and the Privacy of Health Information: The HIPAA Privacy Rule, on the impact of the HIPAA Privacy Rule on pharmaceutical research.

Kaiser, J. 2006. Rule to protect records may doom long-term heart study. *Science* 311:1547–1548.

Kolata, G. 2007. States and V.A. at odds on cancer data. *The New York Times*, October 10.

Kompanje, E. J. O., and A. I. R. Maas. 2006. Is the Glasgow coma scale score protected health information? The effect of new United States regulations (HIPAA) on completion of screening logs in emergency research trials. *Intensive Care Medicine* 32:313–314.

Lydon-Rochelle, M., and V. L. Holt. 2004. HIPAA transition: Challenges of a multisite medical records validation study of maternally linked birth records. *Maternal & Child Health Journal* 8(1):35–38.

McCarthy, D. B., D. Shatin, C. R. Drinkard, J. H. Kleinman, and J. S. Gardner. 1999. Medical records and privacy: Empirical effects of legislation. *Health Services Research* 34(1):417–425.

National Committee on Vital and Health Statistics, Subcommittee on Privacy and Confidentiality. *Susan Ehringhaus's testimony on behalf of the Association of American Medical Colleges.* November 19, 2003.

Ness, R. 2005. A year is a terrible thing to waste: Early experience with HIPAA. *Annals of Epidemiology* 15(2):85–86.

Ness, R. 2007. Influence of the HIPAA Privacy Rule on health research. *JAMA* 298(18):2164–2170.

Newgard, C. D., S. H. Hui, P. Stamps-White, R. J. Lewis, C. D. Newgard, S.-H. J. Hui, P. Stamps-White, and R. J. Lewis. 2005. Institutional variability in a minimal risk, population-based study: Recognizing policy barriers to health services research. *Health Services Research* 40(4):1247–1258.

Nosowsky, R., and T. J. Giordano. 2006. The Health Insurance Portability and Accountability Act of 1996 (HIPAA) Privacy Rule: Implications for clinical research. *Annual Review of Medicine* 57(1):575–590.

O'Herrin, J. K., N. Fost, and K. A. Kudsk. 2004. Health Insurance Portability and Accountability Act (HIPAA) regulations: Effect on medical record research. *Annals of Surgery* 239(6):772–778.

Ramirez, A. G., and J. E. Niederhuber. 2003 (November 5). Letter to the Honorable Tommy G. Thompson, Secretary of the Department of Health and Human Services.

Ring, J. 2007 (October 1–2). PowerPoint presentation to the Institute of Medicine Committee on Health Research and the Privacy of Health Information: The HIPAA Privacy Rule, on the American Heart Association survey results.

Rose, B. S., and V. Lodato. 2004. The role of class actions in litigation involving human research subjects. *BNA Class Action Litigation Report*, March 12.

Russell, S. 2004a. Dispute on medical record access settled: Cancer researchers wanted UC data on new cases quicker. *San Francisco Chronicle*, December 7, B1.

Russell, S. 2004b. Medical privacy law said to be chilling cancer studies: Scientists fight for fast access to patient files. *San Francisco Chronicle*, September 26, A4.

Shaffer, D. 2006. Privacy laws jeopardize heart study: Researchers have put a well-known stroke and heart disease study on hold. *Star Tribune*, February 12.

Shalowitz, D., and D. Wendler. 2006. Informed consent for research and authorization under the Health Insurance Portability and Accountability Act Privacy Rule: An integrated approach. *Annals of Internal Medicine* 144(9):685–688.

Shaul, R. Z., S. Birenbaum, and M. Evans. 2005. Legal liability in research: Early lessons from North America. *BMC Medical Ethics* 6(4):1–4.

Shen, J. J., L. F. Samson, E. L. Washington, P. Johnson, C. Edwards, A. Malone, J. J. Shen, L. F. Samson, E. L. Washington, P. Johnson, C. Edwards, and A. Malone. 2006. Barriers of HIPAA regulation to implementation of health services research. *Journal of Medical Systems* 30(1):65–69.

Trevena, L., L. Irwig, and A. Barratt. 2006. Impact of privacy legislation on the number and characteristics of people who are recruited for research: A randomized controlled trial. *Journal of Medical Ethics* 32:473–477.

Tu, J. V., D. J. Willison, F. L. Silver, J. Fang, J. A. Richards, A. Laupacis, and M. K. Kapral. 2004. Impracticability of informed consent in the registry of the Canadian stroke network. *New England Journal of Medicine* 350(14):1414–1421.

Walker, D. K. 2005. *Impact of the HIPAA Privacy Rule on health services research.* Philadelphia, PA: Abt Associates, Inc.

Ward, H. J. T., S. N. Cousens, B. Smith-Bathgate, M. Leitch, D. Everington, R. G. Will, and P. G. Smith. 2007. Obstacles to conducting epidemiological research in the UK general population. *British Medical Journal* 329:277–279.

Williams, B. A., J. J. Irrgant, M. T. Bottegal, K. A. Francis, and M. T. Vogt. 2007. A post hoc analysis of research study staffing: Budgetary effects of the Health Insurance Portability and Accountability Act (HIPAA) on research staff workload during a prospective, randomized clinical trial. *Anesthesiology* 107(5):860–861.

Wolf, M. S., and C. L. Bennett. 2006. Local perspective of the impact of the HIPAA Privacy Rule on research. *Cancer* 106(2):474–479.

Woolf, S. H., S. F. Rothemich, R. E. Johnson, and D. W. Marsland. 2000. Selection bias from requiring patients to give consent to examine data for health services research. *Archives of Family Medicine* 9:1111–1118.

6

A New Framework for Protecting Privacy in Health Research

In the previous chapters of this report, the committee put forth several recommendations that aim to improve the Privacy Rule and associated guidance in order to ease the impact on health research while still protecting patient privacy. However, in the process of developing these recommendations, the committee recognized that the Privacy Rule's research provisions have many serious limitations and concluded that a new, more uniform approach is needed to accomplish the dual challenge of protecting privacy while facilitating beneficial and responsible research. In this chapter, the committee recommends that the U.S. Department of Health and Human Services (HHS) exempt health research from the Health Insurance Portability and Accountability Act (HIPAA) Privacy Rule and lays out the details of a bold and innovative framework for protecting privacy in health research.

The overall purpose of this Institute of Medicine (IOM) study was to examine the effects of the HIPAA Privacy Rule on health research and to recommend improvements to the legislative and regulatory system accordingly. To achieve this task, the IOM convened a committee to include individuals with a broad range of expertise and experience relevant to the stated goal of the project, including individuals with knowledge of the various fields of health research, privacy and human research protections, health law, health center administration, use and protection of electronic health information, and patient advocacy (see Chapter 1 for complete statement of task and the Front Matter for committee membership).

The committee held a number of information-gathering meetings that were open to the public. During those meetings, the committee heard presentations on privacy in research and public health; the use of information systems to protect privacy; the effect of the Privacy Rule on various research disciplines, including those that are exclusively information based, such as health services research; the Ontario health privacy law; harmonization of the Privacy Rule and the Common Rule (see Chapter 3); challenges associated with the Privacy Rule's regulation of biorepositories, databases, and future research; and the relationship between privacy and autonomy in health research. The committee also reviewed the information presented in an earlier IOM workshop on the same topic (IOM, 2006) and conducted an extensive review of the literature. Members of the public were permitted to submit relevant references and written comments on their experiences with the Privacy Rule's regulation of research and to speak at the committee's public meetings. In addition, because there was a paucity of quantitative and systematic data on the effect of the Privacy Rule on research, the committee commissioned a number of large-scale, evidence-gathering projects to inform the committee's deliberations (see Chapter 5 and Appendix B).

After reviewing the available evidence, the committee concluded that a new framework for protecting privacy in health research is needed. The current system of regulating research and protecting privacy under the Privacy Rule is not working as well as it should to protect patient privacy in research, and as currently implemented, it impedes important research. The committee believes a different system could work better and provide improved privacy protections and stronger data security while also facilitating beneficial and responsible research.

In thinking about a new framework, the committee recognized that the goals of safeguarding privacy and enhancing health research are sometimes in tension. Stringent measures to safeguard privacy can make it harder to conduct high-quality research, and research itself can pose a threat to privacy. Yet the committee believes that there is a synergy between the two, that facilitating both is desirable, and that it is possible to strengthen certain privacy protections while still facilitating important health research.

For that reason, the committee's intent in developing the new framework was to advance both privacy and health research interests to the greatest extent possible. The committee understands that the lines are not neat, the questions are complex, and the challenges are formidable. Nevertheless, the new framework aims to strengthen health research regulations and practices that effectively safeguard personally identifiable health information, and to facilitate data collection and use for beneficial and high-quality health research, with appropriate oversight, to advance knowledge about human health.

This chapter reviews the major goals the committee agreed on during its deliberations and describes how they should be incorporated into a new regulatory system for health research and privacy. First, the chapter will highlight the major problems with the Privacy Rule's regulation of health research, as identified in the earlier chapters of the report. Second, the chapter will lay out the details of the new framework that the committee is recommending. Third, the committee will explain its rationale for developing the proposed framework, address potential criticism of this model, and explain how the new framework avoids many of the problems associated with the Privacy Rule.

REVIEW OF THE LIMITATIONS OF THE PRIVACY RULE

In the earlier chapters of this report, the committee identified three overarching goals on which to ground the recommendations: (1) improve the privacy and data security of health information, (2) improve the effectiveness of health research, and (3) improve the application of privacy protections for health research (see Box 6-1). In the process of recommending changes to the HIPAA Privacy Rule to achieve these three goals, the committee identified many serious problems with the current regulatory system. This section reviews the most serious problems with the Privacy Rule's regulation of health research and protection of privacy in terms of these overarching goals.

Improve the Privacy and Data Security of Health Information

In the context of health research, the privacy goal entails the commitment to handle personal information of patients and research participants in accordance with meaningful privacy protections. These protections should include strong security measures, disclosure of the purposes for which personally identifiable health information[1] is used (transparency), and legally enforceable obligations to ensure information is secure and used appropriately (accountability). The Privacy Rule falls short of the privacy goal for health research in two important ways: (1) it overstates the ability of informed consent (authorization[2]) to protect privacy, and (2) it does not provide other meaningful methods of protecting privacy, such as effective security, accountability, and transparency.

Overemphasis on Informed Consent

The principle of autonomy currently dominates the ethical landscape for both medical care and clinical research in the United States and serves as

---

[1] The term "personally identifiable health information" is used when discussing individual's health data in a context independent of the HIPAA Privacy Rule or any other body of law.

[2] In the Privacy Rule, the informed consent concept is referred to as "authorization."

BOX 6-1
The Committee's Three Overarching Goals

Improve the Privacy and Data Security of Health Information

In the context of health research, protection of privacy includes a commitment to handle personal information of patients and research participants with meaningful privacy protections, including strong security measures, transparency, and accountability. This commitment extends to everyone who collects, uses, or has access to personally identifiable health information of patients and research participants.

Practices of security, transparency, and accountability take on extraordinary importance in the health research setting: Researchers and other data users should disclose clearly how and why personally identifiable health information is being collected, used, and secured, and should be subject to legally enforceable obligations to ensure that personal information is used appropriately and securely. In this manner, privacy protection will help to ensure research participant and public trust and confidence in medical research.

Improve the Effectiveness of Health Research

Research discoveries are central to achieving the goal of extending the quality of healthy lives. Research into causes of disease, methods for prevention, techniques for diagnosis, and new approaches to treatment has increased life expectancy, reduced infant mortality, limited the toll of infectious diseases, and improved outcomes for patients with heart disease, cancer, diabetes, and other chronic diseases. Patient-oriented clinical research that tests new ideas makes rapid medical and public health progress possible.

Today the rate of discovery is accelerating, and we are at the precipice of a remarkable period of investigative promise made possible by new knowledge about the genetic underpinnings of disease. Genomic research is opening new possibilities for preventing illness and for developing safer, more effective medical care that can be tailored for specific individuals. Further advances in relating genetic information to predispositions to disease and responses to treatments will require use of large amounts of existing health-related information and stored biological specimens. The increasing use of electronic medical records will further facilitate the generation of new knowledge through research and accelerate the pace of discovery. These efforts will require broad participation of patients in research to ensure that the results are valid and applicable to different segments of the population. Collaborative partnerships among communities of patients, their physicians, and teams of researchers to gain new scientific knowledge will bring tangible benefits for people in this country and around the world.

Improve the Application of Privacy Protections for Health Research

The HIPAA Privacy Rule was written to provide consistent standards in the United States for the use and disclosure of protected health information (PHI) by covered entities, including the use and disclosure of such information for research purposes. In its current state, however, the HIPAA Privacy Rule is difficult to reconcile with other federal regulations, including U.S. Department of Health and Human Services (HHS) regulations for the protection of human subjects (the Common Rule), Food and Drug Administration regulations pertaining to human subjects, and other applicable federal or state laws.

Inconsistencies, for example, in federal regulations governing the deidentification of personally identifiable health information, obtaining individuals' consent for future research, and the recruitment of research volunteers make it challenging for health researchers seeking to comply with all these regulations to undertake important research activities. In addition, there is substantial variation in the way in which institutions interpret and apply the Privacy Rule. For example, the way in which Institutional Review Boards (IRBs) interpret the provisions when making decisions about authorization requirements varies across institutions, and often is quite conservative. Especially for multisite research and studies that are reviewed by both IRBs and Privacy Boards, the inconsistent interpretation and application of the Privacy Rule's provisions pertaining to research can create barriers to research and even lead to the discontinuation of ongoing research studies. Adding yet another layer of complexity and variability for health researchers is a lack of clarity in the way the Privacy Rule applies to various types of health research or closely related health care practices. Moreover, there are significant gaps in who and what is covered by current federal research regulations. Whether a research activity is subject to the provisions of the Privacy Rule or the Common Rule depends on a number of factors, including the source of funding, the source of the data, and whether the researcher meets the definition of a covered entity.

The situation in the United States is in stark contrast to the situation in most other countries, where uniform regulations apply to all research conducted in the country. The committee believes a new direction is needed, with a more uniform approach to patient protections, including privacy, in health research. Improved clarity, harmonization, and uniform application of regulations governing health research are needed to align the interests and understandings of the research community, the custodians of PHI, and other stakeholders, so that implementation of the privacy protections in health research can be achieved with acceptability by all.

the justification for the doctrine of informed consent (i.e., authorization) in the Privacy Rule. Historically, informed consent was based on the idea that "every human being of adult years and sound mind has a right to determine what shall be done with his own body."[3] It was primarily considered a protection against physical harm, permitting informed, competent patients to refuse unwanted medical interventions, to choose among medically available alternatives, and to make choices that conflict with the wishes of family members or the recommendations of physicians (Buchanan, 1999; Lo, in press). Under this system, a great deal of information-based health research was conducted using personally identifiable health records without the informed consent of the persons whose records were used.

Several recent developments have brought attention to this practice, and have focused attention on the historical absence of patient autonomy in information-based research. First, the increased used of electronic health records has made it significantly easier for researchers to access large quantities of personally identifiable data. Second, the move towards personalized medicine, and the potential improvements to population health and health care that could be developed based on a better understanding of the determinants of health and illness, have increased researchers' needs for personally identifiable health information.

Under the Privacy Rule the concept of informed consent is extended beyond control of one's body, to control of one's health information in an attempt to address the historical lack of informational autonomy, and with the goal of protecting individuals against the nonphysical harm of unauthorized uses or disclosures of their protected health information. However, consent (authorization) itself cannot achieve the separate aim of privacy protection. The Privacy Rule, as currently defined and operationalized in practice, does not provide effective privacy safeguards for information-based research because of an over-reliance on informed consent, rather than comprehensive privacy protections.

The Limitations of Relying on Consent to Protect Privacy

As has been described above, the protection of medical privacy in the data processing environment requires the adoption of comprehensive privacy protections, which establish a variety of obligations on entities that collect and use personal information. These obligations to safeguard privacy, such as security, transparency, and accountability, are independent of patient consent. In fact, preventing the secondary use of personal data is the only privacy obligation that consent can potentially address. However,

---

[3] Stated by Justice Benjamin Cardozo in *Schloendorff v. Society of New York Hospital*, 105 N.E. 92 (N.Y. 1914).

informed consent has recently been put forward as an alternative to the adoption of comprehensive privacy protections, with the practical consequence that many privacy obligations are ignored (Allen, 2007; Rotenberg, 2001; Solove et al., 2006) (see the section on Other Federal Actions for examples of currently proposed bills). This section describes some of the major limitations of relying heavily on informed consent to protect informational privacy, as is done in the HIPAA Privacy Rule, rather than requiring the implementation of a full range of privacy protections.

With a primary focus on informed consent in privacy laws, many entities that hold personal health data may have insufficient incentives to implement comprehensive privacy protections. If compliance with consent requirements frees the data holders from further privacy obligations, some organizations and researchers may be less likely to invest in privacy-enhancing technologies or the infrastructure necessary to truly protect data. This emphasis also creates few reasons for organizations to make their activities transparent or to create institutional accountability (AHIC, 2008; Cate, 2008; CDT, 2008a,b; U.S. Congress, 2008a).

In addition, although informed consent can allow patients to control whether their information is used for any secondary purposes, such as research, few patients are sufficiently informed to make educated decisions about how their data should be used (Schneider, 2006). Studies indicate that many consumers do not read the details of informed consent forms, which are often lengthy documents, and even when they do read the forms they often do not comprehend all the details (Cate, 2008). Two separate studies have found that many consumers mistake the existence of any privacy policy for a guarantee that information will be strongly protected and withheld from outside persons, even if the consent says differently (Good et al., 2005; Turow et al., 2007). This difficulty is magnified by the fact that often patients are asked to give informed consent at a time when they are not in good health and are not motivated or lack the ability to make these kinds of complicated decisions (CDT, 2008b; U.S. Congress, 2008a).

Relying heavily on informed consent rather than comprehensive privacy obligations may also lead to a shift from substantive privacy protections toward costly procedural requirements that actually provide consumers with few meaningful choices, especially if informed consent is required as a condition of obtaining services (Cate, 2008; Thomas and Walport, 2008). Data holders may offer blanket consents to shield themselves from liability without actually providing any substantial privacy protection. In these situations patients lack reasonable alternatives and are forced to relinquish control over how their health information is used (CDT, 2008a,b; Thomas and Walport, 2008; U.S. Congress, 2008a,b).

In the case of medical records research, it is questionable as to whether a reliance on informed consent actually fosters patient confidentiality and protection (AMS, 2006, 2008; Casarett et al., 2005; Thomas and Walport, 2008). For example, if individuals must be contacted each time their records may be used in a particular study in order to obtain informed consent, as the Privacy Rule requires, such contact could be considered intrusive and counter to the tenets of confidentiality. Also, a common methodological approach to studying disease is to compare people with a particular disease to people who do not have that disease—known as a case-control study. But people may become alarmed if they are asked to consent to their records being used in such a study on a particular disease (e.g., cancer) for which they have not been diagnosed (Casarett et al., 2005).

Because of these limitations, the committee believes it is important to shift the focus in privacy protections toward a set of more comprehensive privacy obligations. This will ensure that health information privacy protections are more robust and more likely to minimize the risks to personal privacy that result from the collection of personally identifiable health information.

Failure to Incorporate Other Meaningful Privacy Protections

Implementation of the Privacy Rule does not ensure that covered entities or the research community will adopt a full range of measures to protect data; the security, transparency, and accountability provisions have proven ineffectual. As highlighted in Chapter 2, the HIPAA Security Rule does lay out a number of security requirements that covered entities must implement for protecting electronic protected health information. However, despite this regulation, there have been a number of highly publicized examples of data security breaches in health research, most often due to stolen or misplaced computers containing health data. A recent survey conducted by Campus Computing Project found that from 2006 to 2007, colleges of all types saw a 3.6 percent increase in the number of stolen computers with sensitive data. This problem was most prevalent at major research universities (Foster, 2008). Also, a report from the Identity Theft Resource Center found that identity thefts are up 69 percent for the first half of 2008, compared to the same time period in 2007, and so the consequences of security breaches are more likely to lead to tangible harm than previously believed (ITRC, 2008). These facts suggest that holders of personally identifiable health data should be required to implement security safeguards beyond what is provided for under the current HIPAA Security Rule.

In addition, as discussed in Chapter 4, it has been argued that the current interpretation of the Privacy Rule has not successfully resulted in accountability for misuses and unauthorized disclosures of protected health information. The regulation provides both civil and criminal penalties for covered entities that breach the Privacy Rule, but enforcement of the Privacy Rule has been criticized as inadequate. To date, there have been no civil penalties imposed against any covered entity and only three criminal prosecutions, despite the fact that between April 2003 and August 2008, more than 38,000 complaints were received by HHS regarding alleged violations of the Privacy Rule. HHS has not provided information on how many of these alleged violations are in the context of health research (HHS, 2008a; Rahman, 2006). On July 18, 2008, HHS required a monetary payment to settle potential violations of the Privacy and Security Rules for the first time, signaling that HHS may start to take a more assertive approach to enforcement of the Privacy and Security Rules in the future (HHS, 2008b). This agreement was in response to the covered entity allowing backup tapes, optical disks, and laptops—containing unencrypted protected health information on 386,000 patients—to be stolen or lost.

Finally, the accounting for disclosures provision of the Privacy Rule was intended to make covered entities' actions open and transparent (discussed in Chapter 4). This provision gives individuals the right to receive a list of certain disclosures that a covered entity has made of their protected health information in the past 6 years, including disclosures made for research purposes.[4] However, this requirement has numerous exceptions. Also, for research involving groups of 50 or more, covered entities are only required to produce a general list of all protocols for which a person's protected health information may have been disclosed, but do not have to provide any more specific information. Therefore, the accounting for disclosures provision does not require covered entities to provide individuals with a clear description of how their health information is used, and does not provide individuals with the detailed information they may want (AHIC, 2007; Pritts, 2008). At the same time, survey data show that this provision is a considerable administrative obligation for covered entities, and is rarely requested by patients (AHIMA, 2006; see also Chapter 4).

Improve the Effectiveness of Health Research

The health research goal emphasizes the importance of research in extending high-quality, healthy lives, and in leading to improved methods for prevention, diagnosis, and treatment. Unfortunately, the available evidence indicates that the current interpretation and implementation of the Privacy Rule has had an unintended negative impact on health research. As discussed in Chapter 5, the Privacy Rule, as interpreted and implemented by covered entities, has:

---

[4]See 45 C.F.R. § 164.528 (2006).

- Increased the cost and time needed to conduct a research project from start to finish
- Made recruitment of research participants more difficult
- Increased the likelihood of selection bias and made it more difficult to produce generalizable findings
- Increased research participants' confusion regarding their rights and protections
- Led researchers to abandon important studies
- Created new barriers to the use of patient specimens collected during clinical trials or treatment
- Failed to create an effective way for researchers to conduct studies using data with direct identifiers removed

These negative consequences are particularly problematic in light of recent trends in health care and research. Since the Privacy Rule was implemented, health data have assumed an even greater role in health research, and will become more essential as health care administration moves toward personalized medicine, in which preventive and therapeutic interventions are tailored to the individual characteristics of patients. Developing drug therapies and treatment protocols that focus on smaller and smaller subsets of the population based on genetic makeup or health history and environmental exposures requires access to more and more personal data to conduct effective health research. In addition, burgeoning health care costs and increasing limitations on expenditures by health care plans highlight the need for health services research to better determine which patients benefit from current approaches and which patients may even be harmed. If the current approach to privacy protection in research under the Privacy Rule continues unchanged, these advances will be burdened and potentially delayed, and opportunities for medical progress may be lost.

Alternative models The challenges described above are causing some leading scientists, legal experts, and privacy advocates to develop new paradigms for determining when personally identifiable health data, including biological samples, can be used for research. The recognition that a primary focus on consent is not always meaningful or protective of privacy, and that it impedes important information-based research, is gaining acknowledgment in the United Kingdom and in other countries in Europe, as well as the United States (AMS, 2006, 2008; Thomas and Walport, 2008). The committee reviewed several alternative models and took them into consideration in the development of the proposed new framework for protecting privacy in health research.

- *Reciprocity, Solidarity, and Mutuality Models.* These models seek to address the situation where there is no consent for future research uses (whether specified or unspecified). Proponents of the reciprocity model argue that by accepting the benefit of past medical research (which is intrinsic in the use of medical services), patients inherently agree to allow the use of their health information in future research for the common good (Knoppers and Chadwick, 2005; Liu, 2007). Critics of this approach argue that voluntary altruism by past research participants imposes no reciprocal obligation on the larger community (Jonas, 1991). Proponents of the solidarity model similarly argue that individual ties to society and social relationships require individuals to participate in research without informed consent for the common good (Chadwick and Berg, 2001). The mutuality model is based on the insurance industry's concept of individuals entering a pool for sharing losses and known risks. In the research context, mutuality requires individuals to pool their health information for the benefit of all, rather than provide for discretionary control of individual information (Knoppers and Chadwick, 2005).

- *Harms-Based Model.* The harms-based model seeks to narrowly tailor the restrictions that are applied to the use of personally identifiable health information based on the specific risks associated with unauthorized use of that information. There are two categories of potential harm commonly cited with respect to unauthorized uses of personally identifiable health information: (1) discrimination and stigmatization and (2) erosion of trust leading to compromises in health care (NCVHS, 2007). For example, such an approach would logically call for the adoption of nondiscrimination legislation and a requirement that entities with a legitimate need for personally identifiable health information secure the information against further unauthorized access. This would arguably address directly the risks of harm to the individuals involved when their personally identifiable health information is used for research, while recognizing the need for researchers' access to information in order to achieve the public's goals of improving individual and public health and advancing scientific knowledge.

Improve the Application of Privacy Protections for Health Research

The goal of improving the application of privacy protections for health research stresses the need for consistent standards for the use and disclosure of personally identifiable health information in health research. The extent of privacy protections should not depend on the holder of the personally identifiable health information, the source of the data, or what type of funding is supporting the research project. In addition, all institutions required to comply with the privacy protections should ideally interpret and implement them in a consistent manner. Major problems identified with the Privacy Rule's regulation of research under this principle include: (1) discrepancies between the Privacy Rule and other rules and regulations relevant to health research, (2) the Privacy Rule's limitation in scope, and (3) large variations in interpretation and implementation by covered entities.

Discrepancies with Other Rules That Regulate Research

The Privacy Rule was intended to provide consistent standards in the United States for the use and disclosure of protected health information, including for research purposes. However, in the current state, the Privacy Rule is difficult to reconcile with HHS regulations for the Protection of Human Subjects (45 C.F.R. 46), the Food and Drug Administration human subjects regulation (21 C.F.R. parts 50 and 56), and other applicable federal and state laws. For example, the provisions governing data deidentification, consent for future research, and recruitment of research volunteers vary among these regulations, making important research activities more challenging to undertake (see Chapter 4).

Limitation in Scope

The Privacy Rule pertains only to covered entities; thus this regulation does not apply uniformly to all health research in the United States (see Chapter 4). Similarly, as described in Chapter 3, the Common Rule only applies to research conducted or supported by the U.S. government (although its influence is broader because most institutions that accept federal funds sign a federalwide assurance to abide by the Common Rule requirements in all research conducted at the institution, regardless of funding source). Because both of these Rules are limited in scope, there are significant gaps in whom and what is covered by current federal research regulations. This is in stark contrast to most other countries, in which research regulations are not limited by provisions regarding funding or particular health care transactions, but instead apply to all research conducted in that country (Casarett et al., 2005).

Differences in Interpretation

Because the Privacy Rule is such a complex regulation, there is substantial variation across institutions in how the Privacy Rule has been interpreted and implemented (see Chapter 5). For example, the way in which Institutional Review Boards (IRBs) and Privacy Boards interpret the concepts of impracticability and minimal risk when making decisions about authorization requirements varies across institutions, and often is quite conservative (see Chapter 4). Inconsistent interpretation and application of the Privacy Rule research provisions by IRBs, Privacy Boards, and covered entities that hold the protected health information, especially for multisite research and studies that are reviewed by multiple IRBs and Privacy Boards, can create barriers to research such as variations in protocol at different institutions and, at times, discontinuation of studies. A lack of clarity in how the Privacy Rule applies to various types of health research or closely related health care practices adds another layer of complexity and variability (see Chapter 3). In fact, some covered entities are reluctant to permit access to data for research even when all provisions of the Privacy Rule are followed, out of fear of misinterpreting the Privacy Rule (Casarett et al., 2005; Rothstein, 2005).

THE NEW FRAMEWORK

Given the clear limitations of the HIPAA Privacy Rule, the committee concluded that a new approach to the regulation of health research is needed. The committee favors an approach in which both individual privacy and the societal value of research are carefully considered and supported. To achieve this goal, the committee identified a number of key concepts (CIHR, 2005; Gostin, 2001) to incorporate into the new framework, including:

- All researchers should be required to follow the same set of privacy rules.
- Whenever possible, information-based research should be done using health data with direct identifiers removed.
- Access to personally identifiable health data without patient consent should require impartial, outside scientific and ethical review that considers:
  — Measures taken to protect the privacy, security, and confidentiality of the data;
  — Potential harms that could result from disclosure of the data; and
  — Potential public benefits of the research.
- Researchers should identify and document research objectives to justify the data they wish to use and/or collect.
- Researchers, institutions, and organizations that store personally identifiable health data should establish security safeguards and set limits on access to data.
- Researchers who violate individuals' privacy should be penalized.

These concepts are intended to support the beneficial use of existing health data, as well as the collection and use of health data for research purposes, while protecting individuals' privacy.

Examples of Informative Models

One informative example that incorporates many of the privacy principles listed above is Ontario's Personal Health Information Protection Act (PHIPA).[5] This provincial law governs the manner in which "personal health information"[6] is collected, used, and disclosed within the Ontario health care system. PHIPA only applies to the province of Ontario (not the entire country) and operates in a universal health care system, so the legislation as a whole may not be easily transferable to the United States. However, many of the major concepts in PHIPA influenced the committee's deliberations regarding the new framework.

PHIPA shares a number of similarities with the Privacy Rule (Table 6-1). In general, both regulations require the holder of personally identifiable health data to obtain informed consent (referred to as authorization in the Privacy Rule)[7] before using any personally identifiable health information for a purpose other than providing services directly related to health care of the patient. If a researcher wishes to use personally identifiable health data without informed consent, both regulations require the researcher to obtain a waiver of informed consent approved by an independent ethics board prior to the start of the study.

Despite these similarities, the Privacy Rule and PHIPA have some key differences that are important in research. One major difference is that unlike the Privacy Rule, which applies privacy obligations unevenly across the health care sector, PHIPA implements a more uniform approach. PHIPA applies to health information custodians (HICs) (e.g., providers, hospitals, and pharmacies) who collect, use, and disclose personal health information and to non-HICs when they receive personal health information from a HIC. This means that the privacy protections follow the data, even after the data are no longer held by a HIC. All health researchers are required to comply with PHIPA when using personal health information. In contrast, the Privacy Rule fails to provide individuals with privacy protections if their information is held by an entity other than a covered entity. Only some researchers qualify as covered entities or are employed by covered entities

---

[5] Personal Health Information Protection Act, Statutes of Ontario 2004, Ch. 3, Schedule A; Ontario Regulation 329/04.

[6] PHIPA defines personal health information as "identifying information about an individual in oral or recorded form" (PHIPA, Section 4).

[7] The remainder of this chapter uses the term "informed consent" to refer to the requirement of obtaining permission to use personally identifiable data.

TABLE 6-1 The HIPAA Privacy Rule Versus PHIPA

	HIPAA Privacy Rule	PHIPA
Entities Regulated	Covered entities: Includes health care providers, health plans, and health care clearinghouses that electronically transmit health information in the course of normal health care practices	• Health information custodians (HICs) that collect, use and disclose personal health information (PHI) • Non-health information custodians who receive personal health information from an HIC
Information Protected	Protected health information (PHI): All personally identifiable health information created or received by a covered entity	PHI: Identifying information about an individual in oral or recorded form that: • Relates to his or her physical or mental health • Relates to providing health care • Relates to the donation of a body part or bodily substance
Consent	Express consent is required for the collection, use, and disclosure of PHI to researchers, except if waived by an International Review Board (IRB) or Privacy Board (express consent must be in writing)	In general, HICs must obtain express consent to share PHI outside the health care system, or to share PHI for any purpose other than one related to providing health care (NOTE: Express consent may be oral or written)
Disclosures to Researchers Without Consent	Covered entities may disclose PHI to researchers without obtaining authorization in the following circumstances: • They have documentation that an IRB or Privacy Board waived the authorization requirement • For activities that are preparatory to research • For research on decedents • Where the data are part of a limited dataset and the researcher enters into a data use agreement • The information is deidentified	Disclosure of PHI for research requires approval of researcher's research plan by a Research Ethics Board (REB) Researchers must agree to: • Comply with the conditions imposed by the REB • Use PHI only for purpose set out in the research plan • Not publish information in a form that could identify an individual • Not disclose information unless required by law and subject to prescribed exceptions and additional requirements • Not make contact or attempt to make contact with the individual unless the HIC first obtains consent • Notify the HIC of any breach • Comply with the agreement entered into with the HIC

continued

TABLE 6-1 Continued

	HIPAA Privacy Rule	PHIPA
Waiver of Informed Consent/ Authorization Standard	The use or disclosure of PHI involves no more than a minimal risk to the privacy of individuals, based on, at least, the presence of the following elements: • An adequate plan to protect the identifiers from improper use and disclosure • An adequate plan to destroy the identifiers at the earliest opportunity consistent with conduct of the research, unless there is a health or research justification for retaining the identifiers • An adequate written assurance that PHI will not be reused or disclosed to any other person or entity And, the research could not practicably be conducted without the waiver or alteration And, the research could not practicably be conducted without access to and use of PHI	An REB shall consider the matters that it deems relevant, including: • Whether the objectives of the research can reasonably be accomplished without using the PHI that is to be disclosed • Whether, at the time the research is conducted, adequate safeguards will be in place to protect the privacy of the individuals whose PHI is being disclosed and to preserve the confidentiality of the information • The public interest in conducting the research and in protecting the privacy of the individuals whose PHI is being disclosed • Whether obtaining the consent of the individuals whose PHI is being disclosed would be impractical
Immunity	None	HICs and their agents are protected from liability for acts done and omissions made in good faith and reasonably in the circumstances in the exercise of powers or duties under PHIPA

TABLE 6-1 Continued

	HIPAA Privacy Rule	PHIPA
Certified Entities	None	HICs may disclose PHI to a "prescribed person or entity" without consent, for purposes of compiling or maintaining a registry of PHI intended to facilitate or improve the provision of health care, and for the purpose of analyzing or compiling statistical information with respect to the management, evaluation, or monitoring of the allocation of resources to, or planning for, all or part of the health system. Information compiled by "prescribed persons and entities" is permitted to be used for research, but must follow the same research rules as HICs in using or disclosing PHI for research
Deidentification	There are two methods to deidentify information: • Under the statistical method, a statistician or person with appropriate training verifies that enough identifiers have been removed that the risk of identification of the individual is very small • Under the safe harbor method data is considered deidentified if the covered entity removes 18 specified personal identifiers from the data	To "deidentify," in relation to the PHI of an individual, means to remove any information that identifies the individual or for which it is reasonably foreseeable in the circumstances that it could be utilized, either alone or with other information, to identify the individual, and "deidentification" has a corresponding meaning. HICs and prescribed persons and entities must exercise their own judgment in removing identifiers

and are directly regulated by the Privacy Rule; for others, the Privacy Rule regulates access to protected health information held by covered entities but the researchers themselves are not subject to the provisions.

A second major difference is the Privacy Rule and PHIPA's treatment of deidentified information. Deidentified information is outside the scope of both rules. However, PHIPA provides a more vague definition of "deidentified" than the Privacy Rule, defining it to mean the removal of "any information that identifies the individual or for which it is reasonably foreseeable in the circumstances that it could be utilized, either alone or with other information, to identify the individual."[8] Because of the lack of specificity in the definition, and the fact that the Ontario Information and Privacy Commissioner has not issued any guidance on the deidentification process, HICs are required to exercise judgment in determining when enough identifiers have been removed that the information is deidentified. Many HICs take a very conservative approach to the disclosure of personal-level, deidentified information for research and require Research Ethics Board approval (Canadian equivalent of an IRB or Privacy Board).[9] In contrast, the Privacy Rule provides two very detailed methods of deidentifying health information: (1) the safe harbor method, and (2) the statistical method (see Chapter 4). If a covered entity complies with either of these methods, it may disclose the deidentified information to researchers without IRB or Privacy Board approval.

A third major difference is that under PHIPA, HICs are permitted to disclose personal health information without consent to "prescribed persons or entities" that are prescribed by the legislation, including registries compiled or maintained for purposes of facilitating or improving the provision of health care or that relate to the storage or donation of body parts or bodily substances. In order to be designated as a prescribed person or entity, the person or entity must have in place practices, policies, and procedures to protect the privacy of individuals whose personal health information it receives and to maintain the confidentiality of such information. These practices, policies, and procedures must be reviewed and approved by Ontario's Information and Privacy Commissioner (IPC), an individual appointed by the Ontario Legislature, every 3 years. Prescribed persons and entities must also make public a description of the functions of the registry and a summary of its practices, policies, and procedures. Currently, five registries are designated as a "prescribed person" under PHIPA.[10]

Once personal health information is held by a prescribed entity, the entity may use and disclose the information for research purposes in accordance with the normal rules and restrictions on HICs disclosing information for research—including the requirement for approval by a Research Ethics Board if the information is in identifiable form. There are several advantages for researchers in obtaining information from prescribed entities, rather than other HICs. Prescribed entities collect personal health information from a wide range of sources and can link and match the per-

---

[8] PHIPA, Section 47(1) (2007).

[9] Personal communication, Ann Cavoukian, Ontario's Office of the Information and Privacy Commissioner, October 20, 2008.

[10] The Cardiac Care Network of Ontario (Registry of Cardiac Services), INSCYTE (Information System for Cytology), The Canadian Stroke Network (Canadian Stroke Registry), Cancer Care Ontario (Colorectal Cancer Screening Registry), and Hamilton Health Sciences Corporation (Critical Care Information System).

sonal health information longitudinally. In addition, there is little danger of selection bias, because informed consent is not required in the collection of the data. Prescribed entities very rarely need to disclose information in identifiable form for research, because researchers are given data that is already aggregated and linked. PHIPA instructs the prescribed entities to use their judgment in determining if information is deidentified. However, as noted above, all prescribed entities must have their policies and practices reviewed by the IPC, including their policies for the deidentification of data. As a result, prescribed entities are confident in their deidentification process, and researchers obtaining data from prescribed persons are rarely required to obtain informed consent or Research Ethics Board approval.

Recently, a similar approach to prescribed entities was recommended in a report commissioned by the United Kingdom's Prime Minister on secondary uses of personal information. This report suggested the creation of "safe harbors," which have three defining characteristics: (1) they provide a secure environment for processing personally identifiable health data, (2) they are restricted to "approved researchers" who meet relevant criteria, and (3) they implement penalties and allow for criminal sanctions against researchers who abuse their access to personally identifiable data (Thomas and Walport, 2008).

The United Kingdom approach is also comparable to PHIPA, because both models incorporate the concept that personally identifiable information should only be disclosed for health research when the research is beneficial to the public and has scientific merit. PHIPA instructs Research Ethics Boards to consider both "the public interest in conducting the research and the public interest in protecting the privacy of the individuals whose PHI is being disclosed" when reviewing research plans. The United Kingdom model identifies the principle of proportionality, defined as "an objective judgment as to whether the benefits outweigh the risks," as a key consideration when deciding whether personal information may or may not be shared for health research (Thomas and Walport, 2008). There is also a precedence for weighing scientific merit in the United States—as previously noted in Box 4-5, Centers for Medicare & Medicaid's (CMS's) Privacy Boards are instructed to "balance the potential risks to the beneficiary confidentiality with the probable benefits gained from the completed research," as well as to consider the researchers' demonstrated expertise and experience in conducting such a study.

The committee believes an approach similar to PHIPA and the recently proposed model from the United Kingdom, combined with strong security measures, offers adequate privacy protections for personally identifiable health information, while greatly expanding research opportunities. In particular, the prescribed entity/safe harbor concept offers a useful way to conduct medical records research and effectively protect patient privacy and confidentiality by facilitating greater use of deidentified data in research. Also, PHIPA, the United Kingdom model, and the CMS focus on only permitting the disclosure of personally identifiable information for socially beneficial research that has scientific merit ensures that approved research projects address important health questions and utilizes a scientifically rigorous methodology. In addition, PHIPA's focus on transparency, by requiring prescribed persons and entities to post their research purpose, policies, and procedures, is consistent with desirable comprehensive privacy protections.

The Committee's Recommendation

The committee recommends that Congress authorize HHS and other relevant federal agencies to develop a new approach to ensuring privacy in health research. When this new approach is implemented, HHS should exempt health research from the Privacy Rule. The committee suggests a two-part practical approach to protecting health information privacy because there are fundamental differences between information-based research and direct, interventional human subjects research. **First, congressional action should be taken to require all interventional research (e.g., Phase I–III clinical trials) to comply with the Common Rule, regardless of funding source.** This would eliminate current gaps in oversight and provide protection for all patients who consent to participate in interventional clinical trials. In addition, all researchers who gain access to personally identifiable health information as part of the interventional research should be required to protect that information with strong security measures, as recommended in Chapter 2. Research participants should be allowed to provide consent for future research uses of data and biological materials collected as part of the interventional study, as long as an IRB reviews and approves the future uses, ensuring that the new study is not incompatible with the original consent (as recommended in Chapter 4).

Second, Congress should authorize HHS and other relevant federal agencies to develop a new approach to uniform, goal-oriented oversight of information-based research, with a focus on best practices in privacy, security, and transparency as in PHIPA and the proposed United Kingdom model (CIHR, 2005; Thomas and Walport, 2008) and minimizing ineffective and burdensome administrative tasks. This new approach should include a mechanism by which some programs or institutions could be certified by HHS or another accrediting body, similar to a prescribed entity as in PHIPA or a "safe harbor" as in the United Kingdom model. Such certified entities could then collect and analyze personally identifiable health information for clearly defined and approved purposes, without individual consent. Because of the administrative requirements in becoming certified, this option is most appropriate for disease registries and other very large scale research databases. The regulations should require specific privacy safeguards for certified entities, including mandatory privacy training for all staff/researchers; signing of confidentiality agreements; privacy breach policies and procedures; and mandatory privacy impact assessments. In addition, the regulations should require certified entities to publicize the scope and purpose of their data collection (e.g., the types of studies that may be undertaken with the data). The regulations could also require entities to provide details on what their database will not be used for, to assure the public that certain types of activities will not be conducted.

Certified entities could also link personally identifiable data from multiple sources (see discussion on linking in Chapter 4) and then provide aggregated datasets to researchers with direct identifiers removed (see discussion on deidentified data and limited datasets in Chapter 4) (AMS, 2008; Thomas and Walport, 2008). Aggregation would generate more complete datasets for analysis and thus lead to more meaningful research results. Data with direct identifiers removed would protect patient privacy in research and would also streamline research efforts by eliminating the need to undergo ethics board review, which is not required for research using deidentified data under the Privacy Rule, PHIPA, or the United Kingdom model. To further protect privacy, unauthorized reidentification of information that has had direct identifiers removed should be prohibited by law, and violators should face legal sanctions. In addition, researchers receiving information with direct identifiers removed should be required to establish security safeguards and to set limits on access to data.

In cases where researchers cannot use data with direct identifiers removed, and personally identifiable health information is needed for research, approval and oversight by an ethics board should be required, partially analogous to what is now done under the HIPAA Privacy Rule and PHIPA. This ethics oversight board could perhaps entail a new body specifically formulated to review medical records research, rather than relying on traditional IRBs that were created to review interventional research. If researchers seek a waiver of informed consent, an ethics oversight board should consider the measures the researchers have proposed to take to protect the privacy, security, and confidentiality of the data, the potential harms that could result from disclosure of the data, and the potential public benefits of the proposed research study. Privacy should not automatically be a more compelling interest than improving health care. However, even research with little risk to privacy should not be conducted if the study has little scientific merit or anticipated public benefit.

Under this new system, HHS should implement real consequences for any researcher or institution that mishandles personally identifiable health information, regardless of whether it is obtained through informed consent or under a waiver of informed consent. In order to facilitate consistent application of this option, HHS should issue clear guidance and best practices (as recommended in Chapter 4) on how to assess the potential harm, the proposed measures to protect privacy and confidentiality, and the potential public benefits of a research study, as has been done under PHIPA. For example, the Canadian Institute for Health Information has developed best privacy practices for research to provide guidance for determining whether or not a waiver of consent is warranted (CIHR, 2005).

The primary focus of many IRBs in reviewing research protocols in the past has been on risks to the physical safety of research participants. There is a great deal of variability in whether and how IRBs consider the public benefit and scientific merit of research proposals. But the first rule of ethical research is that the research must have scientific value—meaning that it addresses an important question of human health and is designed and conducted using methodology that is appropriate and rigorous. The scientific merit of research varies by project, just as the potential risk to privacy of research varies across different protocols. The committee believes that when making decisions about whether a research protocol that entails the disclosure of personally identifiable information should go forward, ethical oversight boards should take all these factors—potential risks/harms to research participants' privacy as well as scientific merit and potential public benefit of the research proposal—into consideration.

In 2001, a previous IOM committee, the Committee on Assessing the System for Protecting Human Research Subjects, recommended that "human research participant protection programs" use distinct mechanisms for initial, focused reviews of scientific merit and financial conflicts of interest and that these reviews should precede and inform the comprehensive ethical review of research studies. Ethical oversight board members themselves may not have the expertise to assess the merit of diverse research studies, but they should have access to evaluations by scientific review committees or funder peer review panels. Input regarding the scientific value of studies from these experts would help ethical oversight boards assess the anticipated benefits of a proposed research project.

The Role of Informed Consent in the New Framework

Informed consent is intended to achieve two purposes: (1) protect research participants from harm and (2) provide respect for the person (including the person's privacy, religious beliefs, cultural preferences, and world views). As outlined above, the framework maintains a requirement for informed consent for all interventional clinical research. The purpose of informed consent in this type of research is mainly to protect research participants from harm by providing a description of the potential risks and benefits of the study and to seek permission to involve the subject. Although privacy protection is a component of the risk/benefit considerations, the main focus traditionally has been on physical harms. One study found that confidentiality is one of the least important considerations for potential research participants in deciding whether to participate in interventional clinical research (Tait et al., 2002).

However, it is important to note that interventional researchers are expected to follow the principles of medical ethics, which require that information disclosed in the course of medical treatment is kept as confidential as possible. Moreover, the committee's framework includes the recommendation that strong security safeguards be required for any data collected in conjunction with an interventional study. The framework's permission of future consent for researchers' use of data and biological materials, actually increases individuals' ability to exercise control over their personally identifiable information. Under the Privacy Rule, the requirement to obtain a new authorization form signed for each research study means that most future studies actually proceed under a waiver of authorization, and individuals are deprived of all input into future uses of their information (Nosowsky and Giordano, 2006). Thus, informed consent in this context addresses protection from both physical harm and dignitary harm.

In contrast, in information-based research that relies solely on medical records and stored biospecimens, the research participant faces no risk of physical harm. In this context, informed consent is intended to ensure that individuals are able to exercise control over their personally identifiable health information that is held by third parties, and to give individuals the right to determine whether their personally identifiable health information can be used in a particular research project (or a series of such projects, if consent for future research is permitted). However, a universal requirement for informed consent can lead to invalid results, because of significant differences between patients who do or do not grant consent, and missed opportunities to advance medical science because it can be prohibitively costly and difficult to obtain consent for studies that require analysis of very large datasets.

As a result, the framework includes two alternatives to requiring informed consent that can be used in certain circumstances (i.e., disclosure to a certified entity and waiver of informed consent by an ethics oversight board), which are intended to facilitate research that is in the public interest. For research that makes use of these two alternatives, the framework counterbalances the absence of informed consent with an increase in security, transparency, and accountability protections by: (1) requiring certified entities to protect the privacy and confidentiality of personally identifiable health information records in a manner that is approved by an outside party (HHS or a different body), (2) requiring certified entities to fully disclose what research is being conducted with its data, (3) requiring ethics oversight review for research that uses personally identifiable data under a waiver of informed consent, (4) implementing clear and consistent consequences for researchers who are responsible for privacy or security breaches, and (5) encouraging the development and use of improved security protections for use in health research.

Public opinion polls indicate that a significant portion of the public would prefer to control all access to their medical records via informed consent. However, as noted above, a universal requirement for informed consent would impede important health research and lead to biased, ungeneralizable results, to the detriment of society. The committee believes that the new framework provides strong protections for data privacy and security, beyond that currently provided under the Privacy Rule, while increasing the opportunities for important health research by offering an alternative to informed consent under certain circumstances.

The Belmont Report, one of the most influential reports on the advancement of human research participant protections, recognizes that principles of respect for persons and autonomy are not absolutes and must be considered along with other ethical principles. It acknowledges that there may be compelling reasons to limit autonomy, providing that "To show lack of respect for an autonomous agent is to repudiate that person's considered judgments, to deny an individual the freedom to act on those considered judgments, or to withhold information necessary to make a considered judgment, *when there are no compelling reasons to do so*" (emphasis added) (HEW, 1979). Similarly, a 1994 IOM report argued that existing health information, stored in medical records and biospecimen banks, should be released to researchers without informed consent if such studies were regarded as being in the public's interest (IOM, 1994).

If society seeks to derive the benefits of medical research in the form of improved health and health care, information should be shared to achieve that societal benefit (Chadwick and Berg, 2001; Knoppers and Chadwick, 2005; Liu, 2007), and governing regulations should support the use of such information. Recent reports from the United Kingdom have come to a similar conclusion and recommend that the law allow the use of personally identifiable health information without consent if the use of that information is necessary and the potential benefits to society outweigh the individual risks (AMS, 2006, 2008; Thomas and Walport, 2008). In the committee's proposed new framework, the greater emphasis on ensuring the security protections of personally identifiable health information, facilitating research using data with direct identifiers removed, and ensuring the scientific merits of any proposed research should help to foster its acceptability. Nonetheless, to implement this new framework, effective communication with the public regarding the value of this model will be important to address concerns and gain acceptance, as recommended in Chapter 3.

THE NEW FRAMEWORK ADDRESSES
THE OVERARCHING GOALS

The committee supports its argument in favor of implementing a new framework for protecting privacy in health research by outlining how this approach achieves the committee's three overarching goals: (1) improving the privacy and data security of health information, (2) improving the effectiveness of health research, and (3) improving the application of privacy protections for health research (see Box 6-1). The committee believes many of the limitations of the current federal regulation of research can be improved or solved by the proposed framework.

Improving the Privacy and Data Security of Health Information

The new framework includes a number of mechanisms to improve the protection of research participants' privacy and security in health research. First, the privacy of research participants is improved because the new framework applies to all institutions and all health researchers who collect, use, and disclose personally identifiable health information. Similar to Ontario's PHIPA, this means that the privacy protections follow the data. No matter what entity or individual holds the personally identifiable data, the same set of privacy safeguards are required.

Second, the new framework maintains the requirement that researchers obtain informed consent for all interventional clinical research and strengthens the security protections of data collected in the course of a clinical trial. The new framework also permits research participants in interventional, clinical research to provide informed consent for future research uses of their data and biological materials collected as part of the study. The privacy of these individuals is protected by requiring an IRB to review any future studies and to determine that the future uses are not incompatible with the original informed consent. This aspect of the new framework actually promotes individuals' ability to exercise control over their personally identifiable information. As stated above, the requirement in the Privacy Rule that researchers must obtain new authorization for every use of protected health information means that most future studies proceed under a waiver of authorization, and individuals are deprived of all input into future uses of their information (Nosowsky and Giordano, 2006).

Third, the new framework protects privacy by maintaining the default requirement that researchers must obtain informed consent to use personally identifiable data for research. If researchers wish to use personally identifiable data without obtaining informed consent for information-based research, they are required to identify and document their research objectives to an ethics oversight board, and they must identify the measures by which they will protect the privacy, security, and confidentiality of the data. The ethics oversight boards provide impartial review, and are only permitted to waive informed consent after considering the measures to protect the privacy, security, and confidentiality of the data; the risk of harm in conducting the research; and the potential public benefit of the research study.

Fourth, the new framework protects privacy by creating certified entities that facilitate researchers use of data with direct identifiers removed. One of the major problems with the deidentification provisions of the Privacy Rule is the difficulty in linking data from multiple sources to generate more complete datasets or to follow patient outcomes longitudinally (see Chapter 5 for more details). The new framework's certified entity concept provides a solution to this problem; certified entities are able to link and match personally identifiable information longitudinally from multiple sources and can then disclose data with direct identifiers removed to researchers. Because the data provided by certified entities with direct identifiers removed has already been linked and aggregated, it is more useful for research. Thus, researchers will be able to make greater use of deidentified datasets and will need access to personally identifiable data in fewer situations. Privacy is improved because there are fewer risks to privacy when researchers do not access or use personally identifiable data.

In addition, the privacy of data held by certified entities is protected because certified entities are required to have their privacy and security policies approved and re-approved on a regular basis by an outside party (HHS or a different body). Certified entities are also required to implement specific privacy safeguards including mandatory privacy training for all staff/researchers, signing of confidentiality agreements, privacy breach policies and procedures, mandatory privacy impact assessments, and security safeguards and limits on access to data.

Finally, the new framework protects privacy in health research by requiring the implementation of comprehensive privacy protections, including transparency, accountability, and security. Transparency is improved by the new framework's requirement that certified entities publicize the scope and purpose of their data collection and provide information on what uses of their data will not be permitted. Transparency is also achieved by requiring researchers to describe in detail their research plans and objectives (either to potential research participants or to the ethics oversight board) and to justify the data they wish to use and/or collect. Accountability is improved by the new framework because it requires Congress and HHS to implement clear and consistent consequences for researchers who are responsible for privacy or security breaches. The new framework also includes provisions for penalizing any individuals who attempt to re-identify data that has had its direct identifiers removed. Security is improved in the new framework because all holders of health data, both personally identifiable data and data with direct identifiers removed, are required to implement security safeguards, as described in Chapter 2, and to set limits on access to data. The committee also believes that the increased emphasis on accountability in the new framework will encourage researchers and other stakeholders to invest money in developing privacy-enhancing technologies for use in research, to reduce the risk of accidental breaches and the associated consequences.

Improving the Effectiveness of Health Research

The new framework is intended to provide a method of regulating health research, including the protection of individual privacy, in a way that minimizes impediments to beneficial research. First, allowing patients to consent to the future use of specimens collected during the course of an interventional study or treatment will reduce many barriers to researchers' use of existing biospecimen banks. Patient privacy is protected by requiring any future uses of these specimens to be approved by an IRB, which should determine whether a proposed study has scientific merit, implements appropriate privacy protections, and is not incompatible with the original consent.

Second, the creation of certified entities that can receive personally identifiable health information for information-based research without patient informed consent, similar to PHIPA's prescribed entities and the United Kingdom's safe harbors (Thomas and Walport, 2008), will result in more complete and representative datasets, and thus will result in more generalizable results. The creation of certified entities will also facilitate research using data with direct identifiers removed. As stated above, under the current system, researchers cannot link datasets from multiple covered entities without a unique identifier. If a certified entity performed this task, researchers could make greater use of data without identifiers.

Third, the goal-oriented framework with a focus on best practices should aid the work of both researchers and IRBs and reduce the variability across different institutions. For example, it should be easier for IRBs to make appropriate decisions regarding waivers of informed consent because the framework's goal is to allow beneficial research to be conducted if comprehensive privacy and security safeguards are in place and privacy risks are minimized. Identification and dissemination of best practices in privacy protection for various types of health research would help delineate what IRBs should do to facilitate responsible research, rather than just defining what is permissible.

Finally, the committee believes this framework will reduce some of the research costs and time that have increased since the Privacy Rule was implemented because the framework is designed to make research oversight more uniform and to reduce administrative burdens.

Improving the Application of Privacy Protections for Health Research

A recent report by the National Committee on Vital and Health Statistics (NCVHS) recognized the importance of having nationally uniform privacy protections for all secondary uses of health data, including research. The report criticized the Privacy Rule's reliance on the covered entity construct and creation of business associate agreements to PHI (NCVHS, 2007). The framework proposed by the IOM committee addresses this criticism of the Privacy Rule, and provides for a comprehensive regulation of research that applies to all researchers and protects all personally identifiable health data in research. It eliminates a primary problem of harmonization of privacy protections because the framework is intended to be the only regulation governing researchers' use of health data. In addition, the implementation of this framework would improve the clarity of privacy protections because currently much of the confusion is due to the Privacy Rule's complicated interactions with other existing privacy regulations, such as the Common Rule.

One potential challenge under the new framework is the need to define health research and to distinguish interventional research from information-based research. HHS will need to develop clear guidelines to help researchers and ethics oversight boards consistently make this distinction. The identification and dissemination by HHS of best practices in research protections (as recommended in Chapter 5) will be important to ensure greater uniformity of goal-oriented research oversight and to ensure that the framework is implemented in a way that facilitates research without undermining individual privacy. In addition, there will be some administrative burden in certifying and overseeing the certified entities.

RELEVANCE OF THE RECOMMENDATION TO OTHER FEDERAL ACTIONS

The committee's recommendation for a new framework to regulate health research is particularly timely because new actions at the federal level are being considered or have already been taken to protect the privacy of electronic health records. These developments raise new concerns about potential impacts on health research. The committee believes this proposal will stimulate fresh ideas about the best ways to protect privacy and improve research as the nation addresses these two interrelated values over the next several years.

An example of one of the recent developments affecting research is the Department of Veterans Affairs' (VA's) August 2007 directive. Outlining new conditions under which it would release data from VA hospitals to state central cancer registries, the directive requires states to sign a data use agreement with the VA and to agree to implement privacy and security protections above and beyond the protections required in the HIPAA Privacy and Security Rules. Among other requirements, state registries must agree not to release VA cancer data to persons outside the registry or to reuse the data for any purpose other than for maintaining cancer statistics (Kolata, 2007b).

Each state has a law establishing cancer surveillance programs that collect information on every patient who is diagnosed with cancer in that state. Also, the National Cancer Institute (NCI) collects cancer statistics from 17 U.S. regions in order to track national cancer rates. Prior to the VA directive, the state cancer surveillance programs and the NCI included information gathered from VA hospitals. However, as of October 10, 2007, only a small percentage of the states had signed the VA directive, and most cancer surveillance programs were missing data on veterans (Kolata, 2007a).

In addition, the VA directive stipulates that researchers who want to use cancer statistics from VA hospitals must either obtain permission from the VA Under Secretary of Health or collaborate with a VA researcher on the project. Health researchers are finding it hard to conduct cancer research under these conditions, which makes it difficult to find VA researchers willing to collaborate on specific projects. The directive also complicates the IRB approval process, often requiring researchers to obtain approval from their local IRB, the cancer registry IRB, and the VA Under Secretary (Kolata, 2007b). In addition, cancer researchers who either cannot meet the VA requirements or choose not to go through the additional procedural requirements, and do not include VA data in their study, risk having their results compromised by selection bias (see Chapter 5, section on Selection Bias).

Several recently proposed bills that address the use of electronic medical records also contain language regarding health privacy and health research (Table 6-2).

In 2004, President Bush issued an executive order calling for the widespread adoption of an interoperable electronic health record system within 10 years, arguing that health information technology (HIT) is a means of addressing rising health care costs and improving the quality and efficiency of health care (Bush, 2004). In response, HHS has awarded a number of HIT grants to gather information on privacy and security issues in HIT, solicited recommendations from NCVHS, and created the American Health

TABLE 6-2 Health Information Technology (HIT) Bills from the 110th Congress

Proposed Bill	Main Purpose(s)	Privacy Provisions	Research Provisions	Status
Wired for Health Care Quality Act (S 1693), sponsored by Sens. Kennedy [D-NY] and Enzi [R-WY]; Promoting Health Information Technology (HR 3800), sponsored by Rep. Eshoo [D-CA]	To enhance the adoption of a nationwide, interoperable health information technology (HIT) system, and to improve the quality and reduce the costs of health care	• Establishes an advisory body to provide policy advice to the U.S. Department of Health and Human Services (HHS) on the protection of personally identifiable health information, including ways to notify individuals if their information is wrongfully disclosed • Organizations competing for federal HIT grants must protect the privacy and security of health information and preserve an audit record • Expands the definition of "covered entity" under HIPAA to include operators of HIT systems	• Gives researchers access to deidentified patient enrollment data, reimbursement claims, and survey data maintained by HHS or its contractors • Also gives researchers access to deidentified data maintained by the federal government or government contractors where feasible • In general, research is still governed by the HIPAA Privacy Rule	In the Senate: • Approved by the Health, Education, Labor and Pensions Committee on 6/07 • Sen. Kennedy filed a written report on 10/07 • Placed on the unanimous consent calendar for a vote without debate or possibility of amendment In the House: Referred to the Committee on Energy and Commerce

continued

| Independent Health Record Trust Act of 2007 (HR 2991), sponsored by Reps. Ryan [D-OH] and Moore [D-KS] | To encourage the creation, use, and maintenance of electronic health records in independent health records trusts (IHRTs), and to provide a secure and privacy-protected framework in which health records are only made available by the affirmative consent of individuals | • Participation in an IHRT must be voluntary
• IHRTs must have privacy protection agreements, which govern the access and transfer of individuals' data
• Requires express informed consent before individuals' information can be disclosed
• Gives IHRTs a fiduciary duty to act for the benefit and interests of its participants; penalties for breach include loss of certification, fines of $50,000 or less, prison terms of 5 years or less
• Requires an audit trail to be maintained
• Provides for individual notification of all breaches | • Researchers may only access an individual's health data stored in an IHRT when given express informed consent, and researchers may only access those portions of the record as specified by the participant | Referred to the House Committee on Energy and Commerce, and to the Committee on Ways and Means |

TABLE 6-2 Continued

Proposed Bill	Main Purpose(s)	Privacy Provisions	Research Provisions	Status
TRUST in Health Information Act of 2008 (HR 5442), sponsored by Rep. Markey [D-MA]	To ensure privacy, security, and confidentiality in the creation of a nationwide, interoperable health information infrastructure, and to provide for the strong enforcement of these rights by creating criminal and civil penalties	• Outlines specific requirements for maintaining a HIT system that is private, secure, and confidential • Provides consumers with specific privacy rights • Requires express informed consent before individuals' information can be disclosed for most purposes • Creates an individual right of action for knowing or negligent violations of the Act • Authorizes states' attorney generals to bring civil actions on behalf of residents	• Leaves the HIPAA Privacy Rule in place for health research • Requires HHS to prepare a Report to Congress on whether informed consent should be required for the use of personal health information in research, and under what circumstances • As soon as reasonably possible, researchers who receives personal health information must remove or destroy information that would enable an individual to be identified, unless otherwise approved by an IRB • HHS will provide IRBs with periodic review and technical assistance	Referred to the House Committees on Energy and Commerce, Ways and Means, Education and Labor, and Financial Services

continued

| Health Information Privacy and Security Act (S 1814), sponsored by Sens. Leahy [D-VT] and Kennedy [D-MA] | To ensure the privacy of health information, to promote the use of deidentified information in health research, and to provide for the strong enforcement of these rights by creating criminal and civil penalties | • Creates the Office of Health Information Privacy to establish privacy and security standards for HIT products and to outline punishments for violations
• Provides consumers with specific privacy rights
• Requires express informed consent before individuals' information can be disclosed for most purposes
• Creates an individual right of action for knowing violations of the Act | • Leaves the HIPAA Privacy Rule in place for health research
• Requires HHS to prepare a Report to Congress on whether informed consent should be required for the use of personal health information in research, and under what circumstances
• As soon as reasonably possible, researchers who receive personal health information must remove or destroy information that would enable an individual to be identified, unless otherwise approved by an IRB
• HHS will provide IRBs with periodic review and technical assistance | Read twice and referred to the Senate Health, Education, Labor and Pensions Committee on 7/18/2007 |

TABLE 6-2 Continued

Proposed Bill	Main Purpose(s)	Privacy Provisions	Research Provisions	Status
Health Information Technology Act (HR 6357), sponsored by Reps. Dingell [D-MI], Barton [R-TX], Pallone [D-NJ], and Deal [R-GA]	To encourage the use of HIT, develop technical standards, and improve the quality and reduce the costs of health care	• Provides for individual notification of all breaches • Requires HHS to designate an individual in each regional office to offer guidance and education to covered entities, business associates, and the public on the rights and responsibilities related to PHI • Encourages the use of limited datasets • Requires an audit trail to be maintained	• Directs the Office of the National Coordinator of Health Information Technology to "facilitate health research and health care quality" • Directs HHS to issue guidance on how to best implement the deidentification standards in the HIPAA Privacy Rule	Currently in draft form

Information Community to provide policy advice (AHIC, 2006; GAO, 2007; NCVHS, 2006).

But privacy concerns are emerging as a primary obstacle to implementing a nationwide HIT system, with many privacy and consumer groups pushing for tighter privacy protections than offered under the Privacy Rule. In a 2006 poll, 62 percent of respondents stated that the use of electronic health records would pose new risks to privacy, and 42 percent answered that the privacy risks of HIT outweigh expected benefits (Harris Interactive, 2007). Another poll found that 80 percent of Americans say they are very concerned about identity theft or fraud in an HIT system (Markle Foundation, 2006). The Government Accountability Office recently released a report that legitimized these concerns and criticized HHS for failing to define an overall approach for protecting privacy in a nationwide HIT system (GAO, 2007).

To address the privacy concerns, Congress has proposed a number of bills intended to advance the implementation of an HIT system and at the same time protect individual privacy[11] (see Table 6-2). Several of these bills include new restrictions and rules governing researchers' access to personally identifiable health information. It is unclear whether any of these bills will pass or what requirements a final law might include. However, because a nationwide HIT system has the potential to facilitate health research by making large amounts of health data available to study, and thus could lead to major advances in medicine, caution is warranted. Adoption of new, restrictive regulations might impede health research, to the detriment of patients and society. Therefore, a closer examination of some concepts that have been incorporated into these proposed bills, including autonomy and informed consent, is warranted. At the same time, it is clear there is a need to develop privacy safeguards that anticipate the risk of extensive electronic recordkeeping, as well as the growing problems of identity theft and security breaches.

CONCLUSIONS AND RECOMMENDATIONS

The primary justification for including research provisions in the HIPAA Privacy Rule was to remedy perceived shortcomings of federal privacy protections in health research under the Common Rule. But the Privacy Rule has numerous limitations of its own. In proposing the Privacy Rule, HHS acknowledged that, ideally, it would have preferred to regulate health researchers directly by extending the protections of the Common

---

[11] A number of bills from the 110th Congress also address the implementation of HIT, but do not include comprehensive privacy or research provisions, including HR 1368, S 1408, and S 1455.

Rule to research that is not federally supported and by imposing additional criteria for the waiver of patient informed consent for the use of personally identifiable health information in research.[12] But HHS recognized it did not have the authority to do this. For that reason, HHS attempted to protect the health information released to researchers indirectly (but within the scope of its limited authority) by imposing restrictions on information disclosures by covered entities. NCVHS and others have noted the limitations of the Privacy Rule and have called for stronger protections of health privacy—notably, by expanding the purview of the Privacy Rule beyond the current covered entities.

However, the IOM committee believes an even bolder change is needed. The number of studies using medical records to address important questions about health and disease will likely increase with the growing availability of electronic health records. As the volume and importance of digital personally identifiable health data increase exponentially, the public can be expected to heighten demands for a legal framework that provides meaningful safeguards to protect health information in the health research setting. **Thus, the IOM committee recommends that Congress authorize HHS and other relevant federal agencies to develop a new framework for ensuring privacy that would apply uniformly to all health research and that will both protect individuals' privacy and facilitate responsible and beneficial health research.**

When this new approach is implemented, HHS should exempt health research from the HIPAA Privacy Rule. The new approach would enhance privacy protections through improved data privacy and security, increased transparency of activities and policies, and greater accountability. The new approach should do all the following:

- Apply to any person, institution, or organization conducting health research in the United States, regardless of the source of data or funding.
- Entail clear, goal-oriented, rather than prescriptive, regulations.
- Require researchers, institutions, and organizations that store health data to establish strong data security safeguards.
- Make a clear distinction between the privacy considerations that apply to interventional research and research that is exclusively information based.

---

[12] U.S. Secretary of Health and Human Services, *Recommendations on the Confidentiality of Individually-Identifiable Health Information to the Committees on Labor and Human Resources* (1997), and Standards for Privacy of Individually Identifiable Health Information: Proposed Rule, 64 Fed. Reg. 59918, 59967 (1999) (for a discussion on the benefits of health records research).

- Facilitate greater use of data with direct identifiers removed in health research, and implement legal sanctions to prohibit unauthorized reidentification of information that has had direct identifiers removed.
- Require ethical oversight of research when personally identifiable health information is used without informed consent. HHS should develop best practices for oversight that should consider:
  — Measures taken to protect the privacy, security, and confidentiality of the data;
  — Potential harms that could result from disclosure of the data; and
  — Potential public benefits of the research.
- Certify institutions that have policies and practices in place to protect data privacy and security in order to facilitate important large-scale information-based research for clearly defined and approved purposes, without individual consent.
- Include federal oversight and enforcement to ensure regulatory compliance.

A new approach to protecting the privacy of personally identifiable information used in health research that emphasizes privacy, security, accountability, and transparency and that is applicable to all health research in the United States would eliminate the research community's confusion, reduce institutional variability in research privacy practices, facilitate responsible research, and enhance the public's trust in the research enterprise. Clear and simple regulations that are less subject to varying interpretation by ethical oversight boards, as well as federal oversight and enforcement of regulatory compliance, will be important to consistently and efficiently ensure privacy and instill trust while enabling important research.

The new framework developed by HHS and other relevant federal agencies should provide strong and effective protection for often-sensitive personally identifiable health information and facilitate scientific discovery and medical innovation necessary to save lives and enhance the quality of the public's health. And it should do so in a way that does not burden individuals with a flurry of health privacy notices and consent forms, or burden our health care system with a new level of bureaucracy and expense.

REFERENCES

AHIC (American Health Information Community). 2006. Letter to Michael Leavitt. http://www.ncvhs.hhs.gov/061030lt.pdf (accessed September 3, 2008).

AHIC. 2007. *Confidentiality, privacy, and security workgroup, summary of the 14th web conference.* http://137.187.25.8/healthit/ahic/materials/summary/cpssum_100407.html (accessed August 27, 2008).

AHIC. 2008. *Confidentiality, privacy & security workgroup draft recommendation letter from September 23, 2008.* http://www.hhs.gov/healthit/ahic/materials/08_08/cps/rec_letter. html (accessed September 19, 2008).

AHIMA (American Health Information Management Association). 2006. *The state of HIPAA privacy and security compliance.* http://www.ahima.org/emerging_issues/ 2006StateofHIPAACompliance.pdf (accessed April 20, 2008).

Allen, A. 2007. *Allen's privacy law and society.* Eagan, MN: Thomson-West.

AMS (Academy of Medical Sciences). 2006. *Personal data for public good: Using health information in medical research.* http://www.acmedsci.ac.uk/images/project/Personal.pdf (accessed August 28, 2008).

AMS. 2008. *Submission to data sharing review.* http://www.acmedsci.ac.uk/download. php?file=/images/publication/120341733123.pdf (accessed September 4, 2008).

Buchanan, A. 1999. An ethical framework for biological samples policy, National Bioethics Advisory Committee commissioned paper. In *Research involving human biological materials: Ethical issues and policy guidance.* Vol. II. Washington, DC: National Bioethics Advisory Commission. Pp. B1–B31.

Bush, G. W. 2004. Executive Order 13335. *69 Fed. Reg. 24059.*

Casarett, D., J. Karlawish, E. Andrews, and A. Caplan. 2005. Bioethical issues in pharmaco-epidemiological research In *Pharmacoepidemiology*, 4th ed., edited by B. L. Strom. West Sussex, England: John Wiley & Sons, Ltd. Pp. 417–432.

Cate, F. 2008 (unpublished). *The autonomy trap.*

CDT (Center for Democracy & Technology). 2008a. *Beyond consumer consent: Why we need a comprehensive approach to privacy in a networked world.* http://www.cdt.org/ healthprivacy/20080221consentbrief.pdf (accessed September 4, 2008).

CDT. 2008b. *Comprehensive privacy and security: Critical for health information technology.* Version 1.0. http://www.cdt.org/healthprivacy/20080514HPframe.pdf (accessed September 4, 2008).

Chadwick, R., and K. Berg. 2001. Solidarity and equity: New ethical frameworks for genetic databases. *Nature* 2:318–321.

CIHR (Canadian Institutes of Health Research). 2005. *CIHR best practices for protecting privacy in health research.* Ottawa, Ontario: Public Works and Government Services Canada.

Foster, A. L. 2008. Increase in stolen laptops endangers data security. *The Chronicle of Higher Education* July 4.

GAO (Government Accountability Office). 2007. *Health information technology: Early efforts initiated but comprehensive privacy approach needed for national strategy.* Washington, DC: GAO.

Good, N., R. Dhamija, J. Grossklags, D. Thaw, S. Aronowitz, D. Mulligan, and J. Konstan. 2005. *Stopping spyware at the gate: A user study of privacy, notice and spyware.* http://cups.cs.cmu.edu/soups/2005/2005proceedings/p43-good.pdf (accessed September 4, 2008).

Gostin, L. O. 2001. Health information: Reconciling personal privacy with the public good of human health. *Health Care Analysis* 9:321.

Harris Interactive. 2007. *The benefits of electronic medical records sound good, but privacy could become a difficult issue.* http://www.harrisinteractive.com/news/printerfriend/index. asp?NewsID=1174 (accessed April 3, 2007).

HEW (Department of Health, Education and Welfare). 1979. *The Belmont Report: Ethical principles and guidelines for the protection of human subjects of research.* http://ohsr. od.nih.gov/guidelines/belmont.html (accessed August 21, 2008).

HHS. 2008a. *Compliance and enforcement: Privacy Rule enforcement highlights.* http://www. hhs.gov/ocr/privacy/enforcement/ (accessed July 23, 2008).

HHS. 2008b. *Resolution agreement.* http://www.hhs.gov/ocr/privacy/enforcement/agreement. pdf (accessed October 3, 2008).

IOM (Institute of Medicine). 1994. *Health data in the information age: Use, disclosure, and privacy.* Washington, DC: National Academy Press.

IOM. 2006. *Effect of the HIPAA Privacy Rule on health research: Proceedings of a workshop presented to the National Cancer Policy Forum.* Washington, DC: The National Academies Press.

ITRC (Identity Theft Resource Center). 2008. *Security breaches.* http://www.idtheftcenter. org/artman2/publish/lib_survey/ITRC_2008_Breach_List_printer.shtml (accessed July 22, 2008).

Jonas, H. 1991. Philosophical reflections on experimenting with human subjects. In *Biomedical ethics*, edited by T. A. Mappes and J. S. Zembaty. New York: Oxford University Press. Pp. 215–219.

Knoppers, B. M., and R. Chadwick. 2005. Human genetic research: Emerging trends in ethics. *Nature Reviews Genetics* 6:75–79.

Kolata, G. 2007a. How data on cancer are collected and used. *The New York Times*, October 10.

Kolata, G. 2007b. States and V.A. at odds on cancer data. *The New York Times*, October 10.

Liu, E. T. 2007. *The importance of research using personal information for scientific discovery and the reduction of disease, in personal information for biomedical research.* Annex A. http://www.bioethics-singapore.org/uploadfile/20013%20PMPI%20Annex%20A-3.pdf (accessed September 4, 2008).

Lo, B. 2009 (in press). *Resolving ethical dilemmas: A guide for clinicians.* 4th ed. Philadelphia, PA: Lippincott Williams & Wilkins.

Markle Foundation. 2006. *Survey finds Americans want electronic personal health information to improve own health care.* http://www.markle.org/downloadable_assets/research_ doc_120706.pdf (accessed September 4, 2008).

NCVHS (National Committee on Vital and Health Statistics). 2006. *Functional requirements needed for the initial definition of a nationwide health information network.* http://www. ncvhs.hhs.gov/061030lt.pdf (accessed September 4, 2008).

NCVHS. 2007. Enhanced protections for uses of health data: A stewardship framework for "secondary uses" of electronically collected and transmitted health data. http://ncvhs.hhs. gov/071221lt.pdf (accessed December 19, 2007).

Nosowsky, R., and T. Giordano. 2006. The Health Insurance Portability and Accountability Act of 1996 (HIPAA) Privacy Rule: Implications for clinical research. *Annual Review of Medicine* 57:575–590.

Pritts, J. 2008. *The importance and value of protecting the privacy of health information: Roles of HIPAA Privacy Rule and the Common Rule in health research.* http://www.iom. edu/CMS/3740/43729/53160.aspx (accessed March 15, 2008).

Rahman, N. 2006. Medical: Reflections on privacy: Recent developments in HIPAA Privacy Rule. *I/S: A Journal of Law and Policy for the Information Society* 2(3):685.

Rotenberg, M. 2001. Fair information practices and the architecture of privacy: (what Larry doesn't get). *Stanford Technology Law Review* 1. http://stlr.stanford.edu/STLR/ Articles/01_STLR_1 (accessed November 6, 2008).

Appendix A

Previous Recommendations to the Department of Health and Human Services

As a result of the reported concerns about the Privacy Rule's effect on health research, several organizations have provided the U.S. Department of Health and Human Services (HHS) with recommendations on how to improve the way the Privacy Rule regulates research. Table A-1 describes the recommendations of the National Committee on Vital and Health Statistics, the Association of American Medical Colleges, the Secretary's Advisory Committee on Human Research Protections, and the National Cancer Advisory Board. A brief explanation of how these organizations generated their recommendations is provided below.

NATIONAL COMMITTEE ON VITAL AND HEALTH STATISTICS

The U.S. Congress gave the National Committee on Vital and Health Statistics (NCVHS) the responsibility of advising the Secretary of HHS on the adoption of the Privacy Rule standards, monitoring its implementation, and reporting annually to Congress on the progress made in its adoption. In accordance with this mandate, NCVHS has held a number of hearings on the Privacy Rule and the problems that the medical community has experienced in implementing the requirements of the Privacy Rule. One of the topics explored during these hearings was the obstacles associated with conducting research under the Privacy Rule. After each hearing, NCVHS subsequently issued a letter to the Secretary of HHS with a set of recommendations for improving the Privacy Rule. The recommendations outlined in Table A-1 are based on the hearings held on August 21–23, 2001, and November 19–20, 2003 (NCVHS, 2001, 2004).

TABLE A-1 Previous Recommendations to HHS Regarding Research and the HIPAA Privacy Rule

Topic	Issues	Recommendations	Organization
Accounting for disclosures of protected health information (PHI) for research purposes	Creates excessive paperwork for covered entities and has resulted in some covered entities refusing to make PHI available to researchers.	1. Eliminate the accounting for disclosures requirement for research (AAMC, SACHRP) *and* instead, inform patients that PHI might be used for research purposes (SACHRP). 2. HHS should issue guidance to provide covered entities with ways to fulfill this requirement in a convenient and practical manner (NCVHS).	NCVHS AAMC SACHRP
Standards for deidentification of data	Loss of ability to carry out research because of loss of information, cost, and administrative burden.	HHS should review standards to reduce the number of categories removed from deidentified data.	NCVHS AAMC SACHRP
Recruitment of research subjects	1. Institutional Review Boards (IRBs) already consider recruitment as part of their study oversight. 2. Artificial distinction between internal and external researchers exists. 3. Identification and contacting potential research participants are considered different activities. 4. Creation of biased populations in studies, especially too few less-educated, low-income individuals.	1. HHS should classify research recruitment as a health care operation, obviating the need for authorization and allaying confusion (SACHRP). 2. If "1" is rejected, HHS should provide additional formal guidance on contacting potential research participants *and* HHS should end differential treatment of internal and external researchers for purposes of identifying and contacting potential participants (SACHRP, NCVHS).	NCVHS SACHRP

Databases and tissue repositories: future uses of research data and biological materials	Loss of future research opportunities; confusion regarding combined authorization.	1. When an IRB has approved a consent form that permits future uses under the Common Rule standard, the same should apply under the Privacy Rule. Permit combining research authorization for a clinical trial and for banking data and materials collected as part of the trial in a single form (NCVHS, SACHRP).	NCVHS SACHRP NCAB
		2. Eliminate the restriction on the use of data for unspecified future research, or allow a less specific description of the intended use (NCAB).	
		3. Clarify how identified datasets collected under a broad authorization to create a database could be released to researchers through the use of a waiver of authorization, a limited dataset, or by deidentifying the information.	
Research exempt under the Common Rule	Discrepancies between the Common Rule and the Privacy Rule create challenges for IRBs and Privacy Boards that must make decisions about such things as waivers of authorization.	1. Revise categories of research not requiring authorization to include research determined by IRB to be exempt from Common Rule requirements (SACHRP).	NCVHS SACHRP
		2. HHS should provide further interpretation, guidance, and technical assistance to help the research community to understand the relationship between the Privacy Rule and the Common Rule (NCVHS).	

continued

TABLE A-1 Continued

Topic	Issues	Recommendations	Organization
Use and disclosure of PHI for research	The process for obtaining an authorization or waiver of authorization is burdensome, and discourages research from being conducted.	1. Authorization and waiver of authorization requirements should be eliminated for research purposes. Research disclosures are adequately protected by the Common Rule (AAMC). 2. Continue to require authorization or waiver of authorization for research, despite the administrative burden (NCVHS).	NCVHS AAMC NCAB
IRB waiver of authorization	Authorization and informed consent can be combined into a single document. Under the Common Rule, IRBs must review informed consent documents. However, the Privacy Rule does not require IRBs to review authorization forms.	HHS should clarify that nothing in the Privacy Rule prevents IRBs from reviewing authorization forms when considering the adequacy of privacy and confidentiality of subjects under the Common Rule.	NCVHS
Genetics research	It is unclear whether DNA samples can ever be deidentified because analyzing the samples could reveal unique DNA identifiers of the individual.	HHS should clarify whether DNA samples can be considered deidentified data.	NCVHS
Types of covered entities	Academic medical centers cannot organize in a manner that reflects the functional operations of the medical school, affiliated practice plans, and teaching hospital.	The covered entity status, hybrid entity status, and affiliated covered entity status should be redefined to reflect the function served by the different parts of the organization, not the organizational form of the organization.	AAMC

Transition provisions	The implementation of the Privacy Rule could hamper studies already under way.	For research begun before the Privacy Rule took effect, grandfather research that did not receive IRB review or oversight because it was exempt under Common Rule.	SACHRP
International research	1. Different interpretations of the Privacy Rule lead to recruitment difficulties. 2. Tendency to abandon U.S. research sites for those with less stringent rules. (NOTE: This is not strictly a problem in international research.)	1. Clarify, if legally possible, that PHI from foreign nationals outside the United States collected by researchers from covered entities is not subject to the Privacy Rule solely because of the relationship with the covered entity. 2. More generally, clarify what the rules are regarding research on foreign nationals.	SACHRP
Public health research	Effect on registries and other public health tools.	Broaden the definition of public health authority to ensure inclusion of federal and state agencies that are primarily responsible for the prevention and control of disease, injury, or disability, or the analysis of data in alliance with public health and public benefits agencies.	SACHRP

NOTE: Association of American Medical Colleges (AAMC), National Cancer Advisory Board (NCAB), National Committee on Vital and Health Statistics (NCVHS), and Secretary's Advisory Committee on Human Research Protections (SACHRP).

ASSOCIATION OF AMERICAN MEDICAL COLLEGES

The Association of American Medical Colleges (AAMC) has publicly opposed the current research provisions of the Privacy Rule since the Final Rule was proposed in 2002. During the Notice of Proposed Rulemaking period, AAMC submitted a lengthy and detailed comment urging HHS not to apply the Privacy Rule to research. AAMC has continued to campaign for a change in the rule's regulation of research since it became law. In spring 2003, AAMC conducted a survey of 331 investigators, Institutional Review Board personnel, privacy officials, research administrators, deans, and others involved in research to gain knowledge about how the Privacy Rule has influenced the research process. AAMC then created a database of qualitative case reports documenting research projects that were affected, delayed, hindered, benefited, abandoned, or foregone because of the Privacy Rule (see also Chapter 5 for survey results). Based on the results of the survey, AAMC came up with a number of recommendations for improving the Privacy Rule's regulation of research (NCVHS, 2003).

SECRETARY'S ADVISORY COMMITTEE ON HUMAN RESEARCH PROTECTIONS

The Secretary's Advisory Committee on Human Research Protections (SACHRP) is charged with advising the Secretary of HHS on human subjects research and the protection of human subjects. On March 30, 2004, SACHRP received presentations from a number of different medical experts on the Privacy Rule's impact on human subjects research. Based on these presentations, SACHRP submitted recommendations to HHS on September 1, 2004, on areas of the Privacy Rule that it deemed in need of clarification or modification (SACHRP, 2005).

NATIONAL CANCER ADVISORY BOARD

The National Cancer Advisory Board (NCAB) is appointed by the President to advise the Secretary of HHS and the Director of the National Cancer Institute with respect to the activities of the Institute. In 2003, NCAB undertook a survey to examine the impact that the Privacy Rule has had on cancer research. It requested the names of Privacy Rule experts from cancer center directors, Clinical Cooperative Group Chairs, and principal investigators of Special Programs of Research Excellence. Through this process 226 Privacy Rule experts were identified. These experts were invited to visit a Website and submit public comments on the effect of the Privacy Rule on cancer research. A total of 89 responses were received (see also Chapter 5 for survey results). On November 5, 2004, NCAB sent a set of recommendations to the Secretary of HHS. The recommendations listed ways to minimize the negative impact of the Privacy Rule on cancer research (NCI, 2003).

REFERENCES

NCI (National Cancer Institute). 2003. *The HIPAA Privacy Rule: Feedback from NCI cancer centers, cooperative groups, and specialized programs of research excellence (spores).*

NCVHS (National Committee on Vital and Health Statistics). 2001. Letter to Secretary Thompson on research recommendations as it relates to the new Privacy Rule. http://www.ncvhs.hhs.gov/011121lt.htm (accessed September 11, 2008).

NCVHS, Subcommittee on Privacy and Confidentiality. 2003. *Susan Ehringhaus's testimony on behalf of the Association of American Medical Colleges.* November 19, 2003.

NCVHS. 2004. Letter to Secretary Thompson, recommendation on the effect of the Privacy Rule. http://ncvhs.hhs.gov/040305l2.htm (accessed August 27, 2008).

SACHRP (Secretary's Advisory Committee on Human Research Protections). 2005. *Summary of SACHRP's recommendations on the HIPAA Privacy Rule.* http://www.hhs.gov/ohrp/sachrp/tableofrecommendations.html (accessed March 10, 2006).

Appendix B

Commissioned Survey Methodology

A review of the literature demonstrated a dearth of systematic data to determine what impact the Health Insurance Portability and Accountability Act (HIPAA) Privacy Rule was having on health research. As a result, the Institute of Medicine (IOM) committee sought larger surveys with national coverage. In consultation with committee members, the IOM took the unusual step of commissioning[1] several surveys to assess current perceptions among health researchers of the effect of the Privacy Rule on research and to measure the public's perception of and expectations for privacy in health research.

The first survey entailed a national web-based survey of U.S. epidemiologists, overseen by Dr. Roberta Ness at the University of Pittsburgh. A second project, undertaken by Sarah Greene and Dr. Ed Wagner at the Group Health Center for Health Studies in Seattle, involved a survey of HMO Research Network (HMORN) investigators and a survey of HMORN Institutional Review Boards (IRBs). The third survey was a Harris Interactive Poll of the public, developed by Alan Westin of the Privacy Consulting Group. The methods used in conducting these surveys are described below. The results are described in Chapters 2 and 5 of this report and are reported in more detail in Ness (2007), Westin (2007), and Greene et al. (2008).

---

[1] The surveys were commissioned with private funding. No federal funds were used to support collection of survey data.

NATIONAL SURVEY OF U.S. EPIDEMIOLOGISTS

Participants

Epidemiologists were surveyed because they are an identifiable professional group of scientists engaged in human subjects research, and their research often involves the use of medical records. Support was enlisted from all professional groups that were known to represent U.S. epidemiologists employed in academia, industry, government, and nongovernment organizations. These included the American Academy of Pediatrics, Section on Epidemiology; American College of Epidemiology; American College of Preventive Medicine; American Diabetes Association, Council on Epidemiology & Statistics; American Public Health Association, Epidemiology Section; International Genetic Epidemiology Society; International Society for Environmental Epidemiology; International Society for Pharmacoepidemiology; Society for Clinical Trials; Society for Epidemiologic Research; Society for Healthcare Epidemiology; Society for Pediatric and Perinatal Epidemiology; and Society for the Analysis of African-American Public Health Issues. Of 14 societies approached, the 13 listed above participated.

Each society e-mailed all its active members and requested that they respond to a web-based survey on the Privacy Rule. E-mail lists are updated annually for dues collection. Identical e-mails requesting participation in the survey were sent to the membership of each society three times, once a month during a 3-month period (January–April 2007). In an effort to avoid response duplication—because a substantial number of epidemiologists belong to more than one organization—respondents were asked, both in the cover e-mail and in the introduction to the survey, to respond only once. Individual responses were submitted anonymously over the Internet so that they could not be linked to any individual. IRB approval as an exempt protocol was obtained at the University of Pittsburgh and reviewed and approved by the National Academies' IRB.

The 13 participating epidemiology societies sent e-mails to a total of 10,347 individual addresses. A cover e-mail asked professionals who are engaged in the conduct of U.S.-based human subjects research and who recognized the term Health Insurance Portability and Accountability Act or HIPAA to respond. A total of 2,805 individuals accessed the Website, and 2,376 individuals answered a screening question that asked, "Since HIPAA was implemented in April 2003, how many new applications involving human subjects have you submitted to a U.S. IRB?" Respondents answering zero were thanked for their time, and no further questions were asked. The 1,527 respondents who provided a response of one or more are the participants in these analyses.

Survey Content

The survey questionnaire was developed by Roberta Ness with input and review by the IOM committee. Questions were asked about both positive and negative potential influences of the HIPAA Privacy Rule, including the influence of the Privacy Rule on participant privacy, confidentiality, and public trust, as well as on research procedures. Four general approaches were used to ascertain information. First, questions with quantitative response categories were asked. These questions addressed issues such as the frequency of various types of data collection undertaken by respondents; changes in participant recruitment before and after the implementation of the Privacy Rule; frequency of IRB modifications secondary to Privacy Rule provisions and their effect; level of difficulty in obtaining deidentified data and waivers; familiarity with covered entities' opting out of research because of the Privacy Rule; studies conceived but not submitted to IRBs because of Privacy Rule concerns; and perceived effect of the Privacy Rule on patient confidentiality. Survey respondents were also asked about their gender, training, employment, and sources of funding.

Second, researchers were asked for their perceptions rated on a 5-point Likert scale about issues such as the ease and difficulty of conducting research under the Privacy Rule and the effect the Privacy Rule has had on participant privacy/confidentiality. Third, respondents were asked whether and under what circumstances their IRB would approve each of five case studies. These involved retrieval of historical identified medical records; access to identified participants in a hospital-based cancer registry; access to deidentified data in a hospital-based tissue bank; review of medical records of deceased individuals; and request for a limited dataset (defined by the Privacy Rule) from a nonaffiliated hospital. Finally, respondents were asked open-ended qualitative questions, including a final request: "Please tell us your stories about HIPAA. These will help us to understand all of the circumstances in which HIPAA has affected your research."

After development of a draft instrument, survey content was vetted and modified by members of the IOM committee. In a pilot phase, questions were distributed to 10 epidemiologists at the University of Pittsburgh. After completing the survey, the respondents were debriefed to identify ambiguities, streamline the instrument, and determine how readily a typical epidemiologist could answer questions. After the instrument was finalized, timed pilot tests took 10 to 15 minutes to complete.

Statistical Analysis

Simple descriptive statistics, retaining each distinctive response category, were used to analyze these data. The 5-point Likert scales that were anchored by "none" and "a great deal" were collapsed into 1 to 2, 3, and 4 to 5. Categories were reported rather than central tendencies in order to retain the full and unedited character of the data. Only univariate analyses were reported because the focus was on a description of the self-reported impact of the Privacy Rule, rather than predictors of responses.

HARRIS INTERACTIVE POLL OF THE PUBLIC

Successive drafts of the survey questionnaire were prepared by Alan Westin, with input and review by the IOM committee members. The final version was then reviewed and edited by David Krane, vice president, Harris Interactive. The survey was conducted online by Harris Interactive between September 11 and 18, 2007, with 2,392 respondents. Both closed and open-ended questions were used. The results were adjusted by Harris to represent the total adult U.S. population in 2007, estimated at 225 million persons, not just those who go online. Figures for age, gender, race/ethnicity, education, region, and household income were weighted where necessary to bring them in line with their actual proportions in the population. Propensity score weighting was also used to adjust for respondents' propensity to using the Internet.

Respondents for this survey were selected from among those who have agreed to participate in Harris Interactive surveys. Because the sample is based on those who agreed to participate in the Harris Interactive panel, no estimates of theoretical sampling error can be calculated. According to Harris Interactive, all sample surveys and polls, whether or not they use probability sampling, are subject to multiple sources of error. These errors are most often not possible to quantify or estimate, including sampling error, coverage error, error associated with nonresponse, error associated with question wording and response options, and postsurvey weighting and adjustments. Therefore, Harris Interactive avoids the term "margin of error" because it is misleading. All that can be calculated are different possible sampling errors with different probabilities for pure, unweighted, random samples with 100 percent response rates. These are only theoretical because no published polls come close to this ideal.

For analytic purposes, standard demographics for cross-tabulations were collected for region, age, generation, gender, race, party affiliation, education, income, marital status, children in the household, sexual orientation, disabilities, political philosophy, and employment. In addition, a set of custom health demographics was created from respondents' answers to questions about their overall health status, whether they have been caregivers, whether they have or have had six specified types of health conditions, and whether they have had a genetic test.

Generally, a group with a 5 percent or higher variation from the total public's response, from one of our demographic, health-aspect, or attitudinal subsets, was reported as a significant demographic variation. When the public total is 18 percent or less, 3 or 4 percent higher variation was used.

SURVEY OF HMORN RESEARCHERS AND IRB ADMINISTRATORS

Researcher Survey

A Web-based survey was used to collect data about researchers' experience with the HIPAA Privacy Rule (e.g., how their research protocols may have been affected by HIPAA, knowledge of and attitudes toward the HIPAA Privacy Rule regulations, and limited demographic information). To be eligible, participants had to be members of the scientific faculty (i.e., assistant, associate, or full investigator level, or the equivalent ranking system, plus research associates or staff scientists) at one of the HMO Research Network sites listed below:

1. Geisinger Health System, Center for Health Research and Rural Advocacy
2. Group Health Center for Health Studies
3. Harvard Pilgrim Health Care, Department of Ambulatory Care & Prevention
4. HealthPartners Research Foundation
5. Henry Ford Health System, Center for Health Services Research & the Research Epidemiology Programs in cancer and biostatistics
6. Kaiser Permanente Colorado, Clinical Research Unit
7. Kaiser Permanente Northern California, Division of Research
8. Kaiser Permanente Northwest, The Center for Health Research (includes investigators from Kaiser Permanente Georgia & Kaiser Permanente Hawaii)
9. Kaiser Permanente Southern California, Department of Research and Evaluation
10. Lovelace Clinic Research Foundation, Health Services Research Division
11. Marshfield Clinic Research Foundation, Epidemiology Research Center
12. Meyers Primary Care Institute
13. Scott & White Health System, Research and Education Department

Successive drafts of the survey questionnaire were prepared by Sarah Greene, with input and review by the IOM committee. An invitation e-mail was sent to all faculty members with a link to a web-based survey. Each respondent received a unique website address taking him/her to the survey, and once a respondent completed the survey the website address could not be reused. The recipients also received two e-mail reminders to complete the web-based survey. A total of 235 investigators were invited to complete the web-based survey. Of those, 26 of the e-mail invitations bounced back, and 2 individuals actively refused to complete the survey. A total of 89 individuals completed the survey, and the remaining 118 individuals never responded to the invitations. The information obtained from the investigators included:

- The degree to which a study protocol was affected by the HIPAA Privacy Rule;
- Characteristics of the affected study;
- Attitudes toward the HIPAA Privacy Rule provisions;
- Specific structures or personnel created at their site to address HIPAA;
- Studies considered, but not implemented due to real/perceived HIPAA-related concerns;
- Open-ended "comments" fields to allow researchers to elaborate on their responses;
- Select demographic items including number of years in research;
- HMORN site membership; and
- Request to contact researcher for follow-up interview if web survey answers warrant it.

Nineteen respondents who reported a HIPAA-affected study in the web survey indicated a willingness to participate in a follow-up interview. These subjects were contacted via e-mail to initiate an appointment for a telephone interview at a mutually convenient time. Three individuals opted out when they were contacted about scheduling the interview, and two could not be reached after 4 weeks of both e-mail and phone attempts. Twelve interviews were completed.

The interviews were semi-structured to ensure systematic collection of key study details, but also to allow each individual to describe his/her unique experience about conducting research under the HIPAA Privacy Rule. At least two members of the study team were present for each interview to assist with note taking and capturing all relevant information. The principal investigator then reviewed the qualitative data for common themes and unique issues. Each response was rated as positive, negative, or neutral. The information obtained from these investigators included:

- A general description of the study (e.g., purpose, design, protocol, data sources, intervention)

- What types of changes were made to the study as a result of the HIPAA regulations
- Whether these changes had a negative impact on the study design or time line
- For multisite studies, whether differences arose across sites, and the nature of those differences
- Perceptions about their site's interpretations of HIPAA

For the web survey, descriptive characteristics were reported as means, medians, or frequencies. Frequencies were generated for categorical variables, and chi square tests were used to analyze continuous variables. Survey responses were stratified by site, years of experience, and number of studies affected by HIPAA provisions.

For the semi-structured interviews, qualitative information provided by the respondents was synthesized to determine the characteristics of the affected studies. The content of the interviews was also analyzed to identify recurrent themes.

IRB Administrator Survey

A mailed survey was used to collect data about IRB administrators' experience with the HIPAA Privacy Rule. The IRB administrators were the 15 who work at the HMO Research Network sites. Responses were received from 11 of the 15 sites. The survey was developed by Sarah Greene, with input and review by the IOM Committee. The survey asked questions regarding:

- The role of the IRB as it relates to HIPAA Privacy Rule compliance
- Knowledge of and attitudes toward the research-related provisions of the HIPAA Privacy Rule
- Procedures in place (or planned) to ensure adherence to HIPAA Privacy Rule provisions
- Approaches (e.g., training, new staff) established at the site to address HIPAA compliance
- Specific type of HIPAA Privacy Rule–related training/education developed by the site's IRB
- Sample scenarios of privacy breaches to see how each IRB would respond
- Impact of HIPAA Privacy Rule on IRB process flow
- Desired training/guidance from federal agencies specifically about the HIPAA Privacy Rule
- Open-ended "comments" fields to allow respondents to elaborate on their responses

Given the small sample size (n_{max} = 11), the analysis was limited primarily to reporting frequencies, means, and medians. If warranted, selected frequencies were stratified based on characteristics (e.g., volume of IRB applications and perceived impact of the Privacy Rule).

REFERENCES

Greene, S. M., S. Bennett, B. Kirlin, K. R. Oliver, R. Pardee, and E. Wagner. 2008. *Impact of the HIPAA Privacy Rule in the HMO Research Network.* Seattle, WA: Group Health Cooperative Center for Health Studies.

Ness, R. 2007. Influence of the HIPAA Privacy Rule on health research. *JAMA* 298(18): 2164–2170.

Westin, A. 2007. *How the public views privacy and health research.* http://www.iom.edu/Object.File/Master/48/528/%20Westin%20IOM%20Srvy%20Rept%2011-1107.pdf (accessed November 11, 2007).

Appendix C

Committee Member and Staff Biographies

COMMITTEE MEMBER BIOGRAPHIES

Lawrence O. Gostin, J.D. (*Chair*) is an internationally recognized scholar in law and public health. He is an elected member of the Institute of Medicine of the National Academies and an elected fellow of the Hastings Center. At the National Academies, he has served on the Board on Population Health and Public Health Practice, as well as many committees, including as Chair of the Committee on Genomics and the Public's Health in the 21st Century and Chair of the Committee on Ethical Considerations for Revisions to HHS Regulations for Protection of Prisoners Involved in Research. Professor Gostin is the Health Law and Ethics Editor of the *Journal of the American Medical Association* and serves on the editorial boards of many other scholarly journals. His recent books have included: *The AIDS Pandemic: Complacency, Injustice, and Unfulfilled Expectations* (2004), *The Human Rights of Persons with Intellectual Disabilities: Different But Equal* (2003, with S. S. Herr, H. H. Koh, eds.), *Public Health Law and Ethics: A Reader* (2002), and *Public Health Law: Power, Duty, Restraint* (2000). He currently works as a Professor of Public Health at Johns Hopkins University, and as Professor of Law and Director of the Center on Law and the Public's Health at the Georgetown University Law Center.

Paul S. Appelbaum, M.D., is the Elizabeth K. Dollard Professor of Psychiatry, Medicine, and Law, and Director, Division of Psychiatry, Law, and Ethics, Department of Psychiatry, College of Physicians and Surgeons of Columbia University. He is the author of many articles and books on law and ethics in clinical practice, including four that were awarded the Manfred S. Guttmacher Award from the American Psychiatric Association and the American Academy of Psychiatry and the Law. Dr. Appelbaum is Past President of the American Psychiatric Association, the American Academy of Psychiatry and the Law, and the Massachusetts Psychiatric Society, and serves as Chair of the Council on Psychiatry and Law for the American Psychiatric Association. He was previously Chair of the Commission on Judicial Action for the American Psychiatric Association and a member of the MacArthur Foundation Research Network on Mental Health and the Law. He is currently a member of the MacArthur Foundation Network on Mandatory Outpatient Treatment. He has received the Isaac Ray Award of the American Psychiatric Association for "outstanding contributions to forensic psychiatry and the psychiatric aspects of jurisprudence," was the Fritz Redlich Fellow at the Center for Advanced Study in the Behavioral Sciences, and has been elected to the Institute of Medicine. Dr. Appelbaum is a graduate of Columbia College, received his M.D. from Harvard Medical School, and completed his residency in psychiatry at the Massachusetts Mental Health Center in Boston.

Elizabeth Beattie, Ph.D., is a Professor, School of Nursing, Faculty of Health Sciences, The Queensland University of Technology. She was formerly a Research Compliance Associate at the Office of Human Research Compliance Review, University of Michigan, and an Adjunct Associate Professor in the Adult and Gerontology Nursing Program, University of Iowa. In her former role in regulatory affairs she was involved in compliance monitoring activities with human research studies in many disciplines, and in human subjects protection education and research. Prior to these positions, she was research faculty at the School of Nursing, University of Michigan. Her primary role was Project Director for several large multisite federally-funded projects focused on wandering behavior associated with dementia in long term care residents. As Project Director, she coordinated all aspects of the projects, including Institutional Review Board and Special Project Assurance requirements, site access, subject recruitment and informed consent procedures, research team training, data collection, and data coding. She served on the Institutional Review Board for Health Sciences for over 3 years. She was formally tenured foundation faculty in Australia at two new schools of nursing: The University of Technology and James Cook University. Dr. Beattie received her Ph.D. (Nursing Science) in a unique arrangement between the University of Michigan School of Nursing and James Cook University in Australia, and completed a fellowship at the Hartford Institute for Gerontological Nursing Research Summer Institute, New York University. She completed her Advanced Psychiatric Nursing Certificate at the Bethlem Royal and Maudsley hospitals, London, United Kingdom. Dr. Beattie is a Fellow of the Gerontological Society of America.

Marc Boutin, J.D., is the Executive Vice President at the National Health Council, an umbrella organization representing approximately 100 million people with chronic conditions. The Council promotes health care for all people, the importance of medical research, and the role of patient-based groups. Throughout Mr. Boutin's career, he has been highly involved in health advocacy, policy, and legislation. He has designed and directed numerous strategies for issues ranging from access to health care to cancer prevention. Before joining the Council, Mr. Boutin served as the Vice President of Government Relations and Advocacy at the American Cancer Society for New England and was a faculty member at Tufts University Medical School. In addition to senior government relations positions at Easter Seals and the Massachusetts Association of Health Boards, he was a civil rights litigator. Mr. Boutin received his Bsc. Econ. in International Politics/Law from the University College of Wales, Aberystwyth, United Kingdom, in 1989, and his J.D. from Suffolk University Law School in 1994.

Thomas W. Croghan, M.D., is a Senior Fellow at Mathematica Policy Research, Inc., where his research concentrates on studying health care access and quality, adequacy of coverage, and outcomes for different groups, in addition to analyzing the capabilities of the health system to provide care for vulnerable populations. Dr. Croghan received his M.D. from West Virginia University School of Medicine and undertook postdoctoral training at Johns Hopkins University and Stanford University. Prior to his position at Mathematica, he was a Senior Natural Scientist at the RAND Corporation. He has directed many studies of health care access, quality, cost, and cost-effectiveness of medical treatments, including projects for the National Institutes of Health, Center for Multicultural Mental Health Research, U.S. Department of the Army, National Defense Research Institute, and Eli Lilly and Company. While at Lilly, he founded the Department of Health Services and Policy Research and served as Principal Project Officer for a National Bureau of Economic Research project that created price indexes for the treatment of depression and other conditions. He also initiated the Schizophrenia Care and Assessment Program, a prospective observational study of 2,400 persons with severe psychosis. In 1999, he received a Robert Wood Johnson Foundation Investigator Award in Health Policy Research for conceptualizing the social, economic, and cultural issues underlying health care outcomes. He has published widely and serves as a reviewer for many publications, including *Health Services Research, Health Affairs, Archives of General Psychiatry*, and the *American Journal of Managed*

Care. Board certified in internal medicine and rheumatology, Dr. Croghan practices primary care medicine at the Washington Free Clinic.

Stanley W. Crosley, Esq., is Chief Privacy Officer at Eli Lilly and Company. Mr. Crosley initiated Lilly's global privacy program, and he currently oversees the company's privacy program on a global basis across all company functions. He is a co-founder and Chairman of the Board of Directors of the International Pharmaceutical Privacy Consortium (IPPC) and is on the Executive Committee of the Center for Information Policy Leadership. He also sits on the Conference Board's Chief Privacy Officers Council. Prior to his arrival at Lilly, Mr. Crosley worked at Armstrong Teasdale Schlafly & Davis in St. Louis, and at Ice Miller Donadio & Ryan where he concentrated on technology, privacy, and eBusiness. Mr. Crosley earned his B.S. in Biology, with a minor in Chemistry, from Hillsdale College and his J.D. from Indiana University.

Sandra J. Horning, M.D., is Professor of Medicine (Oncology and Bone Marrow Transplantation) at Stanford University School of Medicine in Stanford, California. She chairs the Lymphoma Committee of the Eastern Cooperative Oncology Group (ECOG), serving as senior investigator for multiple Phase II and III clinical trials. Her patient-oriented research in Hodgkin's disease and lymphoma is supported by National Institutes of Health (NIH) and other peer-reviewed funding. Dr. Horning is active in a number of professional societies including the American Society of Clinical Oncology, where she is the Immediate Past President. She is a member of the NCI Clinical Trials Advisory Committee to the Director of the National Cancer Institute and served as a member of the NIH Clinical Oncology Study Section. Dr. Horning chairs the Scientific Review Committee at Stanford Cancer Center and she co-leads the program in lymphoma for the Cancer Center. She lectures nationally and internationally and serves on the steering committees for several international consortia. An advocate of new drug development, Dr. Horning has served on the Oncology Drug Advisory Board for the Federal Drug Administration. She currently serves on the editorial boards of *Annals of Internal Medicine, Leukemia and Lymphoma, Clinical Lymphoma,* and *C.U.R.E.* Dr. Horning earned her medical degree at the University of Iowa, after which she completed internal medicine training at the University of Rochester. She also completed a medical oncology fellowship at Stanford University.

James S. Jackson, Ph.D., is a Daniel Katz Distinguished University Professor of Psychology, Professor of Health Behavior and Health Education, School of Public Health, and Director of the Institute for Social Research; past Director of the Research Center for Group Dynamics, past Director of the

Program for Research on Black Americans, and past Director of the Center for Afroamerican and African Studies, all at the University of Michigan.

He is past-Chair of the Section on Social, Economic, and Political Sciences of the American Association for the Advancement of Science (AAAS). He is a former Chair of the Section on Social and Behavioral Sciences and the Task Force on Minority Issues of the Gerontological Society of America, Committee on International Relations; Association for the Advancement of Psychology, and American Psychological Association. He was a recipient of a Fogarty Senior Postdoctoral International Fellowship, 1993–1994, for study in France and Western Europe. He has conducted research and published numerous books, scientific articles, and chapters on international, comparative studies on immigration, race and ethnic relations, physical and mental health, adult development and aging, attitudes and attitude change, and African American politics. He is former National President of the Black Students Psychological Association and the Association of Black Psychologists. He is a Fellow of the Gerontological Society of America, the American Psychological Association, the Association of Psychological Sciences, and the American Association for the Advancement of Science. He is an elected a member of the Institute of Medicine.

Dr. Jackson has been the principal investigator of more than two dozen NIH-funded and National Science Foundation (NSF) grants. He is currently directing the most-extensive social, political behavior, and health surveys on the American and Caribbean populations ever conducted; the National Institute of Mental Health, the National Institute on Aging, and the National Institute on Drug Abuse supported "National Survey of American Life" and "Family Survey Across Generations and Nations," and NSF-supported "National Study of Ethnic Pluralism and Politics."

Mary Beth Joublanc, J.D., is the Chief Privacy Officer for the State of Arizona, Arizona Government Technology Agency. She was formerly the Chief HIPAA Compliance Officer for the Arizona Department of Health Services, Phoenix, Arizona. She is also the Chair for the Department's Human Subjects Research Board. Ms. Joublanc is an active member of the State Bar of Arizona. Her legal practice focuses on regulatory compliance, health care law, risk management, and professional liability claims management. Ms. Joublanc has lectured on a variety of topics related to health law and risk management. She holds a B.S. in Health Information and, prior to law school, was a health information manager with experience in primary, secondary, and tertiary care.

Bernard Lo, M.D., is Professor of Medicine and Director of the Program in Medical Ethics at the University of California, San Francisco (UCSF). He is National Program Director for the Greenwall Faculty Scholars Program in Bioethics. He is Co-Chair of the Standards Working Group of the California Institute of Regenerative Medicine, which will recommend regulations for stem cell research funded by the state of California. He also serves on the Data and Safety Monitoring Committees for diabetes prevention trials and a HIV vaccine trial at the National Institute of Allergy and Infectious Disease. He is a member of the Ethics Working Group of the NIH-sponsorsed HIV Prevention Trials Network, which carries out clinical trials in developing countries. Dr. Lo is Co-Director of the Policy and Ethics Core of the Center for AIDS Prevention Studies at UCSF, which provides technical advice and consultation to researchers carrying out clinical research, including research in resource-poor nations. He is a member of the IOM and serves on the IOM Council. He has been involved in a number of studies on ethical issues in human participants research carried out by the IOM and the National Academy of Science (NAS). He chaired an IOM panel on confidentiality in health services research. He developed a course on Responsible Conduct of Research that 120 postdoctoral fellows and junior faculty take each year. He also carries out research on ethical issues in human participants research, end-of-life decisions, and stem cell research. He is a practicing general internist and attends on the inpatient medical service at UCSF.

Andrew F. Nelson, M.P.H., is Executive Director of the HealthPartners Research Foundation and Vice President of HealthPartners. Mr. Nelson has provided leadership for this nonprofit, medical/health care research organization since its inception in 1990. He also serves as a Corporate Officer for HealthPartners, Inc. HealthPartners is an integrated health delivery system servicing over 725,000 people in Minnesota through a medical group of 650 providers, a large clinic system, and a 450-bed hospital. HealthPartners Research Foundation conducts more than 200 laboratory, clinical, and health services research projects annually, through 90 full-time staff, 25 full-time career researchers, and more than 45 clinical researchers. More than 350 of HealthPartners 10,000 employees are engaged in research and represent a broad array of medical, scientific, and administrative disciplines.

Prior to the HealthPartners Research Foundation position, Mr. Nelson was a Research Development Officer for the University of Minnesota's Health Sciences and Executive Director of the Day Community and Connections Programs at the University of Minnesota's programs that serve emotionally and behaviorally disturbed adolescents. Mr. Nelson is a founding member and serves as Immediate Past Chair of the Board of Directors for the HMO Research Network, 15 research organizations with funding of more than $100 million. He serves on a wide range of professional and community committees and boards.

Marc Rotenberg, J.D., is president of the Electronic Privacy Information Center and Adjunct Professor of Law, Georgetown Law. He was counsel to Senator Patrick J. Leahy on the Senate Judiciary Committee, specializing in technology and law. Professor Rotenberg has testified before Congress on many issues, including access to information, computer crime, computer security, and privacy. In 2003, he testified before the 9-11 Commission on Security and Liberty. He is the Editor (with Daniel J. Solove and Paul Schwartz) of *Information Privacy Law* (Aspen Publishing, 2006), is the Editor (with Phil Agre) of *Technology and Privacy: The New Landscape* (MIT Press, 1998), *The Privacy Law Sourcebook: United States Law, International Law and Recent Developments* (Epic, 2005), and is on the editorial boards of *BNA Electronic Commerce and Law* and *Computer Law and Security Reporter*. Professor Rotenberg has served on advisory panels for the American Bar Association Section on Criminal Justice, the American Association for the Advancement of Science, the Austrian Institute for Law and Policy, the National Academy of Sciences, UNESCO, and the Organization for Economic Cooperation and Development. He chairs the American Bar Association Committee on Privacy and Information Protection. He is also Former Chair of the Public Interest Registry, which manages .ORG domain. He was a Teaching Fellow in computer science at Harvard University from 1980 to 1982 and an instructor at Stanford University from 1986 to 1987. He received his A.B. cum laude from Harvard University and his J.D. from Stanford University.

Wendy Visscher, Ph.D., is Director of RTI International's Office of Research Protection and Ethics, where she oversees the operation of the three Institutional Review Boards and chairs one of these committees. She maintains RTI's Federalwide Assurance with HHS's Office for Human Research Protections. She earned her Certified IRB Professional rating in 2002. In addition to her knowledge of human subjects protection, Dr. Visscher trains researchers on HIPAA and other data privacy requirements and regulations, and consults with RTI management on these and related issues. Dr. Visscher is also a trained epidemiologist with more than 20 years of health research experience. Her areas of expertise include: heart disease and diabetes in minority communities, drug use in pregnant women, children's mental health, global burden of influenza, HIV, reproductive epidemiology, radiation and cancer, and patient outcomes studies. She received her Ph.D. in 1987 from the University of Minnesota.

Fred Wright, M.D., has served as Associate Chief of Staff for Research (director of the research program) since 1984. He is a Staff Physician at the VA Connecticut Healthcare System and has also been Acting Chief of Staff in 1995 and 1998. He is a Professor in the Departments of Internal Medicine and Cellular & Molecular Physiology at the Yale University School of Medicine. Dr. Wright received his A.B. and M.D. from the University of Michigan. He trained as a resident in medicine at the Johns Hopkins Hospital in Baltimore and as a postdoctoral trainee in kidney physiology at the National Institutes of Health in Bethesda, Maryland. He was then appointed to the faculty at Yale University where his research continued to focus on the structure and function of the kidney, with an emphasis on mechanisms of ion transport by kidney tubules in health and disease. He joined the medical staff at the West Haven VA Medical Center in 1997 and continued to be involved in laboratory research and teaching of medical students and advanced trainees.

Clyde W. Yancy, M.D., is a cardiologist and heart failure/heart transplant specialist at Baylor University Medical Center at Dallas, where he is the medical director of the Baylor Heart and Vascular Institute, and chief of cardiothoracic transplantation at Baylor University Medical Center at Dallas. Previously, Dr. Yancy was a professor of internal medicine and cardiology and holder of the Carl Westcott Chair in Medical Research at the University of Texas Southwestern Medical Center in Dallas where he served as director of its heart transplant program. He also is credited with establishing the medical center's heart failure program and cardiovascular institute. He holds fellowships in the American College of Cardiology, the American Heart Association, and the American College of Physicians. He is an active member of the American Heart Association, the American College of Cardiology, the International Society of Heart and Lung Transplantation, and the American Society of Hypertension. Presently, he serves on the executive committee of the Heart Failure Society of America. He also sits on the editorial board of a number of professional journals. In 2003, he was recognized as physician of the year by the American Heart Association for leadership in programs related to its mission. He currently serves on the Cardiovascular Device Panel for the Food and Drug Administration and is a consultant to the National Heart, Lung, and Blood Institute. His research interests include the broad areas of heart transplantation, heart failure, and heart disease in special populations. Dr. Yancy received his M.D. from Tulane University School of Medicine and completed post-graduate training at the University of Texas Southwestern Medical Center.

STAFF BIOGRAPHIES

Sharyl Nass, Ph.D., is a Study Director and Senior Program Officer at the Institute of Medicine, where she has worked with the Board on Health Sciences Policy, Board on Health Care Services, and the National Cancer Policy Board and Forum. Her previous work at the IOM has focused on topics that include developing cancer biomarkers, strategies for large-scale biomedical science, developing technologies for the early detection of breast cancer, improving breast imaging quality standards, and contraceptive research and development. Her current position at the IOM combines her dual interests in biomedical research and health science policy. With a Ph.D. in Cell and Tumor Biology from Georgetown University and post-doctoral training at the Johns Hopkins University School of Medicine, she has authored numerous papers on the cell and molecular biology of breast cancer. She also holds a B.S. in Genetics and an M.S. in Endocrinology/Reproductive Physiology, both from the University of Wisconsin–Madison. In addition, she studied developmental genetics and molecular biology at the Max Planck Institute in Germany under a fellowship from Fulbright and the German Heinrich Hertz-Stiftung Foundation. Dr. Nass was the 2007 recipient of the Cecil Award for Excellence in Health Policy Research.

Laura Levit, J.D., is an Associate Program Officer for the Board on Health Care Services and the National Cancer Policy Forum. She started at the IOM as a Christine Mirzayan Science and Technology Graduate Fellow in winter 2007. In 2007, she received the IOM rookie award for her work with the National Cancer Policy Forum. She graduated from the University of Virginia School of Law in May 2006, and was admitted into the Virginia Bar Association in October 2006. She completed her undergraduate studies at the College of William and Mary, receiving a B.S. in Psychology. In law school, Ms. Levit worked for several different nonprofit organizations that focused on health and mental health care policy, including the World Federation for Mental Health, the Treatment Advocacy Center, the Bazelon Center, and the National Research Center for Women & Families.

Roger Herdman, M.D., received his undergraduate and medical school degrees from Yale University. Following an internship at the University of Minnesota and a stint in the U.S. Navy, he returned to Minnesota where he completed a residency in pediatrics and a fellowship in immunology and nephrology and served on the faculty at the University of Minnesota. He served as Professor of Pediatrics at Albany Medical College until 1979.

In 1969, Dr. Herdman was appointed Director of the New York State Kidney Disease Institute in Albany, New York, and shortly thereafter was appointed Deputy Commissioner of the New York State Department of Health (1969–1977) and in 1977 was named New York State's Director of Public Health. From 1979 until joining the U.S. Congress's Office of Technology Assessment (OTA), he served as a Vice President of the Memorial Sloan-Kettering Cancer Center in New York City.

In December 1983, Dr. Herdman was named Assistant Director of OTA where he subsequently served as Director (1993–1996). He later joined the

IOM as a Senior Scholar and directed studies on graduate medical education, organ transplantation, silicone breast implants, and the Veterans Administration national formulary. Dr. Herdman was appointed Director of the IOM/National Research Council National Cancer Policy Board from August 2000 through April 2005. Beginning in May 2005, he has directed the IOM National Cancer Policy Forum, which includes federal and private-sector cancer relevant agencies or organizations in addition to academic/industry members. In October 2007, he was also appointed Director of the IOM Board on Health Care Services. During his work at the IOM, Dr. Herdman has worked closely with the U.S. Congress on a wide variety of health care policy issues.

Andrew Pope, Ph.D., is Director of the IOM Board on Health Sciences Policy. He has a Ph.D. in Physiology and Biochemistry from the University of Maryland and has been a member of the National Academies staff since 1982 and of the IOM staff since 1989. His primary interests are science policy, biomedical ethics, and environmental and occupational influences on human health. During his tenure at the National Academies, Dr. Pope has directed numerous studies on topics that range from injury control, disability prevention, and biologic markers to the protection of human subjects of research, NIH priority-setting processes, organ procurement and transplantation policy, and the role of science and technology in countering terrorism. Dr. Pope is the recipient of IOM's Cecil Award and the NAS President's Special Achievement Award.

Michael Park is a Senior Program Assistant for the Board on Health Care Services and the National Cancer Policy Forum. Before arriving at the IOM in September of 2007, Mr. Park worked for the National Academy of Education and the International Law Group in Washington, DC. He earned his B.A. in German and Italian Studies from the University of Maryland at College Park. He is fluent in Spanish, Italian, and German.

Abbrevations and Acronyms

AAHRPP	Association for the Accreditation of Human Research Protection Programs
AAMC	Association of American Medical Colleges
ACC	American College of Cardiology
AHA	American Heart Association
AHIMA	American Health Information Management Association
AHRQ	Agency for Healthcare Research and Quality
AOD	Accounting of disclosure
ASCO	American Society for Clinical Oncology
BA	Business associate
CaBIG	Cancer Biomedical Informatics Grid
CCW	Chronic Conditions Warehouse
CDC	Centers for Disease Control and Prevention
CMS	Centers for Medicare & Medicaid Services
DES	Diethylstilbestrol
DUA	Data use agreement
ELSO	Extracorporeal Life Support Organization
EPHI	Electronic protected health information
EPHR	Electronic personal health records
EU	European Union

FDA	Food and Drug Administration
FOIA	Freedom of Information Act
GAO	Government Accountability Office
GINA	Genetic Information Nondiscrimination Act
HAS	Health Assessment Survey
HEW	U.S. Department of Health, Education and Welfare
HHS	U.S. Department of Health and Human Services
HIC	Health information custodians
HIPAA	Health Insurance Portability and Accountability Act
HIT	Health information technology
HMAC	Keyed-hash message authentication code
HMO	Health maintenance organization
HMORN	HMO Research Network
ICMJE	International Committee of Medical Journal Editors
ICU	Intensive care units
INTERMACS	Interagency Registry for Mechanically Assisted Circulatory Support
IOM	Institute of Medicine
IPC	Information and Privacy Commissioner
IRB	Institutional Review Board
JHU	Johns Hopkins University
NAACCR	North American Association of Central Cancer Registries
NCAB	National Cancer Advisory Board
NCI	National Cancer Institute
NCVHS	National Committee on Vital and Health Statistics
NIH	National Institutes of Health
NIST	National Institute of Standards and Technology
NPDB	National Practitioner Data Bank
NTD	Neural tube birth defects
OCR	Office for Civil Rights
OECD	Organisation for Economic Co-operation and Development
OHRP	Office for Human Research Protections
PCPS	Partners for Child Passenger Safety
PDA	Personal digital assistant

PHI	In HIPAA, protected health information; in PHIPA, personal health information
PHIPA	Personal Health Information Protection Act
PRIM&R	Public Responsibility in Medicine and Research
REB	Research ethics board
SACHRP	Secretary's Advisory Committee on Human Research Protections
SELECT	Selenium and Vitamin E Cancer Prevention Trial
SMOG	Simple Measure of Gobbledegook
UDE	Unique data elements
UNOS	United Network for Organ Sharing
VA	U.S. Department of Veterans Affairs

Glossary

Accounting of Disclosures: This provision of the Privacy Rule gives individuals the right to receive a list of certain disclosures that a covered entity has made of their protected health information in the past 6 years, including disclosures made for research purposes.

Association for the Accreditation of Human Research Protection Programs, Inc. (AAHRPP): An independent, nonprofit entity that accredits organizations' human research protection programs.

Authorization: An individual's written permission to allow a covered entity to use or disclose specified protected health information (PHI) for a particular purpose. Authorization states how, why, and to whom the PHI will be used and/or disclosed for research, and seeks permission for that use or disclosure.

Autonomy: The capacity of a *rational individual* to make an informed, uncoerced decision.

Business Associate: A person or entity who, on behalf of a covered entity, performs or assists in performance of a function or activity involving the use or disclosure of protected health information, such as data analysis, claims processing or administration, utilization review, and quality assurance reviews, or any other function or activity regulated by the HIPAA Administrative Simplification Rules, including the Privacy Rule. Business associates are also persons or entities performing legal, actuarial, accounting, consulting, data aggregation, management, administrative, accreditation, or financial services to or for a covered entity where performing those services involves disclosure of protected health information by the covered entity or another business associate of the covered entity to that person or entity.

Chronic Conditions Warehouse: Section 723 of the Medicare Prescription Drug, Improvement, and Modernization Act of 2003 instructed the Secretary of the U.S. Department of Health and Human Services to make Medicare data more readily available to researchers studying chronic illness in the Medicare population, with the intent to help "identify areas for improving the quality of care provided to chronically ill Medicare beneficiaries, [and] reduce program spending." The Chronic Conditions Warehouse implements this requirement of the Act and contains fee-for-services claims, enrollment/eligibility, and assessment data. Researchers can efficiently access data on 21 predefined chronic health conditions, such as diabetes, breast cancer, Alzheimer's, and depression.

Common Rule: The federal rule that governs most federally funded research conducted on human beings and aims to ensure that the rights of human subjects are protected during the course of a research project, historically focusing on protection from physical and mental harm by stressing autonomy and consent.

Confidentiality: Addresses the issue of how personal data that have been collected for one approved person may be held and used by the organization that collected the data, what other secondary or further uses may be made of the data, and when the permission of the individual is required for such uses.

Covered Entity: A health plan, a health care clearinghouse, or a health care provider that transmits health information in electronic form in connection with a transaction for which the U.S. Department of Health and Human Services has adopted a standard.

Data Use Agreement: An agreement into which the covered entity enters with the intended recipient of a limited dataset that establishes the ways in which the information in the limited dataset may be used and how it will be protected.

Deidentified Information: The Privacy Rule provides for two methods to deidentify personally identifiable health information. Under the statistical method, a statistician or person with appropriate training verifies that enough identifiers have been removed that the risk of identification of the individual is very small. Under the safe harbor method, data are considered deidentified if the covered entity removes 18 specified personal identifiers from the data.

Effectiveness: The extent to which a specific test or intervention, when used under *ordinary* circumstances, does what it is intended to do.

Efficacy: The extent to which a specific test or intervention produces a beneficial result under *ideal* conditions (e.g., a clinical trial).

Fair Information Practices: Principles affording individuals the meaningful right to control the collection, use, and disclosure of information, and imposing affirmative responsibilities to safeguard information on those who collect it.

Food and Drug Administration (FDA) Protection of Human Subjects Regulations: Regulations intended to protect the rights of human subjects enrolled in research involving products that the FDA regulates (i.e., drugs, medical devices, biologicals, foods, and cosmetics).

Health Care Clearinghouse: A public or private entity, including a billing service, repricing company, community health management information system or community health information system, and value-added networks and switches, that either process or facilitate the processing of health information received from another entity in a nonstandard format or containing nonstandard data content into standard data elements or a standard transaction, or receive a standard transaction from another entity and process or facilitate the processing of health information into a nonstandard format or nonstandard data content for the receiving entity.

Health Care Provider: A provider of services (as defined in Section 1861(u) of HIPAA, 42 U.S.C. 1395x(u)), a provider of medical or health services (as defined in Section 1861(s) of HIPAA, 42 U.S.C. 1395x(s)), and any other person or organization who furnishes, bills, or is paid for health care in the normal course of business.

Health Information: Any information, whether oral or recorded in any form or medium, that (1) is created or received by a health care provider, health plan, public health authority, employer, life insurer, school or university, or health care clearinghouse; and (2) relates to the past, present, or future physical or mental health or condition of an individual; the provision of health care to an individual; or the past, present, or future payment for the provision of health care to an individual.

Health Insurance Portability and Accountability Act of 1996 (HIPAA): An Act that requires, among other things, under the Administrative Simplification subtitle, the adoption of standards for protecting the privacy and security of personally identifiable health information.

Hybrid Entity: A single legal entity that is a covered entity, performs business activities that include both covered and non-covered functions, and designates its health care components as provided in the Privacy Rule. If a covered entity is a hybrid entity, the Privacy Rule generally applies only to its designated health care components. However, non-health care components of a hybrid entity may be business associates of one or more of its health care components, depending on the nature of the relationship.

Informed Consent: A legal form required by the Common Rule that describes the potential risks and benefits of research and seeks permission to involve the subject.

Institutional Review Boards (IRBs): "An administrative body established to protect the rights and welfare of human research subjects recruited to participate in research activities conducted under the auspices of the institution with it is affiliated. The IRB has the authority to approve, require modification in, or disapprove all research activities that fall within its jurisdiction as specified by both the federal regulations and local institutional policy" (Department of Health and Human Services IRB Guidebook).

Limited Dataset: Refers to protected health information that excludes 16 categories of direct identifiers and may be used or disclosed, for purposes of research, public health, or health care operations, without obtaining either an individual's authorization or a waiver or an alteration of authorization for its use and disclosure, with a data use agreement.

Nonmaleficence: The ethical principle of doing no harm, based on the Hippocratic maxim, primum non nocere, first do no harm.

Privacy: In this report, the privacy of personal health information pertains to the collection, storage, and use of personal information and addresses the question of who has access to personal information and under what conditions.

Privacy Board: A board that is established to review and approve requests for waivers or alterations of authorization in connection with a use or disclosure of protected health information as an alternative to obtaining such waivers or alterations from an Institutional Review Board. A Privacy Board consists of members with varying backgrounds and appropriate professional competencies as necessary to review the effect of the research protocol on an individual's privacy rights and related interests. The board must include at least one member who is not affiliated with the covered entity, is not affiliated with any entity conducting or sponsoring the research, and is not related to any person who is affiliated with any such entities. A Privacy Board cannot have any member participating in a review of any project in which the member has a conflict of interest.

Protected Health Information: Protected health information is personally identifiable health information created or received by a covered entity.

Public Health: The Privacy Rule defines a public health authority as any "federal, tribal, or local agency or person or entity acting under a grant of authority or contract with the agency, including state and local health departments, the Food and Drug Administration, the Centers for Disease Control and Prevention, and the Occupational Safety and Health Administration."

Public Health Practice: "The collection and analysis of identifiable health data by a public health authority for the purpose of protecting the health of a particular community, where the benefits and risks are primarily designed to accrue to the participating community" (Hodge, 2005; Hodge and Gostin, 2004).

Public Health Research: "The collection and analysis of identifiable health data by a public health authority for the purpose of generating knowledge that will benefit those beyond the participating community who bear the risks of participation" (Hodge, 2005; Hodge and Gostin, 2004).

Public Responsibility in Medicine and Research (PRIM&R): An organization whose mission is to promote ethical research in both humans and animals.

Quality Improvement: "Systematic, data-guided activities designed to bring about immediate, positive change in the delivery of health care in a particular setting" (Baily et al., 2006).

Research: A systematic investigation, including research development, testing, and evaluation, designed to develop or contribute to generalizable knowledge.

Respect for Persons: The ethical principle requiring that individuals be treated as autonomous agents, and that individuals with diminished autonomy are entitled to protection (HEW, 1979).

Security: "The procedural and technical measures required (a) to prevent unauthorized access, modification, use, and dissemination of data stored or processed in a computer system, (b) to prevent any deliberate denial of service, and (c) to protect the system in its entirety from physical harm" (Turn and Ware, 1976).

Selection Bias: This phenomenon occurs when data are more likely to be collected from one subset of the population than from a representative sample of the entire population. This can cause systematic differences between the characteristics of the individuals included in a study and the individuals not included.

Waiver of Authorization: The documentation that the covered entity obtains from a researcher or an IRB or a Privacy Board that states that the IRB or Privacy Board has waived or altered the Privacy Rule's requirement that an individual must authorize a covered entity to use or disclose the individual's protected health information for research purposes.

REFERENCES

Baily, M. A., M. Bottrell, J. Lynn, and B. Jennings. 2006. The ethics of using QI methods to improve health care quality and safety. *A Hastings Center Special Report* 36(4):S1–S40.
HEW (Department of Health, Education and Welfare). 1979. *The Belmont Report: Ethical principles and guidelines for the protection of human subjects of research.* http://ohsr.od.nih.gov/guidelines/belmont.html (accessed August 21, 2008).
Hodge, J. G., Jr. 2005. An enhanced approach to distinguishing public health practice and human subjects research. *Journal of Law, Medicine & Ethics* 33(1):125–141.
Hodge, J. G., and L. O. Gostin. 2004. *Public health practice vs. Research: A report for public health practitioners including cases and guidance for making distinctions.* Atlanta, GA: Council of State and Territorial Epidemiologists.
Turn, R., and W. H. Ware. 1976. Privacy and security issues in information systems. *The RAND Paper Series.* Santa Monica, CA: The RAND Corporation.